Peripheral Neuropathy

Peripheral Neuropathy

Edited by Conor Clayton

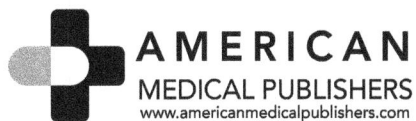

AMERICAN
MEDICAL PUBLISHERS
www.americanmedicalpublishers.com

American Medical Publishers,
41 Flatbush Avenue,
1st Floor, New York,
NY 11217, USA

Visit us on the World Wide Web at:
www.americanmedicalpublishers.com

ISBN: 978-1-63927-327-0

Cataloging-in-Publication Data

Peripheral neuropathy / edited by Conor Clayton.
    p. cm.
Includes bibliographical references and index.
ISBN 978-1-63927-327-0
1. Nerves, Peripheral. 2. Nerves, Peripheral--Diseases. 3. Nervous system.
4. Neuropathy. I. Clayton, Conor.
RC409 .P47 2022
616.856--dc23

Table of Contents

Preface

Peripheral neuropathy is a disease that affects the nerves beyond the brain and spinal cord, known as peripheral nerves. Damage to these nerves causes a lack of sensation, movement, organ function, etc. It also depends on which nerves are damaged. Neuropathy affects the motor, sensory or automatic nerves. It is classified into mononeuropathy, polyneuropathy, mononeuritis multiplex, autonomic neuropathy and neuritis. Its symptoms depend on the types of nerve fiber affected. In the case of sensory function, symptoms include numbness, tremor, impairment of balance, tingling, crawling, pain, etc. Motor symptoms include weakness, tiredness, muscle atrophy or twitch and cramps. Some of its primary causes include genetic diseases, vitamin deficiency, effects of chemotherapy, and metabolic and endocrine diseases. Electromyography, a comprehensive metabolic panel screening and nerve conduction studies some of the techniques used for the diagnosis of peripheral neuropathy. The treatment of peripheral neuropathy depends on the cause of the condition. The topics included in this book on peripheral neuropathy are of utmost significance and bound to provide incredible insights to readers. It presents researches and studies performed by experts across the globe. This book is appropriate for students seeking detailed information in this area as well as for experts.

Various studies have approached the subject by analyzing it with a single perspective, but the present book provides diverse methodologies and techniques to address this field. This book contains theories and applications needed for understanding the subject from different perspectives. The aim is to keep the readers informed about the progresses in the field; therefore, the contributions were carefully examined to compile novel researches by specialists from across the globe.

Indeed, the job of the editor is the most crucial and challenging in compiling all chapters into a single book. In the end, I would extend my sincere thanks to the chapter authors for their profound work. I am also thankful for the support provided by my family and colleagues during the compilation of this book.

Editor

Pregabalin versus gabapentin in the management of peripheral neuropathic pain associated with post-herpetic neuralgia and diabetic neuropathy: a cost effectiveness analysis for the Greek healthcare setting

Kostas Athanasakis[1*], Ioannis Petrakis[1], Eleftheria Karampli[1], Elli Vitsou[2], Leonidas Lyras[2] and John Kyriopoulos[1]

Abstract

Background: The anticonvulsants pregabalin and gabapentin are both indicated for the treatment of peripheral neuropathic pain. The decision on which treatment provides the best alternative, should take into account all aspects of costs and outcomes associated with the two therapeutic options. The objective of this study was to examine the cost – effectiveness of the two agents in the management of patients with painful diabetic neuropathy or post – herpetic neuralgia, under the third party payer perspective in Greece.

Methods: The analysis was based on a dynamic simulation model which estimated and compared the costs and outcomes of pregabalin and gabapentin in a hypothetical cohort of 1,000 patients suffering from painful Diabetic Peripheral Neuropathy (DPN) or Post-Herpetic Neuralgia (PHN). In the model, each patient was randomly allocated an average pretreatment pain score, measured using an eleven-point visual analogue scale (0 – 10) and was "run through" the model, simulating their daily pain intensity and allowing for stochastic calculation of outcomes, taking into account medical interventions and the effectiveness of each treatment.

Results: Pregabalin demonstrated a reduction in days with moderate to severe pain when compared to gabapentin. During the 12 weeks the pregabalin arm demonstrated a 0.1178 (SE 0.0002) QALY gain, which proved to be 0.0063 (SE 0.0003) higher than that in the gabapentin arm. The mean medication cost per patient was higher for the pregabalin arm when compared to the gabapentin arm (i.e. €134.40) over the 12 week treatment period. However, this higher cost was partially offset by the reduced direct medical costs (i.e. the cost of specialist visits, the cost of diagnostic tests and the other applied interventions). Comparing costs with respective outcomes, the ICERs for pregabalin versus gabapentin were €13 (95%CI: 8 – 18) per additional day with no or mild pain and €19,320 (95%CI: 11,743 – 26,755) per QALY gained.

Conclusions: Neuropathic pain carries a great disease burden for patients and society and, is also, associated with a significant economic burden. The treatment of pain associated with DPN and PHN with pregabalin is a cost-effective intervention for the social security in Greece compared to gabapentin. Thus, these findings need to be taken into consideration in the decision – making process when considering which therapy to use for the treatment of neuropathic pain.

Keywords: Peripheral neuropathic pain, Post-herpetic neuralgia, Diabetic neuropathy, Pregabalin, Gabapentin, Cost-effectiveness analysis

* Correspondence: kathanasakis@esdy.edu.gr
[1]Department of Health Economics, National School of Public Health, Athens, Greece
Full list of author information is available at the end of the article

Background

Neuropathic pain (NeP) is defined by the International Association for the Study of Pain (IASP) as "Pain caused by a lesion or disease of the somatosensory nervous system". NeP can be a result of a variety of conditions associated with impairing the functioning of the nervous system, such as diabetes, multiple sclerosis, trauma and herpes zoster infections [1]. It is a common condition with an overall prevalence between 0.9 and 8.0% [1,2]. Previous literature suggests that individuals with NeP were known to experience more severe pain when compared to non-NeP chronic pain sufferers [1]. Despite the plethora of etiologies associated with NeP, the scientific focus lies mainly on painful diabetic peripheral neuropathy (DPN) and post-herpetic neuralgia (PHN), extrapolating any outcomes on other causes of NeP [3]. Painful DPN is a common complication of diabetes with a prevalence of up to 25% among diabetic patients [3]. PHN is in turn the most common chronic complication of herpes zoster infection (10 – 75% of cases) [4,5]. Neuropathic pain has been associated with impaired quality of life, reduced individual productivity and increased patient and healthcare resource expenditure [3,6]. Co-morbid conditions include sleep disturbances, depression and anxiety disorders [6], increasing even further the economic burden to the healthcare system. In a recent review, the average pain severity associated with painful DPN and PHN was identified to be 5.0/10 and 4.4/10 (Visual Analog Scale) and the average EQ-5D values, for patients with severe pain, equal to 0.2 and 0.26 respectively [3].

The anticonvulsants pregabalin and gabapentin are indicated for the treatment of neuropathic pain. Treatment with the third generation anticonvulsant - pregabalin can be started at a dose of 150 mg per day given as two to three divided doses. Based on individual patient response and tolerability, the dose may be gradually increased, if needed, to a maximum dose of 600 mg per day. Clinical trials using pregabalin for both peripheral and central NeP, showed a reduction in pain scores within the first week, which was maintained throughout the treatment period [7,8]. Alternatively, the starting dose of gabapentin is 900 mg/day given as three equally divided doses, increasing gradually up to a maximum daily dose of 3,600 mg. Clinical trials have shown that the optimal daily dosing for pain control exceeded 1,800 mg [9,10].

A cohort study by Toth et al. [11] investigated the utility associated with the substitution of gabapentin with pregabalin therapy in patients with peripheral NeP. Results showed that both previous responders and non-responders to gabapentin had additional pain relief of approximately 25%, six or twelve months after initiation of pregabalin. Another study by Tarride et al. showed that following a twelve-week regime, therapy with pregabalin was associated with nine additional days with no or mild pain, against six additional days with gabapentin therapy [11].

Along with the previously mentioned high incidence, chronicity, maladaptivity and co-morbidities associated with NeP, comes the significant economic burden to the national health system. In an attempt to estimate the costs associated with NeP, Dworkin et al. (2010) calculated the excess healthcare costs associated with peripheral NeP between $1,600 and $7,000 [12]. In the same context, Berger and colleagues estimated [13], that the excess expenditure of patients with NeP, can reach a threefold increase compared to their non-NeP peers ($17,355 versus $5,715, 2000 values). When investigating costs associated with painful DPN, Gordois et al. found that direct medical costs exceeded $10billion per year in the United States [14]. Another study, found that the average medical costs due to PHN following herpes zoster infections ranged from $760 to $1300 per patient for the first year after infection (2004 values) [15]. Apart from the direct costs mentioned above, another dimension of costs, the societal costs from NeP also need to be taken into account. Characteristically, in a cross-sectional European study, researchers identified that 43% of patients reported work absence and even change in employment status and 17% were disabled due to NeP [16].

Thus, the benefit of treatment for patients with chronic neuropathic pain is dual, including both the effects of reduced morbidity as well as their subsequent contribution in societal and health care costs. However, the decision on which treatment provides the best alternative, should take into account all aspects of treatment costs included. In this decision – making process, pharmacoeconomic tools, such as economic evaluation, are deemed pivotal. In light of the above, the purpose of this study was to examine the cost – effectiveness of pregabalin versus gabapentin in the management of patients with painful diabetic neuropathy or PHN in view of the third party payer in Greece.

Methods

Study model

The cost – effectiveness analysis was based on a dynamic simulation model [17,18] which estimated the costs and outcomes of pregabalin and gabapentin in a hypothetical cohort of 1,000 patients suffering from painful DPN or PHN.

In the model, each patient was randomly allocated an average pretreatment pain score, measured using an eleven-point visual analogue scale, with 0 referring to "no pain" and 10 to "the worst pain imaginable", which was derived from the actual distribution of pain levels in a randomized, double-blind controlled trial of pregabalin in patients with chronic NeP, defined as subjects with DPN or PHN [7]. Following that, every patient in the cohort was "run through" the model, which used a

Markovian process to simulate their daily pain intensity and allow for stochastic calculation of outcomes taking into account medical interventions and the effectiveness of each treatment. Three different health states relative to NeP were adopted from clinical practice for the purposes of the model. Specifically, days with "no or mild pain" reflected a pain intensity of "0 to < 4", whereas days with "moderate" and "severe" pain were associated with pain scores "4 to < 7" and "7 to 10", respectively. The randomly allocated pretreatment scores ranged from 4 to 10 (moderate to severe pain). As the patient progressed through treatment with pregabalin or gabapentin, the model projected the estimated efficacy of the two pharmacotherapies on the assigned daily pain scores, and, thus, the "journey" of patients and the respective outcomes. Default estimates, model assumptions and further description of the model have been previously presented elsewhere [3,11,19]. An outline of the model is presented in Figure 1.

The time frame of interest in the model was twelve weeks and all NeP-associated direct costs were considered. Several outcomes were derived from the above dynamic simulation model. The number of days with no or mild pain was the primary measure in the model, but also the mean number of days with 30% and 50% reduction in pain score were estimated. Other outcomes of interest included Quality Adjusted Life Years (QALYs) gained and the cost per QALY gained along with costs of medication and NeP-related healthcare services.

Pharmacotherapies

In the model, the cost effectiveness of pregabalin at a daily dose of 150 – 600 mg (average maintenance dose of 457 mg [7]) was compared against gabapentin mean dose 2,400 mg daily (900 – 3,600 mg). The two therapies were considered to have similar side-effect profiles and therefore no discontinuation of treatment or added costs due to unwanted effects were assumed. The efficacy of the two anticonvulsants in reducing weekly pain scores (Table 1) was derived from three randomized, double-blind, controlled studies [7,9,10]. The model allows for variations in week to week reductions in pain scores in accordance to

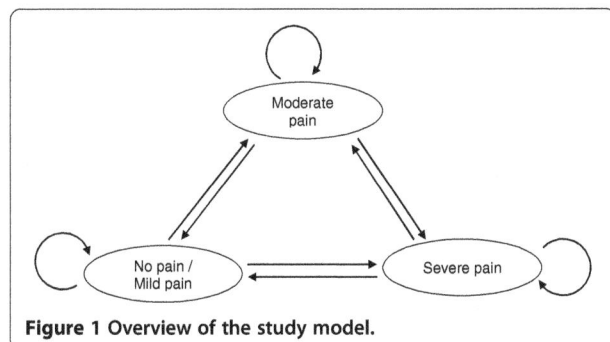

Figure 1 Overview of the study model.

Table 1 Percentage weekly change in pain severity among patients with painful DPN or PHN receiving treatment with pregabalin or gabapentin

	Pregabalin n = 141	Gabapentin n = 193
Mean dose mg/day	457	2400
Mean total weekly reduction versus baseline in daily pain scores %		
Week 1	13.7	17.2
Week 2	23.2	25.1
Week 3	29.9	29.7
Week 4	39.1	32.1
Week 5	44.4	33.7
Week 6	44.2	34.9
Week 7	45.0	35.8
Week 8	46.3	36.4
Week 9	49.8	36.9
Week 10	51.1	37.2
Week 11	53.3	37.4
Week 12	54.1	37.6

Data obtained from Protocol 1008–155 for pregabalin [7], and Protocols 945–210 and 945–211 for gabapentin [9,10].

the actual distribution of change as presented in the above controlled trials.

Healthcare resource use and medication costs

Medication costs were calculated using the latest price catalogue of medicinal products, as published in the price bulletin issued by the Ministry of Health (generic preparations of gabapentin were not included in the analysis due to their low penetration in the Greek healthcare market). Moreover, for the purposes of the analysis, it was assumed that no cost variations would result from prescribing divided doses of the comparator therapies. The costs per health service and diagnostic tools were derived from the official NHS price lists.

To identify healthcare resource utilization data according to pain severity, a survey, was conducted in a group of 100 general practitioners and 20 specialized pain clinics in Greece. General practitioners were requested to provide the percentage of patients that were referred to pain clinics, according to pain score, whereas data on utilization of diagnostic tests and other health services arose from the survey of referable specialized pain clinics (Table 2).

The time frame of interest in the model was twelve weeks and all NeP-associated direct costs were considered, and calculated from a third party payer (social insurance) perspective and reported in year 2011 values.

Sensitivity analyses

To address parameter uncertainty, a series of one-way sensitivity analyses, were performed, by recalculating the results, after a ±20% change in baseline values, for selected

Table 2 Probability of healthcare resource use and unit costs per utilized service

Healthcare service	Probability of utilization	Unit cost (Euros)
Referral to specialist		
Pain score		
0 to < 4	0.13	20.00
4 to < 7	0.24	20.00
7 to 10	0.57	20.00
Diagnostic tests		
CAT	0.10	71.11
MRI	0.30	236.95
Nerve conduction studies	0.17	8.63
Doppler sonograph	0.12	27.00
EMG	0.19	8.28
Blood testing (Basic Haematology Biochemistry)	0.74	34.56
X-Ray	0.30	4.05
γ-Ray	0.05	60.16
Other interventions		
Physical therapy	0.33	25.00
Drug infiltrations	0.63	20.00
Nerve block	0.39	14.67
TENS	0.36	54.18
Spinal stimulator implant	0.03	4610.90

CAT – computerized axial tomography. *MRI* – magnetic resonance imaging. *EMG* – electromyogram. *TENS* – transcutaneous electric nerve stimulation. Physical therapy and drug infiltrations – prices per session.

parameters. The sensitivity analysis focused on the cost of pregabalin, the weekly probability of physician visiting due to NeP and the health utility values in association with neuropathic pain. Additional scenarios of calculations included alternating daily dosages of gabapentin (1800 mg and 1200 mg) as well as the exclusion of non-medication related health-resource use (i.e. consideration of medication costs only).

Results

The clinical outcomes at endpoint (t = 12 weeks) are presented in Table 3. Mean pretreatment pain scores were identical (6.9) for both pregabalin and gabapentin. Post-treatment pain score mean values were 4.1 for pregabalin and 4.8 for gabapentin, with the differences in the simulations being statistically significant at the 0.05 level. Pregabalin also demonstrated a statistically significant reduction in days with moderate to severe pain when compared to gabapentin. That was also apparent when measuring percentage reduction in pain scores. During the 12 weeks treatment period, the pregabalin arm demonstrated a 0.1178 (SE 0.0002) QALY gain, which proved to be 0.0063 (SE 0.0003) higher than that in the gabapentin arm (p < 0.05).

The mean medication cost per patient was higher for the pregabalin arm when compared to the gabapentin arm (i.e. €134.40 higher) over the 12 week treatment period. However, as presented in Table 4, this cost was partially offset by the reduced direct medical costs, such as the cost of specialist visits, the costs of diagnostic tests and the other applied interventions, which were €12 lower Comparing costs with respective outcomes, the ICERs for pregabalin versus gabapentin were €13 (95%CI: 8 – 18) per additional day with no or mild pain and €19,320 (95%CI: 11,743 – 26,755) per QALY gained. Results are summarized in Table 5.

The sensitivity analysis showed that parameters with the greatest impact on results were the daily cost of pregabalin and the utilities associated with pain severity (Table 6). The incremental costs per additional day with no or mild pain ranged between 7(95%CI: 2, 14) and 24

Table 3 Expected clinical outcomes per patient after treatment with Pregabalin or Gabapentin

	Treatment		
	Pregabalin (150–600 mg/d)	Gabapentin (2400 mg/d)	Difference (Pregabalin - Gabapentin)
Pain score			
Pre-treatment	6.9 (0.0)	6.9 (0,0)	0.0 (0.0)
Post-treatment	4.1 (0.0)	4.8 (0,0)	−0.6 (0.0)
Days with			
No or mild pain	36 (0.3)	27 (0.3)	9 (0.5)
Moderate pain	32 (0.3)	38 (0.3)	−6 (0.5)
Severe pain	15 (0.2)	19 (0.3)	−4 (0.3)
Days with			
≥30% reduction in pain score	50 (0.3)	42 (0.4)	8 (0.5)
≥50% reduction in pain score	36 (0.3)	26 (0.4)	10 (0.5)
Quality-adjusted life-years (QALYs)	0.1178 (0.0002)	0.1115 (0.0002)	0.0063 (0.0003)

Results presented as Mean (SE) for the 12 – week duration of modeling.

Table 4 Expected medical care costs per patient

	Treatment		Difference (Pregabalin - Gabapentin)
	Pregabalin (150–600 mg/d)	Gabapentin (2400 mg/d)	
Medication	306.60 (0.00)	172.20 (0.00)	134.40 (0.00)
Outpatient care			
Primary care provider	36.12 (0.70)	37.45 (0.74)	−1.33 (1.04)
Specialist referral	9.89 (0.33)	10.52 (0.33)	−0.63 (0.47)
Diagnostic tests	56.86 (3.13)	60.57 (2.90)	−3.72 (4.01)
Other interventions	90.88 (18.52)	97.22 (17.12)	−6.34 (24.15)
Total	500.35 (19.08)	377.96 (17.73)	122.39 (25.26)

Values in Euros mean (SE).
For the 12 – week treatment period.

(95%CI: 18, 34), while the corresponding cost per QALY gained ranged between 11,075 (95%CI: 2,944, 23,040) and 39,073 (95%CI: 28,704, 54,620). Both values refer to a 20% lowering and a 20% rise, respectively, to the baseline daily cost of pregabalin. A 1200 mg reduction in the mean gabapentin daily dose caused the ICER value per QALY gained to exceed the €30,000 threshold.

Discussion

The present study aimed at estimating the cost-effectiveness of pregabalin, versus gabapentin for the treatment of DPN or PHN, taking into account the perspective of a social security organization in Greece. For that purpose, a previously presented and validated health economic model was adapted for the Greek healthcare setting, taking into account direct costs of treatment and follow up for a hypothetical cohort of 1,000 patients that were treated under the two alternatives for a 12 week period, based on the efficacy profile of each intervention as recorded in the results of published clinical trials.

The results of the analysis indicate that pregabalin is a more costly but also a more effective treatment option compared to gabapentin. The excess costs of pharmaceutical treatment for pregabalin are partially offset by its improved clinical profile in terms of reductions in resource utilization and its improved outcomes in the patient level, thus leading to incremental cost-effectiveness

Table 5 Incremental cost-effectiveness ratios of pregabalin vs. gabapentin in the treatment of painful DPN and PHN

Cost per additional (€)	Pregabalin vs Gabapentin Mean (95% CI)
Day with no or mild pain	
Mean estimate	13
95% confidence interval	(8, 18)
QALY gained	
Mean estimate	19,320
95% confidence interval	(11,743 - 26,755)

ratios of €13 per additional day with mild/no pain and €19,320 per QALY gained.

In Greece there are currently no established thresholds under which interventions can be classified as cost-effective. In general, the accepted willingness to pay per QALY gained falls within £20,000 – £30,000 in the UK and $50,000 – $100,000 in the US [20], whereas older studies in other healthcare settings have placed this limit at a lower level (e.g. 20,000$ per QALY gained in Canada [21]). A generally acknowledged criterion (a "rule of thumb") states that interventions costing less than 30,000€/QALY gained are "good value for money", from an economic evaluation point of view [22], a principle that the results of the present study fulfil. Moreover the study results also meet the criteria for cost-effective interventions recommended by the WHO Commission on Macroeconomics and Health [23]. Specifically, based on the Commission's recommendations, interventions with an ICER (expressed in cost per Disability Adjusted Life Year averted) that is lower than three times the Gross National Income (GNI) per capita can be classified as cost-effective, whereas ICERs lower than $1 \times$ GNI indicate highly cost effective interventions. Taking into account a GNI per capita of €19,801 in Greece (2010 values) and extending the criterion to a per QALY decision, treatment of painful DPN or PHN with pregabalin falls within the range of highly cost-effective interventions.

The findings of this study are in accordance to previously published literature [3,11] that aimed to estimate the cost – effectiveness of the two pharmacotherapies. The outcomes of the Rodriguez et al. study in Spain [3] estimated an ICER (euros per QALY gained and per day with no or mild pain) of €20,535 (1,607 – 40,345) and €12 (1 – 24) respectively. The Canadian study of Tarride et al. [11] examined the two disorders separately and provided two sets of results, indicating in both cases that pregabalin was cost-effective. More specifically, regarding painful DPN, pregabalin had an ICER of $13 per day with no or mild pain and $15,708 per QALY gained respectively, whereas, for the PHN outcomes the equivalent values were $3 and $3,325, respectively

Table 6 Sensitivity analysis of the incremental cost effectiveness of pregabalin versus gabapentin in the treatment of painful diabetic neuropathy and post herpetic neuralgia

Parameter	Baseline	Sensitivity analysis	Cost per additional day with no or mild pain	Cost per QALY gained
Gabapentin dose (mg)	2400	1800	14 (8,19)	23 786 (14266,33498)
Gabapentin dose (mg)	2400	1200	16 (9,24)	30 241 (18086,44056)
Costs considered	All healthcare costs	Medication cost only	16 (14,18)	25 683 (22812,29829)
Pregabalin daily cost	3.65	↑20%	24 (18,34)	39 063 (28704,54620)
Pregabalin daily cost	3.65	↓20%	7 (2,14)	11 075 (2944,23040)
Weekly probability of PCP visit in relation to NeP	No/mild: 0.25 Moderate: 0.31 Severe: 0.48	↑20%	14 (8,20)	21 025 (11592,30710)
Weekly probability of PCP visit in relation to NeP	No/mild: 0.25 Moderate: 0.31 Severe: 0.48	↓20%	13 (7,19)	19 773 (10531,28687)
Health utility associated with pain severity	No/mild: 0.64 Moderate: 0.48 Severe: 0.27	↑20%	13 (9,18)	17 017 (10296,23936)
Health utility associated with pain severity	No/mild: 0.64 Moderate: 0.48 Severe: 0.27	↓20%	14 (8,20)	27 505 (15418,40596)

Mean values in € (SE) 95% CI.
NeP – Neuropathic pain.
PCP – primary care physician.

(all values reported in year 2004 Canadian dollars). Moreover, the results of this study are in accordance with findings from a recent systematic review on the effectiveness and cost-effectiveness of pregabalin in the management of DPN . Meshkini et al. (2012) [24] concluded that higher doses of pregabalin (300 mg – 600 mg daily), appear highly cost-effective treatment options.

As with any study of its kind, the present one has some limitations that should be acknowledged. Firstly, the data on efficacy of the treatments under comparison are based on clinical trial data, which considered patients in a different healthcare setting than that in Greece. Thus, the trial cohorts might not be fully representative for patients with painful DPN or PHN in Greece, Nevertheless, the magnitude of this (possible) discrepancy is extremely difficult to quantify and to include in the calculations of the analysis. Moreover, the perspective of the analysis (third-party payer, i.e. the Greek Social Insurance Funds) does not include other costs, such as the indirect expenses due to productivity losses. If the societal perspective had been adopted, there is evidence that the ICERs would probably be more favourable (i.e. lower). For example, a recent cost analysis of adding pregabalin or gabapentin to the management of community – based patients with peripheral NeP, which estimated also the indirect costs, showed that although the pharmaceutical costs of pregabalin were significant, the overall patient cost was

lower in the pregabalin group due to reduced sick leave and lower healthcare costs, and thus was compensated the higher treatment acquisition cost of pregabalin [25]. A limitation also arises from the fact that calculations do not include variations of cost that could arise from divided dosing regimens due to the design of the model. The same approach was used in other adaptations of the model, in different health care settings [3,11].

Another limitation of the analysis that should be considered is the source of data regarding the resource use incorporated in the calculations, i.e., the elicitation of some data via a questionnaire survey. Although an ideal approach would be to review actual patient data, the absence of centralized patient records or databases containing relevant data in the Greek NHS, rendered necessary the use of a questionnaire survey. Inevitably, the above mentioned approach introduces uncertainty in the calculations, whose extent, however, is quite difficult to quantify. Nevertheless, the magnitude of the study sample, the simplicity of the data that were requested and the extensive sensitivity analysis on the baseline values, enhance the robustness of outcomes.

Finally, the present study concludes that the intervention under investigation was followed by favourable incremental cost-effectiveness ratios, compared to other treatment strategies on pain management. However, the discussion on the adoption of such a policy by the Social Insurance

Pregabalin versus gabapentin in the management of peripheral neuropathic pain associated with post-herpetic...

7

will be complete, in economic terms, when accompanied by estimations of this intervention to insurance budgets, i.e. a budget impact analysis. This issue certainly constitutes an area of future research.

Conclusion

Neuropathic pain carries a great disease burden for patients and society and, also, a significant economic burden. From a third part payer perspective, the treatment of pain associated with painful DPN and PHN with pregabalin is a cost-effective intervention for the social security in Greece compared to gabapentin. Notwithstanding its limitations, the study's findings need to be taken into consideration in the decision – making process when considering which therapy to use for the treatment of neuropathic pain.

Abbreviations
DPN: Diabetic peripheral neuropathy; EQ-5D: Euroqol-5D; GBP: Gabapentin; IASP: International association for the study of pain; ICER: Incremental cost effectiveness ratio; NeP: Neuropathic pain; NHS: National health service; PHN: Post herpetic neuralgia; PGB: Pregabalin; QALY: Quality adjusted life years; WHO: World health organization.

Competing interests
EV and LL are employees of Pfizer Hellas. KA has received funding in the past from Pfizer with the purpose of data analyses and manuscript revision. The authors declare no other financial or non-financial competing interests.

Authors' contribution
KA and IP performed the calculations and analyses reported in the text. EV and LL reviewed the literature for relevant data and documentation. IP and EK drafted the manuscript which was edited and critically revised by KA and JK. All authors read and approved the final manuscript.

Acknowledgments
This study does not fall into the types of research for which an ethics evaluation by a REC (Research Ethics Committees) is recommended as confirmed by the National School of Public Health Ethics committee. This study was sponsored by Pfizer Ltd.
Athanasakis K, Petrakis I., Karampli E., Kyriopoulos J are employees of the National School of Public Health, which received financial support from Pfizer in connection with the development of this manuscript.

Author details
[1]Department of Health Economics, National School of Public Health, Athens, Greece. [2]Pfizer Hellas, Athens, Greece.

References
1. O' Connor A: Neuropathic pain; quality of life impact, costs and cost effectiveness of therapy. *PharmacoEcon* 2009, **27**(2):95–112.
2. Toth C: Substitution of Gabapentin therapy with pregabalin therapy in neuropathic pain due to peripheral neuropathy. *Pain Med* 2010, **11**:456–465.
3. Rodriguez MJ, Diaz S, Vera–Llonch M, Dukes E, Rejas J: Cost – effectiveness analysis of pregabalin versus gabapentin in the management of neuropathic pain due to diabetic polyneuropathy or post – herpetic neuralgia. *Curr med res opin* 2007, **23**(10):2585–2596.
4. Dubinsky RM, Kabbany H, El-Chami Z, Butwell C, Ali H: Practice parameter: treatment of postherpetic neuralgia: an evidence-based report of the quality standards subcommittee of the American academy of neurology. *Neurology* 2004, **63**:959–965.

5. Kost RG, Straus SE: Postherpetic neuralgia: pathogenesis, treatment and prevention. *N Engl J Med* 1996, **335**:32–42.
6. Navarro A, Saldana MT, Perez C, Torrades S, Rejas J: A cost – consequenses analysis of the effect of pregabalin in the treatment of peripheral neuropathic pain in routine medical practice in primary care settings. *BMC Neurol* 2011, **11**:7.
7. Freynhagen R, Strojek K, Griesing T, Whalen E, Balkenohl M: Efficacy of pregabalin in neuropathic pain evaluated in a 12 – weeks, randomised, double – blind, multicentre, placebo-controlled trial of flexible- and fixed dose regimens. *Pain* 2005, **115**:254–263.
8. Strojek K, Flöter T, Balkenohl M, et al: Pregabalin in the management of chronic neuropathic pain (NeP): a novel evaluation of flexible and fixed dosing. *J Pain* 2004, **5**(3 Suppl 1):S59.
9. Backonja M, Beydoun A, Edwards KR, et al: Gabapentin for the symptomatic treatment of painful neuropathy in patients with diabetes mellitus: a randomized controlled study. *JAMA* 1998, **280**:1831–1836.
10. Rowbotham M, Harden N, Stacey B, et al: Gabapentin in the treatment of post-herpetic neuralgia: a randomized controlled trial. *JAMA* 1998, **280**:1837–1842.
11. Tarride JE, Gordon A, Vera-Llonch M, Dukes E, Rousseau C: Cost – effectiveness of pregabalin for the management of neuropathic pain associated with diabetic peripheral neuropathy and postherpetic neuralgia: a Canadian perspective. *Clin Ther* 2006, **28**(11):1922–1934.
12. Dworkin RH, Malone DC, Panarites CJ, Armstrong EP, Pham SV: Impact of postherpetic neuralgia and painful diabetic peripheral neuropathy on health care costs. *J Pain* 2010, **11**(4):360–368.
13. Berger A, Dukes EM, Oster G: Clinical characteristics and economic costs of patients with painful neuropathic disorders. *J Pain* 2004, **5**:143–149.
14. Gordois A, Schuffham P, Shirer A, Oglesby A: The health care costs of diabetic neuropathy in the United States. *Diabetes Care* 2003, **26**:1790–1795.
15. Dworkin RH, White R, O'Connor AB, Baser O, Hawkins K: Health care costs of acute and chronic pain associated with a diagnosis of herpes zoster. *J Am Geriatr Soc* 2007, **55**:1168–1175.
16. McDermott AM, Toelle TR, Rowbotham DJ, Schaefer CP, Dukes EM: The burden of neuropathic pain: results of a cross-sectional survey. *Eur J Pain* 2006, **10**:127–135.
17. Halpern EF, Weinstein MC, Hunink MGM, Gazelle GS: Representing both first and second order uncertainties by Monte Carlo simulation for groups of patients. *Med Decis Making* 2000, **20**:314–322.
18. Craig B, Black M, Sendi P: Uncertainty in decision models analyzing cost-effectiveness. *Med Decis Making* 2000, **20**:135–137.
19. Vera-Lonch M, Dukes E, Delea TE, Wang ST, Oster G, Neuropathic pain outcomes modeling working group: Treatment of peripheral neuropathic pain: a simulation model. *Eur J Pain* 2006, **10**:279–285.
20. Shiroiwa T, Sung YK, Fukuda T, Lang HC, Bae SC, Tsutani K: International survey on willingness-to-pay (WTP) for one additional QALY gained: what is the threshold of cost effectiveness? *Health Econ* 2010, **19**:422–437.
21. Laupacis A, Feeny D, Detsky AS, Tugwell PX: How attractive does a new technology have to be to warrant adoption and utilization? Tentative guidelines for using clinical and economic evaluations. *CMAJ* 1992, **15**:473–481.
22. Eichler HG, Kong SX, Gerth WC, Mavros P, Jonsson B: Use of cost-effectiveness analysis in health-care resource allocation decision-making: how are cost-effectiveness thresholds expected to emerge? *Value in Health* 2004, **7**:518–528.
23. World Health Organization: *Macroeconomics and health: investing in health for economic development-report of the commission on macroeconomics and health. Report of the commission on Macroeconomics and Health, chaired by J. Sachs.* Geneva, Switzerland: WHO Library Cataloguing-in-Publication Data; 2001.
24. Meshkini AH, Keshavarz K, Gharibnaseri Z, Nikfar S, Abdollahi M: The effectiveness and cost-effectiveness of pregabalin in the treatment of diabetic peripheral neuropathy: a systematic review and economic model. *Int J Pharmacol* 2012, **8**:490–495.
25. Sicras-Mainar A, Rejas-Gutierrez J, Navarro-Artieda R, Planas-Comes A: Cost analysis of adding pregabalin or gabapentin to the management of community-treated patients with peripheral neuropathic pain. *J Eval Clin Prac* 2012, **18**:1170–1179.

2

Differences in peripheral myelin antigen-specific T cell responses and T memory subsets in atypical versus typical CIDP

M. Staudt[1], J. M. Diederich[1], C. Meisel[2], A. Meisel[1] and J. Klehmet[1]*

Abstract

Background: Chronic inflammatory demyelinating polyneuropathy (CIDP) is presented by a large heterogeneity of clinical phenotypes. Around 50% of patients suffer from typical CIDP and show better therapy response than atypical variants. The goal of our study was to search for cellular immunological differences in typical versus atypical CIDP in comparison to controls.

Methods: We evaluated 26 (9 typical, 17 atypical) patients with mainly active-unstable CIDP using clinical and immunological examinations (enzyme-linked immunospot assay ELISPOT, fluorescence-activated cell sorting FACS) in comparison to 28 healthy, age-matched controls (HC). Typical or atypical CIDP measurements were compared with HC using Kruskal-Wallis test.

Results: Atypical CIDP patients showed increased frequencies of T cell subsets, especially CD4+ effector memory T cells (TEM) and CD4+ central memory T cells (TCM) as well as a tendency of higher T cell responses against the peripheral myelin antigens of PMP-22, P2, P0 and MBP peptides compared to typical CIDP. Searching for novel auto-antigens, we found that T cell responses against P0 180-199 as well as MBP 82-100 were significantly elevated in atypical CIDP patients vs. HC.

Conclusions: Our results indicate differences in underlying T cell responses between atypical and typical CIDP characterized by a higher peripheral myelin antigen-specific T cell responses as well as a specific altered CD4+ memory compartment in atypical CIDP. Larger multi-center studies study are warranted in order to characterize T cell auto-reactivity in atypical CIDP subgroups in order to establish immunological markers as a diagnostic tool.

Keywords: Chronic inflammatory demyelinating polyneuropathy, T memory subsets, MBP protein, P0 protein, Atypical, Typical

Background

Chronic inflammatory demyelinating polyneuropathy (CIDP) is the most common autoimmune peripheral neuropathy but remains a rare disease with a prevalence of 0.8-8.9 cases per 100.000 [1, 2]. The disorder causes severe disability in more than 50% of the patients in a chronic-progressive course [1]. Diagnosis can be difficult given the heterogeneity of CIDP phenotypes. About 50% of the patients suffer from so-called atypical variants including *Distal Acquired Demyelinating Polyneuropathy* (DADS) in 25-35% of the cases, *Multifocal Acquired Demyelinating Sensory And Motor Polyneuropathy* (MADSAM) in 15% and rare variants such as pure sensory CIDP (10-13%), pure motor CIDP (<10%) and focal CIDP (2%) [3]. These CIDP subtypes are likely to differ with respect to underlying pathomechanisms and may necessitate different treatment approaches.

Despite recent progress, the underlying immunopathogenetic mechanisms remain poorly understood [4]. Both humoral as well as cellular immune responses are likely to play a role in the induction of autoimmune neuroinflammation, which leads to demyelination and axonal degeneration [4–7].

---

* Correspondence: juliane.klehmet@charite.de
[1]Department of Neurology, Charité University Medicine, Charitéplatz 1, 10117 Berlin, Germany
Full list of author information is available at the end of the article

Peripheral myelin antigens are promising auto-antigens in CIDP pathogenesis. Recently, we demonstrated higher frequencies of auto-reactive IFN-γ responses directed against the peripheral myelin antigens PMP-22 and P2 in treatment naïve patients who responded subsequently well to intravenous immunoglobulin (IVIG) treatment. Clinical improvement under IVIG-treatment correlated with the reduction of antigen-specific responses against PMP-22 and P2 [8].

Experimental studies in the EAN model of Guillain-Barré-Syndrom (GBS) support a pathogenic role of another compact myelin P0. Immunization with P0 180-199 is capable to induce EAN in wildtype-, IFN-γ *knockout* and TNF-α *knockout* mice [9–11]. However, an evaluation in CIDP patients remains to be done.

Myelin basic protein (MBP) is a major constituent of the myelin sheath in the central and peripheral nervous system [12]. Whereas it has been established as an immunodominant auto-antigen for demyelination in the immunopathogenesis of Multiple Sclerosis (MS) its auto-reactive potential in CIDP remains elusive [13].

T cells can be differentiated into CD45RA+ CCR7+ naïve, CD45RA- CCR7- effector memory (TEM), CD45RA- CCR7+ central memory (TCM) and CD45RA+ CCR7- terminally differentiated effector memory (TEMRA) T cells [14]. Especially CD4+ T cells play a major role in CIDP immunopathogenesis [15–17]. In blood and CSF of CIDP patients, significantly elevated frequencies of CD4+ TEM and CD4+ TCM were demonstrated, whereas long-term treated CIDP patients showed significantly reduced CD4+ memory subsets in contrast to untreated CIDP patients [17–19].

Here, we hypothesize that autoreactive myelin-specific T cell responses as well as T cell memory subsets differ between atypical and typical manifestations of CIDP.

Methods

Patients

We evaluated 26 CIDP patients using clinical and immunological (enzyme-linked immunospot assay ELISPOT, fluorescence-activated cell sorting FACS) examinations in comparison to 28 healthy, age-matched controls. CIDP patients who met the diagnostic criteria of European Federation of Neurological Sciences (EFNS) 2010 were divided into "typical" vs. "atypical" according to EFNS 2010 [20]. Therapy response was defined as an improvement of ≥2 in Medical Research Council (MRC) sum score in 2 different muscle groups, an improvement of ≥1 in Inflammatory Neuropathy Cause and Treatment (INCAT) score (excluding changes in arm function from 0 to 1) or alternatively an improvement of ≥50% of the walking distance as described previously [8]. Patients and controls were recruited in the outpatient clinic of the Department of Neurology, Charité University Medicine Berlin.

Peripheral myelin antigens

ELISPOT assay was performed using peptides of seven peripheral myelin antigens and CEF as positive control for T cell responses (Table 1). CEF is a peptide pool containing 23 MCH class 1 restricted viral antigens [21]. Peripheral myelin antigens were provided by Dr. R. Volkmer, Institute of Medical Immunology, Charité University Medicine Berlin. CEF was provided by JPT Peptide Technologies GmbH, Berlin.

Cryopreservation of Peripheral Blood Monocytes (PBMC)

To evaluate T cell responses efficiently we preserved PBMC in liquid nitrogen over a maximum of 6 months. Blood was sampled in CPT tubes for ELISPOT and in EDTA tubes for flow cytometry. PBMC were isolated within 2 h after venipuncture by 1500 g centrifugation for 20 min. After washing, we diluted the PBMC at a concentration of $2x10^7$cells/ml in freezing medium A (60% FCS; 40% RPMI, Biochrom, Berlin, Germany) at 4 °C. The same volume of freezing medium B (20% DMSO, 80% FCS) at 4 °C was added before cell suspensions were transferred into cryovials (Sarstedt, Nürnbrecht, Germany) and set in one at 4 °C prechilled Nalgene Cryogenic Freezing Container (Fisher Scientific, Hannover, Germany) which was placed in –80 °C overnight. After 12-24 h, cryovials were transferred into liquid nitrogen tanks for storage until ELISPOT.

Thawed cell suspensions were transferred into a 15 ml tube containing 10 ml of ice cold PBS. After two washing steps, cells were pipetted in complete RPMI medium (93% RPMI-1640. 5% heat-inactivated FCS, 1% L-glutamin, 1% penicillin-streptomycin) and counted manually using Trypan blue-staining and light microscopy.

ELISPOT

IFN-γ ELISPOT assay in this study was performed on human PBMC as previously described [8]. We plated 4×10^5cells/well in triplicates for each antigen and positive (CEF) or negative control (medium). CEF, a peptide pool containing viral antigens functioning as a positive control for T cell responses, was added at 9 μg/ml [21].

Table 1 ELISPOT-antigens

antigen	Sequence
PMP-22 32–51	NGHATDLWQNCSTSSSGNVH
PMP-22 51–64	HHCFSSSPNEWLQS
PMP-22120–133	RHPEWHLNSDYSYG
P2 14–25	ENFDDYMKALGV
P2 61–70	EISFKLGQEF
P0 180-199	ASKRGRQTPVLYAMLDHSRS
MBP 82-100	DENPVVHFFKNIVTPRTPP
CEF	peptide pool

The peripheral myelin antigens PMP-22 32-51, PMP-22 51-64, PMP-22 120-133, P2 14-25, P2 61-70 were used at 40 μg/ml and P0 180-199, MBP 82-100 were used at 20 μg/ml. Spot counts were analyzed via ELISPOT Reader Immunospot (CTL Analyzers, Cleveland, Ohio, USA) and custom software. Spot forming units (SFU) for each antigen were subtracted by SFU of spontaneous IFN-γ secretion (usually <5) and then calculated for a cell amount of 10^6 cells.

FACS

Flow cytometry analyses were performed on lymphocyte- and T cell-subpopulations in EDTA whole blood within 12 h after venipuncture.

Flow cytometric analysis was performed as we described recently [17]. Briefly, mouse anti-human fluorescently labelled monoclonal antibodies allowed to quantifying the frequencies of lymphocyte and T cell subpopulations. The following antibodies were used: CD3 Allophycocyanine-Alexa Fluor 750 (APC-A750), CD4 energy coupled dye (ECD), CD8 APC, CD14 Fluorescein isothiocyanate (FITC), CD16 Phycoerythrine (PE), CD19 PE-Cy5.5, CD56 PE, CD45RA Pacific-Blue (PB), CD45 Krome-Orange (KrO) (all by Beckman Coulter) and CCR7 Phycoerythrine (PE) (R&D Systems). Stained samples were evaluated on a ten-colour Navios flow cytometer and were analyzed using Navios Software (Beckman Coulter).

Statistics

All statistical tests were performed using GraphPadPrism 6.0 software. The study was assessed as an exploratory analysis. Typical or atypical CIDP measurements were compared with healthy, age-matched controls (HC) using Kruskal-Wallis test followed by post-hoc unpaired t-test or Mann-Whitney-test when $p < 0.05$. For group differences with regard to sex, prior treatment, disease activity and therapy response, Fisher's exact test was used. For age and INCAT score, unpaired t-test was used. For time since diagnosis, Mann-Whitney-test was used. Level of significance was defined as $p < 0.05$ for all comparative tests.

Results

Clinical characterization of typical and atypical CIDP patient group (Table 2)

We recruited 17 (65.4%) male and nine (35.6%) female patients. Mean age was 59 years (range 32-78). 20/26 (76.9%) patients were included in active-unstable stages of the disease, 1 (3.8%) with active-stable CIDP and five (19.2%) in clinical remission [22]. 12 (46.2%) patients were treatment naïve whereas 10 (38.5%) received IVIG therapy and four (15.4%) glucocorticosteroids (GS) prior to our study. We classified 9 (38.5%) as typical and 17 (61.5%) as atypical CIDP patients, including 6

with pure sensory CIDP, 4 with MADSAM, 5 with DADS, 1 with pure motor CIDP and 1 with a sensory-ataxic course of disease.

Therapy-responders were classified as 9/9 (100%) typical and only 8/17 (47%) atypical CIDP patients. As controls we used age-matched, healthy patients (HC). For ELISPOT-analyses 14 HC (mean age 70, range 53-83) and for FACS-analyses 28 HC (mean age 61, range 42-83) were evaluated.

T cell IFN-γ- responses to P0 180-199 and MBP 82-100 were elevated in CIDP patients compared to healthy controls

T cell responses against the peripheral myelin antigens, P0 180-199 and MBP 82-100 were measured by IFN-γ ELISPOT in a cohort of 26 CIDP patients. Due to spontaneous IFN-γ-production, 6 patients (1 typical, 5 atypical) were excluded for further ELISPOT analysis.

T cell responses against P0 180-199 as well as MBP 82-100 were significantly elevated in CIDP patients vs. HC: P0 180-199 ($p < 0.05$), MBP 82-100 ($p < 0.001$) (Fig. 1). CEF-specific IFN-γ-production in CIDP did not differ from HC excluding unspecific T cell activation in CIDP.

Increased myelin antigen-specific T cell responses in atypical CIDP

Atypical CIDP variants tended to have increased IFN-γ responses to all 7 tested peripheral myelin antigens compared to both, typical CIDP patients and HC (Fig. 2). This difference between typical and atypical CIDP patients was more pronounced for PMP-22 32-51 ($p = 0.0621$), PMP-22 51-64 ($p = 0.1050$), PMP-22 120-130 ($p = 0.1451$), P0 180-199 ($p = 0.1894$) and MBP 82-100 ($p = 0.1841$) (Fig. 2). In comparison to HC, atypical CIDP patients showed significantly higher SFU for the following peripheral myelin antigens: PMP-22 32-51 ($p_{atypical} < 0.05$), PMP-22 51-64 ($p_{atypical} < 0.01$), PMP-22 120-130 ($p_{atypical} < 0.01$), P2 14-25 ($p_{atypical} < 0.01$), P0 180-199 ($p_{atypical} < 0.05$), MBP 82-100 ($p_{atypical} < 0.01$) (Fig. 2). CEF responses did not differ between tested groups.

Atypical CIDP variants have significantly higher levels of Cd4+ memory T cells

Frequencies of T cells ($p < 0.01$) and CD4+ T cells ($p < 0.001$) were higher in patients with atypical CIDP variants in comparison to typical CIDP patients (Fig. 3a).

Investigating CD4+ T cell subpopulations, CD4+ memory T cell subsets were significantly increased in atypical vs. typical CIDP patients, as shown for CD4+ TEM ($p < 0.05$) and CD4+ TCM ($p < 0.01$) in Fig. 3b.

Likewise CD8+ TEM ($p = 0.1745$) and CD8+ TCM ($p = 0.1475$) tended to be increased in atypical compared to typical CIDP patients. Further compared to HC, atypical CIDP patients had significantly elevated CD8+ TCM-frequencies ($p < 0.05$) (Fig. 3c).

Table 2 Clinical information (n = 26; IVIG intravenous immunoglobulins, CIDP chronic inflammatory demyelinating polyneuropathy, INCAT Inflammatory Neuropathy Cause and Treatment, GS glucocorticosteroids)

		typical	atypical	p-values atypical vs. typical
Sex	male	3/9 (33%)	14/17 (82%)	0.013
	female	6/9 (66%)	3/17 (18%)	
Age (years)	mean	61.0	57.2	0.512
	range	32-78	33-74	
Previous treatment	None	3/9 (33%)	9/17 (53%)	0.429[a]
	IVIG	4/9 (44%)	6/17 (35%)	0.652[a]
	Steroid	2/9 (22%)	2/17 (12%)	0.547[a]
Time since diagnosis	mean	4.1	4.2	0.860
(years)	range	1-8	1-7	
INCAT	mean	3.2	2.3	0.045
	Range	<1-8	<1-7	
Disease activity	range	1-5	1-3	
	active-unstable	6/9 (66%)	14/17 (82%)	1.000[b]
	active-stable	1/9 (11%)	0/17 (0%)	0.333[b]
	in remission	2/9 (22%)	3/17 (18%)	1.000[b]
Therapy response	responder	9/9 (100%)	8/17 (47%)	0.022
	non-responder	0/9 (0%)	9/17 (53%)	

Fishers exact test for sex, previous treatment, disease activity and therapy response

[a]compared versus treatment naïve patients

[b]compared versus remission state; unpaired t-test for age and INCAT score; Mann-Whitney test for time since diagnosis

Discussion

In the present study, typical CIDP differed from the group of atypical variants. Here, we found a stronger activated immune system in patients suffering from atypical variants of CIDP defined by a trend towards increased peripheral myelin antigen-specific (PMP-22, P0 180-199, MBP 82-100) T cell responses associated with a specific altered

CD4+ memory compartment of increased CD4+ TEM and CD4+ TCM counts in the blood. Further we detected elevated T cell responses against antigens P0 180-199 and MBP 82-100 in CIDP patients which have not described before.

We confirmed or previous findings that changes of the T memory compartment is a common finding especially

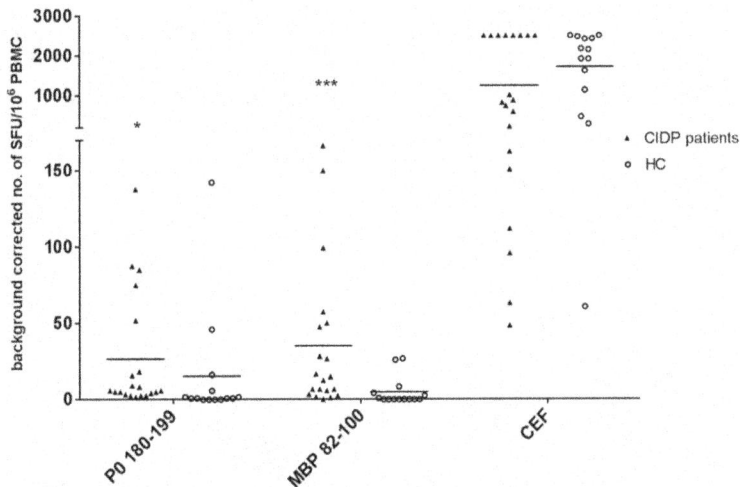

Fig. 1 Frequency of P0 and MBP specific T cells in CIDP patients. Frequencies of peripheral myelin antigen-specific T cell responses in CIDP patients (n = 20) vs. HC (n = 14) measured by IFN-γ ELISPOT. Background corrected SFU per 10^6 PBMC were significantly elevated for P0 180-199 as well as MBP 82-100 in CIDP patients vs. HC. Maximum value defined due to methodical limitations (CEF = 2500). (*p < 0.05, **p < 0.01, ***p < 0.001). Scatter dot plot with line at mean

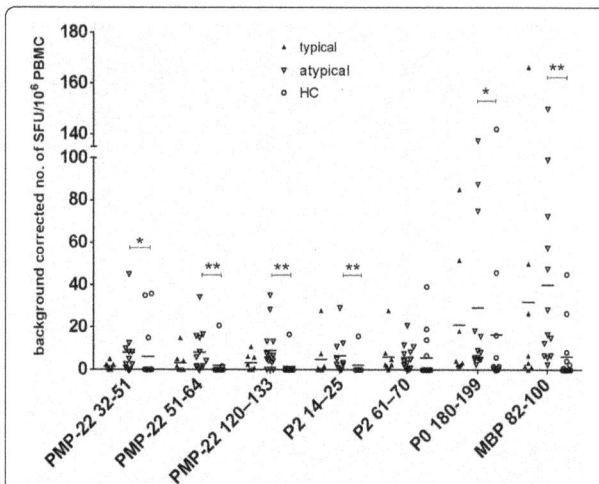

Fig. 2 Frequencies of peripheral myelin antigen-specific T cell responses in typical versus atypical CIDP patients. Typical ($n = 8$) vs atypical CIDP patients ($n = 12$) vs. HC ($n = 14$) were measured by IFN-γ ELISPOT. Background corrected SFU per 10^6 PBMC. Significantly, elevated SFU were observed in atypical CIDP patients vs. HC for PMP-22 32-51, PMP-22 51-64, PMP-22 120-133, P2 14-25, P0 180-199, MBP 82-100. (*$p < 0.05$, **$p < 0.01$, ***$p < 0.001$). Scatter dot plot with line at mean. For P0 180-199, a cut-off value of 5 SFU/10^6 PBMC in T cell-Elispot having a sensitivity of 91,7% (11/12) and a specificity of 62,5% (5/8) with AUC 0.69. For MBP 82-100 using a cut-off value of 10 SFU per 10^6 PBMC in a T cell-Elispot assay had a sensitivity of 75,0% (9/12) and a specificity of 62,5% (5/8) with AUC 0.68

higher specific immune responses against myelin-derived peptides in atypical compared to typical variants may be a cause for the lower treatment-responses. Likewise, the increased immune reactivity in atypical CIDP patients could result from insufficient treatment.

Recently, it has been demonstrated that CIDP patients show a diminished pro-regenerative function of Schwann cells leading to the axonal loss and therefore incomplete clinical recovery after treatment which is probably caused by inflammatory mediators [25]. Thus, differences in immune responses between typical and atypical CIDP we have demonstrated might also influence Schwann cell function resulting in different treatment responses and long-term outcome. The INCAT score was significantly lower in atypical cases. However, there was no difference in the time since diagnosis so that a longer disease course and hence pronounced disability and/or altered immune response is not the cause of this difference. Yet, we included mainly atypical case with mild motoric disability (6 patients with sensory CIDP [35.3%] and 5 patients with DADS [29.4%]) who are less often dependent on walking aids leading to lower INCAT disability scores.

Since we included mainly clinically unstable patients who had partly received treatment before, we are not able to answer this question at present. Based on previous results of reduced CD4+ memory subsets in GS-treated patients [17], it might be further argued that GS treatment may be efficient for this patient group. In contrast to Sanvito et al. [26], we identified higher IFN-γ responses to P2 and PMP22 peptides which have been more pronounced in the atypical compared to the typical CIDP subgroup. A higher number and proportion of atypical patients might explain this discrepancy as well as the fact that we included mainly clinically unstable and newly diagnosed patients.

in untreated patients [8, 17], which is in contrast to Sanvito and colleagues who showed no differences in T cell subpopulation [23]. In the present study, we detected elevated TEM and TCM primarily in atypical CIDP patients. Clinical experience and studies suggest that typical CIDP patients respond better to therapy than atypical CIDP variants, especially DADS [24], which is in line with our presented data showing that 100% (9/9) of typical compared to 47% (8/17) of atypical CIDP patients were therapy-responders. The reason for different treatment responses of CIDP subtypes remains unknown. The

Earlier publications detected P0 IgG-antibodies in CIDP patients and P0 180-199 specific T cell responses in spontaneous autoimmune polyneuropathy-

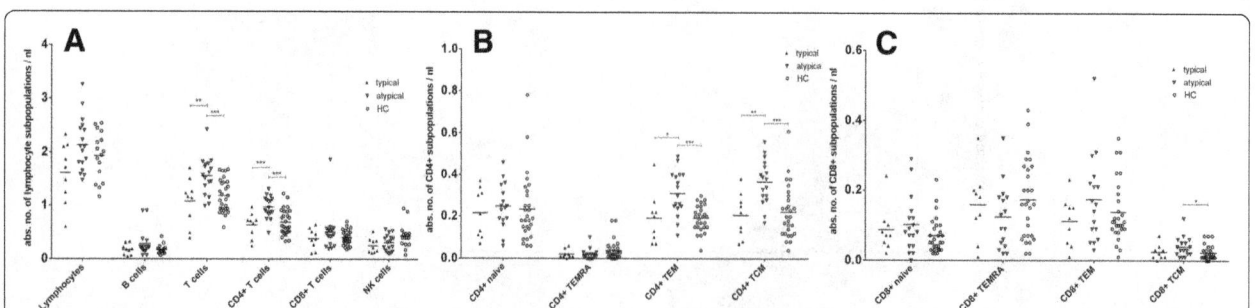

Fig. 3 Quantitative analysis of lymphocyte subpopulations in typical versus atypical CIDP. Lymphocyte subpopulations of typical ($n = 9$) vs. atypical CIDP patients ($n = 17$) vs. HC ($n = 28$) were measured by flow cytometry. In atypical CIDP patients significantly higher frequencies of T cells and CD4+ T cells were seen compared to vs. typical CIDP patients and HC (**a**). Significantly higher frequencies for CD4+ TEM and TCM in atypical vs. typical CIDP patients and HC (**b**). Significantly higher frequencies for CD8+ TCM in atypical CIDP patients vs. HC (**c**). (*$p < 0.05$, **$p < 0.01$, ***$p < 0.001$). Scatter dot plot with line at mean

mice [11]. Although EAN resembles Guillain-Barré-Syndrom (GBS) much more than CIDP, we regarded P0 as possible further candidate autoantigen of compact myelin for CIDP. Here, we detected elevated P0 180-199 specific T cell responses primarily in atypical CIDP.

Up to now, only little is known about the role of MBP 82-100 in the pathogenesis of CIDP even though MBP has been detected as part of the myelin sheath of peripheral nerves. Nevertheless, there is long-standing evidence that MBP 82-100 can induce neuroinflammation in autoimmune diseases [27]. Glatirameracetat, known antagonist of MBP 82-100 specific T cell receptor and part of MS therapy has been demonstrated to alleviate symptoms also in EAN- mice [28, 29]. Here, we demonstrated significantly elevated MBP 82-100 specific T cell responses in CIDP patients, again primarily in patients with atypical manifestations.

There is growing evidence for the autoimmune potential of antigens which are derived from non-compact myelin of the nodal/paranodal region such as neurofascin 155 of 186 leading to antibody response in distinct subgroups of CIDP or multifocal motoric neuropathy (MMN) [30–33]. Thus, antigenic targets derived from both compact and non- compact myelin leading to humeral and/or cellular immune response may define underlying immune mechanism of different clinical phenotypes of CIDP.

Several limitations may have affected our results. First, our clinically heterogeneous group of atypical patients was too small to distinguish between subgroups of atypical CIDP, which would be necessary to characterize atypical subtypes and to define specific cut offs for our immunological parameters. Second, differences in gender and INCAT score between typical and atypical CIDP patients might have influenced our immunological findings. Third, we aimed to recruit treatment-naïve patients in active-unstable stages of the disease. However, only 46% of patients (12/26) were treatment-naïve at enrollment. Previous immunosuppressive and –modulating therapy might have influenced our immunological findings.

Conclusions

Higher myelin-antigen specific T cell responses together with elevated T cell memory subsets were found in atypical compared to typical CIDP patients suggesting different patterns of immune responses in clinically distinctive CIDP subgroups. Myelin as well as nodal/paranodal proteins might serve as candidate autoantigens to establish robust immune markers for CIDP subtype differentiation. Given the clinical diversity of CIDP a larger cohort study is warranted in order to establish those markers with reliable cut-off values.

Abbreviations
CIDP: Chronic inflammatory demyelinating polyneuropathy; DADS: Distal acquired demyelinating polyneuropathy; EAN: Experimental autoimmune neuritis; EFNS: European Federation of Neurological Sciences; ELISPOT: Enzyme-linked immunospot assay; FACS: Fluorescence-activated cell sorting; GBS: Guillain-Barré-Syndrom; GS: Glucocorticosteroids; HC: Healthy control; IFN-γ: Interferon-gamma; INCAT: Inflammatory neuropathy cause and treatment; IVIG: IV immunoglobulin; MADSAM: Multifocal Acquired Demyelinating Sensory And Motor Polyneuropathy; MBP: Myelin basic protein; MGUS: Monoclonal gammopathy of uncertain significance; MRC: Medical Research Council Scale; MS: Multiple sclerosis; PBMC: Peripheral blood mononuclear cells; SFU: Spot forming unit; TCM: Central memory T cells; TEM: Effector memory T cells; TEMRA: Terminally differentiated T cells

Acknowledgment
The authors thank Sandra Bauer, Sonya Becker and Maik Stein for technical assistance.

Funding
The study was funded by a research grant from Grifols and supported by the Deutsche Forschungsgemeinschaft = German Research Foundation (NeuroCure Cluster of Excellence, Exc. 257). The funder had no role in the design of the study and collection, analysis, and interpretation of data and in writing the manuscript.

Author's contributions
MS recruited the patients, performed the experiments, analyzed and interpreted the data, and wrote the manuscript. JD recruited patients and analyzed the data. CM performed the experiments and revised the manuscript. AM analyzed the data and revised the manuscript. JK designed the study, was involved in ethical approval, recruited the patients, analyzed the data, revised the manuscript and supervised the study. She is the guarantor of the study. All authors gave their final approval to the study to be published and agree to be accountable for all aspects of the work.

Competing interests
J. Klehmet and A. Meisel have received personal compensation outside the submitted work for activities with Grifols, Octapharma and CSL Behring. M. Staudt, JM. Diederich, C. Meisel report no relevant financial activities outside the submitted work from any organisation for the submitted work; no financial relationships with any organisations that might have an interest in the submitted work in the previous 3 years, no other relationships or activities that could appear to have influenced the submitted work disclosures.
Parts of this work has been presented as a poster at the Inflammatory Neuropathy Consortium (INC) in Glasgow, UK in June 2016.

Author details
[1]Department of Neurology, Charité University Medicine, Charitéplatz 1, 10117 Berlin, Germany. [2]Department of Clinical Immunology, Charité University Medicine, Charitéplatz 1, Berlin, Germany.

References
1. Lunn MP, Manji H, Choudhary PP, Hughes RA, Thomas PK. Chronic inflammatory demyelinating polyradiculoneuropathy: a prevalence study in south east England. J Neurol Neurosurg Psychiatry. 1999;66:677–80.
2. Mahdi-Rogers M, Hughes RA. Epidemiology of chronic inflammatory neuropathies in southeast England. Eur J Neurol. 2014;1:28–33.
3. Latov N. Diagnosis and treatment of chronic acquired demyelinating polyneuropathies. Nat Rev Neurol. 2014;8:435–46.
4. Dalakas MC. Pathophysiology of autoimmune polyneuropathies. Presse Med. 2013;6:181–92.

5. Trebst C, Brunhorn K, Lindner M, Windhagen A, Stangel M. Expression of chemokine receptors on peripheral blood mononuclear cells of patients with immune-mediated neuropathies treated with intravenous immunoglobulins. Eur J Neurol. 2006;12:1359–63.

6. Tackenberg B, Nimmerjahn F, Lunemann JD. Mechanisms of IVIG efficacy in chronic inflammatory demyelinating polyneuropathy. J Clin Immunol. 2010; 30:65–9.

7. Ritter C, Förster D, Albrecht P, Hartung HP, Kieseier BC, Lehmann HC. IVIG regulates BAFF expression in patients with chronic inflammatory demyelinating polyneuropathy (CIDP). J Neuroimmunol. 2014;274:225–7.

8. Klehmet J, Goehler J, Ulm L, Kohler S, Meisel C, Meisel A, Harms H. Effective treatment with intravenous immunoglobulins reduces autoreactive T-cell response in patients with CIDP. J Neurol Neurosurg Psychiatry. 2015;6:686–91.

9. Zhu Y, Ljunggren H, Mix E, Li HL, van der Meide P, Elhassan AM, et al. CD28-B7 costimulation: a critical role for initiation and development of experimental autoimmune neuritis in C57BL/6 mice. J Neuroimmunol. 2001; 1:114–21.

10. Zhang HL, Azimullah S, Zheng XY, Wang XK, Amir N, Mensah-Brown EP, et al. IFN-gamma deficiency exacerbates experimental autoimmune neuritis in mice despite a mitigated systemic Th1 immune response. J Neuroimmunol. 2012;2:18–26.

11. Yan WX, Archelos JJ, Hartung HP, Pollard JD. P0 protein is a target antigen in chronic inflammatory demyelinating polyradiculoneuropathy. Ann Neurol. 2001;3:286–92.

12. Nave KA, Werner HB. Myelination of the nervous system: mechanisms and functions. Annu Rev Cell Biol. 2014;30:503–33.

13. Wucherpfennig KW, Catz I, Hausmann S, Strominger JL, Steinman L, Warren KG. Recognition of the immunodominant myelin basic protein peptide by autoantibodies and HLA-DR2-restricted T cell clones from multiple sclerosis patients. Identity of key contact residues in the B-cell and T-cell epitopes. J Clin Invest. 1997;5:1114–22.

14. Sallusto F, Langenkamp A, Geginat J, Lanzavecchia A. Functional subsets of memory T cells identified by CCR7 expression. Curr Top Microbiol Immunol. 2000;251:167–71.

15. Van den Berg LH, Mollee I, Wokke JH, Logtenberg T. Increased frequencies of HPRT mutant T lymphocytes in patients with Guillain-Barre syndrome and chronic inflammatory demyelinating polyneuropathy: further evidence for a role of T cells in the etiopathogenesis of peripheral demyelinating diseases. J Neuroimmunol. 1995;1:37–42.

16. Hughes RA, Allen D, Makowska A, Gregson NA. Pathogenesis of chronic inflammatory demyelinating polyradiculoneuropathy. J Peripher Nerv Syst. 2006;1:30–46.

17. Klehmet J, Staudt M, Ulm L, Unterwalder N, Meisel A, Meisel C. Circulating lymphocyte and T memory subsets in glucocorticosteroid versus IVIG treated patients with CIDP. J Neuroimmunol. 2015;283:17–22.

18. Mausberg AK, Dorok M, Stettner M, Müller M, Hartung HP, Dehmel T, et al. Recovery of the T-cell repertoire in CIDP by IV immunoglobulins. Neurology. 2013;3:296–303.

19. Giunti D, Borsellino G, Benelli R, Marchese M, Capello E, Valle MT, et al. Phenotypic and functional analysis of T cells homing into the CSF of subjects with inflammatory diseases of the CNS. J Leukoc Biol. 2003;5:584–90.

20. Van den Bergh PY, Hadden RD, Bouche P, Cornblath DR, Hahn A, Illa I, et al. European Federation of Neurological Societies; Peripheral nerve society. European Federation of Neurological Societies/peripheral nerve society guideline on management of chronic inflammatory demyelinating polyradiculoneuropathy: report of a joint task force of the European Federation of Neurological Societies and the peripheral nerve society - first revision. Eur J Neurol. 2010;3:356–63.

21. Currier JR, Kuta EG, Turk E, Earhart LB, Loomis-Price L, Janetzki S, et al. A panel of MHC class I restricted viral peptides for use as a quality control for vaccine trial ELISPOT assays. Journal Immunol Methods. 2002;1-2:157–72.

22. Gorson KC, van Schaik IN, Merkies IS, Lewis RA, Barohn RJ, Koski CL, et al. Chronic inflammatory demyelinating polyneuropathy disease activity status: recommendations for clinical research standards and use in clinical practice. J Peripher Nerv Syst. 2010;4:326–33.

23. Sanvito L, Makowska A, Gregson N, Nemni R, Hughes RA. Circulating subsets and CD4(+)CD25(+) regulatory T cell function in chronic inflammatory demyelinating polyneuropathy. Autoimmunity. 2009;42(8):667–77.

24. Nobile-Orazio E. Chronic inflammatory demyelinating polyradiculoneuropathy and variants: where we are and where we should go. J Peripher Nerv Syst. 2014;19(1):2–13.

25. Joshi AD, Holtmann L, Bobylev I, Schneider C, Ritter C, Weis J, Lehmann HC. Loss of Schwann cell plasticity in chronic inflammatory demyelinating polyneuropathy (CIDP). J Neuroinflammation. 2016;13(1):255.

26. Sanvito L, Makowska A, Mahdi-Rogers M, Hadden RD, Peakman M, Gregson N, Nemni R, Hughes RA. Humoral and cellular immune responses to myelin protein peptides in chronic inflammatory demyelinating polyneuropathy. J Neurol Neurosurg Psychiatry. 2009;80(3):333–8.

27. Mannie MD, Paterson PY, U'Prichard DC, Flouret G. Induction of experimental allergic encephalomyelitis in Lewis rats with purified synthetic peptides: delineation of antigenic determinants for encephalitogenicity, in vitro activation of cellular transfer, and proliferation of lymphocytes. Proc Natl Acad Sci U S A. 1985;16:5515–9.

28. Schrempf W, Ziemssen T. Glatiramer acetate: mechanisms of action in multiple sclerosis. Autoimmun Rev. 2007;7:469–75.

29. Zhang CJ, Zhai H, Yan Y, Hao J, Li MS, Jin WN, Su N, Vollmer TL, Shi FD. Glatiramer acetate ameliorates experimental autoimmune neuritis. Immunol Cell Biol. 2014;2:164–9.

30. Ng JK, Malotka J, Kawakami N, Derfuss T, Khademi M, Olsson T, et al. Neurofascin as a target for autoantibodies in peripheral neuropathies. Neurology. 2012;79:2241–8.

31. Querol L, Nogales-Gadea G, Rojas-Garcia R, Diaz-Manera J, Pardo J, Ortega-Moreno A, et al. Neurofascin IgG4 antibodies in CIDP associate with disabling tremor and poor response to IVIg. Neurology. 2014;82:879–86.

32. Devaux JJ, Miura Y, Fukami Y, Inoue T, Manso C, Belghazi M, et al. Neurofascin-155 IgG4 in chronic inflammatory demyelinating polyneuropathy. Neurology. 2016;86:800–7.

33. Notturno F, Di Febo T, Yuki N, Fernandez Rodriguez BM, Corti D. Nobile-Orazio et al. Autoantibodies to neurofascin-186 and gliomedin in multifocal motor neuropathy. J Neuroimmunol. 2014;276:207–12.

3

Changes in lymphocyte subsets in patients with Guillain-Barré syndrome treated with immunoglobulin

Hui Qing Hou[1], Jun Miao[2], Xue Dan Feng[1], Mei Han[3], Xiu Juan Song[1] and Li Guo[1*]

Abstract

Background: Guillain-Barré syndrome (GBS) is an autoimmune condition characterized by peripheral neuropathy. The pathogenesis of GBS is not fully understood, and the mechanism of how intravenous immunoglobulin (IVIG) cures GBS is ambiguous. Herein, we investigated lymphocyte subsets in patients with two major subtypes of GBS (acute inflammatory demyelinating polyneuropathy, AIDP, and acute motor axonal neuropathy, AMAN) before and after treatment with IVIG, and explored the possible mechanism of IVIG action.

Methods: Sixty-four patients with GBS were selected for our study and divided into two groups: AIDP (n = 38) and AMAN (n = 26). Thirty healthy individuals were chosen as the control group. Relative counts of peripheral blood T and B lymphocyte subsets were detected by flow cytometry analysis.

Results: In the AIDP group, the percentage of $CD4^+CD45RO^+$ T cells was significantly higher, while the percentage of $CD4^+CD45RA^+$ T cells was notably lower, than in the control group. After treatment with IVIG, the ratio of $CD4^+/CD8^+$ T cells and the percentage of $CD4^+CD45RA^+$ T cells increased, while the percentages of $CD8^+$ T cells and $CD4^+CD45RO^+$ T cells decreased significantly, along with the number of $CD19^+$ B cells. However, there were not such obvious changes in the AMAN group. The Hughes scores were significantly lower in both the AIDP and AMAN groups following treatment with IVIG, but the changes in Hughes scores showed no significant difference between the two groups.

Conclusions: This study suggested that the changes in T and B-lymphocyte subsets, especially in $CD4^+$T-lymphocyte subsets, might play an important role in the pathogenesis of AIDP, and in the mechanism of IVIG action against AIDP.

Keywords: Acute inflammatory demyelinating polyneuropathy, Acute motor axonal neuropathy, Guillain-Barré syndrome, Intravenous immunoglobulin, Lymphocyte subsets

Background

Guillain-Barré syndrome (GBS) is an acute, immune-mediated attack on the peripheral nervous system that leads to flaccid paralysis, with a case fatality rate of 5–10% [1]. Both cellular and humoral immunity participate in the onset of GBS, though cellular immunity is the primary cause [2]. Based on clinical, electrophysiological, and pathologic characteristics, GBS can be divided into two major subtypes: AIDP (acute inflammatory demyelinat-ing polyneuropathy, AIDP) and AMAN (acute motor axonal neuropathy, AMAN) [3]. At present there is no specific treatment for GBS; intravenous immunoglobulin (IVIG) has been the drug of choice for GBS treatment because it provides the most effective clinical results [4,5], with almost no contraindications.

Lymphocyte function is related to the numerous complex superficial cell membrane proteins on the cell surface. As a result, lymphocyte immune phenotype analysis can be used as an important reference index for evaluating the body's immune status. In recent years, much work has been undertaken to study the distribution of lymphocyte subsets in GBS, but the results are variable [6-9]. Our team found that the distribution of lymphocyte subsets differs greatly between individuals; therefore, it is important

* Correspondence: guoli6105@163.com
[1]Department of Neurology, the Second Hospital of Hebei Medical University, Key laboratory of Hebei Neurology, Shi jia zhuang, Hebei 050000, China
Full list of author information is available at the end of the article

to test individual GBS patients both before and after IVIG treatment [5]. In the current study, we examined GBS in a population of individuals from northern China who developed AIDP or AMAN. This study used a matched-pairs design using each patient's own pre- and post-treatment data. We detected changes in T and B lymphocyte subset distribution, allowing us to explore the pathogenesis of GBS and speculate on the mechanism of IVIG in treating GBS.

Methods
Patients
All subjects (patients with AIDP or AMAN and healthy controls) were from northern China and were referred to the Second Hospital of Hebei Medical University in Shijiazhuang from 2010–2013. All patients fulfilled accepted diagnostic criteria [10], and were studied within 2 weeks of the onset of GBS. Sixty-four cases underwent electrophysiological examination, being recorded for motor conductive velocity (MCV), distal latency, F wave, and motor evoked amplitude [10-13], and were classified into two groups: AIDP (n =38) and AMAN (n =26). The primary outcome parameter was GBS disability (Hughes) scale score at discharge. Thirty subjects (age- and sex-matched controls) from the same area were also included in the study. Controls had no personal or family history of GBS, and no sign of any peripheral neuropathy. Controls were chosen randomly.

Peripheral blood was collected and T and B lymphocyte subset relative counts were detected by flow cytometry both before and after treatment with IVIG. This study protocol was approved by the Research Ethics Committee of the Second Hospital of Hebei Medical University and followed the ethical guidelines of the 1975 Declaration of Helsinki and all subsequent modifications [14]. All patients provided a written informed consent to participate in this research.

Therapeutic method
Patients were treated with IVIG (0.4 g·kg^{-1}·d^{-1}) continuously for 5 days. At 3 weeks post-therapy, patients were again graded using the Hughes scale [15,16].

Flow cytometry
Prior to therapy, and again within 24 hours of the final therapy with IVIG, whole blood was collected in EDTA vacutainer tubes. Cyflow reagents and consumables were used according to the manufacturer's protocol. The set comprised the following antibodies: CD4-APC/CD8-PE/CD3-FITC; CD4-APC/CD45RA-FITC/CD45RO-PE; CD19-FITC (Becton Dickinson, San Jose, CA, USA). Meanwhile, IgG1-FITC/IgG2a-PE was replied as isotype control. 100 μl of the blood was incubated in tubes together with 20 μl of the antibodies. The incubation was performed in the dark, at room temperature for 15 min. After incubation, erythrocytes were subsequently lysed, and the cell suspension was centrifuged, washed three times, and resuspended in an appropriate volume of flow staining buffer. A minimum of 10,000 cells was accepted for FACS (BD Biosciences, San Jose, CA, USA) analysis. Cells were gated based on morphological characteristics.

Analysis
Statistical analyses were conducted using SPSS18.0 software, and continuous variables are expressed as mean ± standard deviation ($\bar{x} \pm s$). The mean differences between the two samples were analyzed using a t-test. The mean differences between the two patient groups before and after treatment were compared using a paired t-test. The inspection level was α =0.05 and differences were considered significant at p <0.05.

Results
The percentage of CD4^{+}CD45RO^{+} T cells (65.60 ± 10.41 vs 55.06 ± 5.48) was significantly higher, while the percentage of CD4^{+}CD45RA^{+} T cells (29.10 ± 10.13 vs 39.24 ± 6.25) was obviously lower (p <0.05), in the AIDP group than in the control group, but there was no significant difference between samples drawn from the AMAN group (Figures 1 and 2).

In the AIDP group, the ratio of CD4^{+}/CD8^{+} T cells (1.85 ± 1.09 vs 1.29 ± 0.80) and the percentage of CD4^{+}CD45RA^{+} T cells (37.56 ± 9.22 vs 29.10 ± 10.13) increased significantly (p <0.05), while the percentage of CD8^{+} T (29.60 ± 7.90 vs 35.12 ± 11.94), CD4^{+}CD45RO^{+} T (57.51 ± 8.45 vs 65.60 ± 10.41), and CD19^{+} B (12.11 ± 4.58 vs 15.89 ± 3.41) cells significantly decreased (p <0.05) after treatment. Again, there was not such a marked change following treatment in the AMAN group (Figures 3, 4, and 5).

The Hughes scores were significantly lower in both the AIDP and AMAN groups following treatment with IVIG (p <0.05) (Table 1).

The change in Hughes scores was 1.95 ± 0.56 in the AIDP group and 1.73 ± 0.80 in the AMAN group, and there was no significant difference between the two groups (p >0.05).

Discussion
Demyelination of motor and sensory nerves occurs in AIDP, whereas motor neurons evoke reduced amplitudes in AMAN, without demyelination. AIDP is an autoimmune disorder mediated by T and B lymphocyte systems. Pathologically, varying degrees of lymphocyte infiltration [17] and myelin sheath depigmentation can be found in AIDP, and the complement-mediated antibody attack on nerves is likely to play an important role in the pathogenesis of AIDP [18]. In AMAN, motor nerve axons, especially in Ranvier's

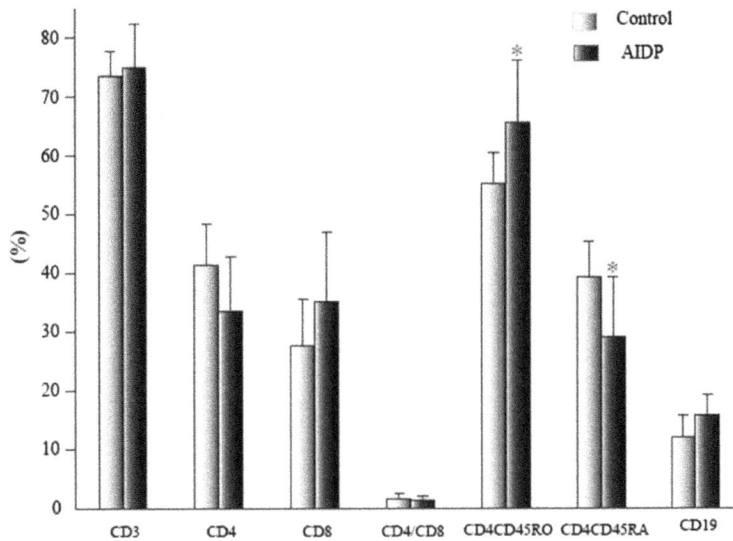

Figure 1 Comparison of lymphocyte subsets in AIDP and control groups before treatment. The data are mean ± S.D. *p <0.05, relative to the control group.

section, are attacked by macrophages, with varying degrees of Wallace degeneration, but rarely with inflammation and demyelination [19,20]. The etiology of GBS is not clear; however, a possible relationship with certain infections and vaccination has been documented in several studies [21-23]. GBS frequently follows a variety of presumed viral and bacterial infections [24,25], and *Campylobacter* gastroenteritis is the single most identifiable agent associated with GBS (AMAN) [26]. In subjects with GBS from northern China who developed AIDP and AMAN, the DNA-based typing of the HLA class II alleles in the two subtypes demonstrated that HLA class II epitopes are not distributed equally [27].

According to their antigen recognition receptors, T lymphocytes can be classified into two groups: TCR α/β T cells and TCR γ/δ T cells. The former make up more than 90% of T cells in peripheral blood. TCR α/β T cells, which are composed of $CD3^+CD4^+CD8^-$ T cells and $CD3^+CD4^-CD8^+$ T cells, play an important role in common immune response. γ/δ T cells were discovered in the past decade, and make up 0.5–10% of T cells in peripheral blood. Most γ/δ T cells express $CD3^+CD4^-CD8^-$T, which can be activated in autoimmune diseases. T lymphocytes include helper T lymphocytes ($CD4^+$T) and killer T lymphocytes ($CD8^+$T). $CD4^+$ T cells are heterogeneous, and include naive T cells and memory T cells, the former predominately expressing CD45RA and the latter expressing CD45RO [28,29]. In different stages of T cell development, different CD45 subtypes are expressed. Studies have shown that during the development of T cells in the thymus, a shift from CD45RO to CD45RA occurs, which

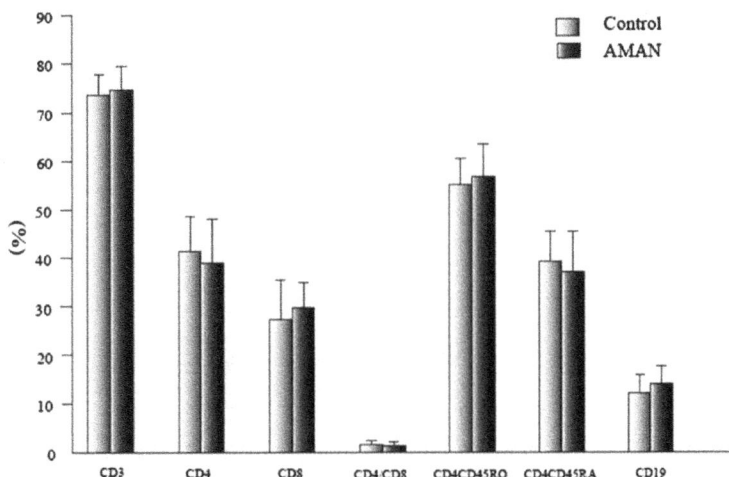

Figure 2 Comparison of lymphocyte subsets in AMAN and control groups before treatment. The data are mean ± S.D.

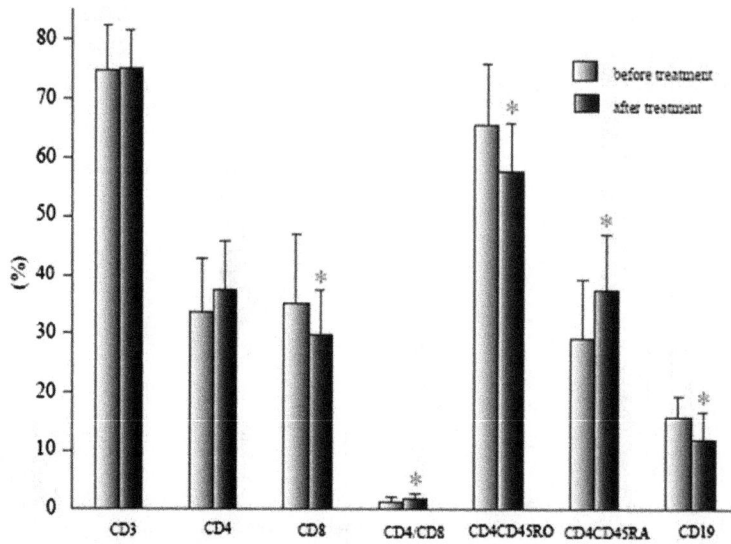

Figure 3 Comparison of lymphocyte subsets in AIDP before and after treatment. The data are mean ± S.D. *p <0.05.

marks the completion of negative selection and helps to eliminate autoreactive T cells and prevent autoimmune disease [30]. In the peripheral blood, CD4+CD45RA+ T cells can convert into CD4+CD45RO+ T cells following stimulation by antigen [30]. CD45RA and CD45RO have distinct effects on the function of B cells, and B cells can also increase the proliferation of CD45RO, in contrast to a decreased proliferation of CD45RA [31]. CD19 is an idioantigen of B lymphocytes, which also participates in their activation and signal conduction.

Our previous investigation found that if the number of CD4+ T or CD8+ T cells, or the ratio between them, changed, then immune functions may become disordered leading to a disease state in patients with GBS [5]. Studies have also shown that the number of CD4+ T cells in patients with GBS decreased while CD8+ T cells increased,

especially in the progressive stage. More specifically, CD4+CD29+ T cells (assist/induction of CD4+ T cells) increased and CD4+CD45RA+ T cells (restrain/induction of CD4+ T cells) decreased [6,7]. In contrast, other studies reported that the number of CD4+ T cells in patients with GBS increased and CD8+ T cells decreased [8,9]. Our previous study showed that following treatment with IVIG, CD8+ T and CD4+CD29+ T cells decreased in patients with GBS, whereas CD4/CD8 and CD4+CD45RA+ T cells increased [5]. To understand the changes in lymphocyte subsets in different subtypes of GBS, we carried out a further study and divided GBS patients into AIDP and AMAN groups.

In AIDP, demyelination and lymphocyte infiltration are observed. However, there is very little inflammation and demyelination in AMAN. Our research showed that

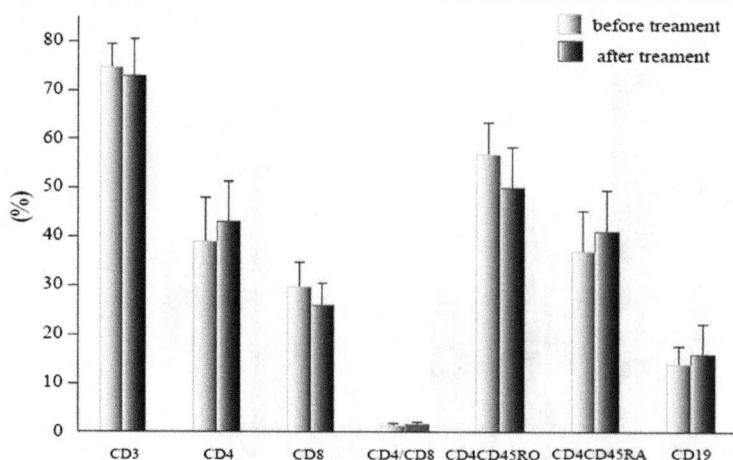

Figure 4 Comparison of lymphocyte subsets in AMAN before and after treatment. The data are mean ± S.D.

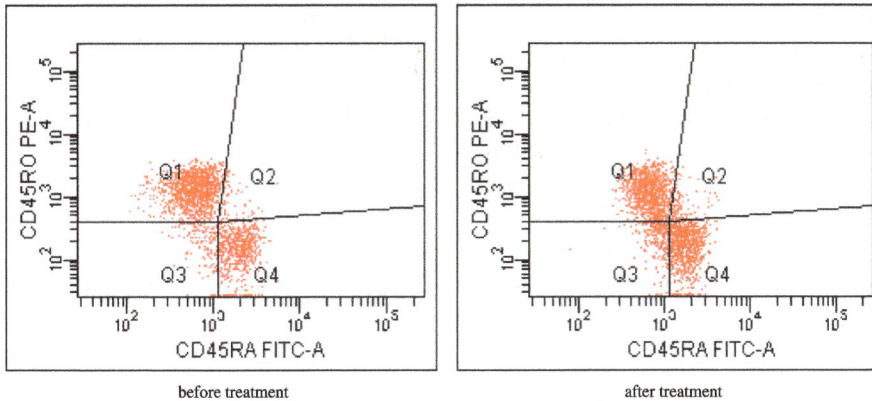

Figure 5 Representative plots from individual patient from AIDP group, gated on CD4+. The number in each quadrant represents CD45RA and CD45RO gated on CD4+.

the changes in lymphocyte subsets in the two GBS groups were different. In the AIDP group, the percentage of CD4+CD45RA+ T cells was markedly lower, whereas the percentage of CD4+CD45RO+ T cells was significantly higher than in the control group. The reason for this may be that CD4+CD45RA+ T cells transformed into CD4+CD45RO+ T cells after activation by antigens in the peripheral blood. This result is consistent with a study that showed that CD45RO enters into the cell cycle earlier than CD45RA stimulated by growth factors [32]. The transformation suggested that cellular immunology, especially the change in CD4+ T cell subsets, might play an important role in the pathogenesis of AIDP.

Cortical hormone has been the drug of choice to treat GBS. However, research has shown that routine hormone treatment cannot prevent the progression of GBS or improve prognosis [33]. At present, large doses of IVIG are the foremost immunoregulatory therapeutic method, and can ameliorate the course of GBS progression [5,34]. After therapy with IVIG, the ratio of CD4+/CD8+ T and the percentage of CD4+CD45RA+ T cells increased, while the percentage of CD8+ T, CD4+CD45RO+ T, and CD19+ B cells significantly declined in the AIDP group.

Table 1 Comparison of Hughes scores before and after treatment in each group ($\bar{x} \pm s$)

Group	Time	Hughes score
AIDP	Before treatment	3.59 ± 0.45
(n = 38)	After treatment	1.32 ± 0.67
	Falling value	2.27
	p	<0.05
AMAN	Before treatment	4.12 ± 0.63
(n = 26)	After treatment	2.47 ± 0.82
	Falling value	1.65
	p	<0.05

We presumed that IVIG inhibited the toxic effects of CD8 killer T cells on the myelin of nerves in AIDP and by altering the distribution of CD8+ T, CD4+CD45RA+ T, and CD4+CD45RO+ T cells, IVIG reduced the total number of B lymphocytes. Therefore, IVIG might affect the production of autoantibodies and decrease inflammatory cell infiltration, and we found Hughes scale score was significantly lower after treatment, this result suggested IVIG could suppress peripheral nerve injury and encourage neurofunctional recovery mediated by increasing CD45RA T cell and decreasing CD45RO T cell.

In the AMAN group, changes were not significant. That is, less inflammation and demyelination were present. Although IVIG suppressed immune reactions to a certain degree and prevented aggravation of the condition, our study showed no association between the immune parameters investigated and IVIG. These findings hint that there might be other changes in immune function, and further studies are needed.

The Hughes scale score was significantly lower both in the AIDP and AMAN groups after therapy with IVIG, and the change in the score was not significantly different between the AIDP and AMAN groups. Although this study cannot explain the pathogenicity of AMAN and the mechanism by which IVIG treats it, the effect of IVIG curing AMAN is evident. Therefore, in our clinical setting, we propose administering full doses of IVIG to patients with AIDP and AMAN at the earliest stage. This might prevent aggravation of the condition, decrease paralysis of respiratory muscle, prevent tracheal incision, preclude complications, and encourage the recovery of function of damaged neurology as soon as possible.

A search of the literature found very different conclusions on lymphocyte subgroup detection in patients with GBS. We designed this study of GBS patients to make patients their own controls, before and after treatment.

Such design can preclude the impact of different individuals who have suffered from infection previously. Furthermore, it can reveal the impact of disease and IVIG intervention on the immune system of an individual. GBS can be classified into two major groups: AIDP and AMAN. These groups differ in their hematological and immunological pathogenesis. Consequently, when studying lymphocyte subsets in GBS, it is important to classify GBS into AIDP or AMAN, and use patients as their own controls, before and after treatment, to minimize the effects of variation on the results.

Conclusions

This study suggested that the changes in CD4$^+$T-lymphocyte subsets might play an important role in the pathogenesis of AIDP. After treatment with IVIG, the changes in T and B-lymphocyte subsets are significant and also might play an important role in the mechanism of IVIG action against AIDP. But there were not such changes in AMAN, this study might infer that the pathogenesis and the mechanism of IVIG action against two subjects of GBS(AIDP and AMAN) are different and further studies are needed to expound these problems.

Competing interests
The authors declare that they have no competing interests.

Authors' contributions
HHQ, MJ, GL: substantially contributed to the drafting and revision of the manuscript, study concept and design, analysis and interpretation of data, and acquisition of data. FXD, SXJ: substantially contributed to the study concept and design and acquisition of data. HM: substantially contributed to the revision of the manuscript, study concept, and design. All authors read and approved the final manuscript.

Author details
[1]Department of Neurology, the Second Hospital of Hebei Medical University, Key laboratory of Hebei Neurology, Shi jia zhuang, Hebei 050000, China. [2]Department of Neurosurgery, the General Hospital of North China Petroleum Administration Bureau, Ren qiu, HeBei 062550, China. [3]Emergency Department, the Second Hospital of Hebei Medical University, Shi jia zhuang, Hebei 050000, China.

References
1. Yuki N: Infectious origins of, and molecular mimicry in, Guillain-Barre and Fisher syndromes. Lancet Infect Dis 2001, 1(1):29–37.
2. Ariga T, Yu RK: Antiglycolipid antibodies in Guillain-Barre syndrome and related diseases: review of clinical features and antibody specificities. J Neurosci Res 2005, 80(1):1–17.
3. Griffin JW, Li CY, Ho TW, Xue P, Macko C, Gao CY, Yang C, Tian M, Mishu B, Cornblath DR: Guillain-Barre syndrome in northern China. The spectrum of neuropathological changes in clinically defined cases. Brain 1995, 118(Pt 3):577–595.
4. Hughes RA, Swan AV, Raphael JC, Annane D, van Koningsveld R, van Doorn PA: Immunotherapy for Guillain-Barre syndrome: a systematic review. Brain 2007, 130(Pt 9):2245–2257.
5. Guo L, Hou HQ, Song XJ, Yang JC, Gao CY: Change of T-Lymphocyte subsets in the patients with Guillain-Barre syndrome between pre and post-therapy with intravenous immunoglobulin and its meaning. Chin J Neurol 2008, 41(2):87–90.
6. Dahle C, Vrethem M, Ernerudh J: T lymphocyte subset abnormalities in peripheral blood from patients with the Guillain-Barre syndrome. J Neuroimmunol 1994, 53(2):219–225.
7. Sindern E, Oreja-Guevara C, Raulf-Heimsoth M, Baur X, Malin JP: A longitudinal study of circulating lymphocyte subsets in the peripheral blood during the acute stage of Guillain-Barre syndrome. J Neurol Sci 1997, 151(1):29–34.
8. Hughes RA, Aslan S, Gray IA: Lymphocyte subpopulations and suppressor cell activity in acute polyradiculoneuritis (Guillain-Barre syndrome). Clin Exp Immunol 1983, 51(3):448–454.
9. Lisak RP, Zweiman B, Guerrero F, Moskovitz AR: Circulating T-cell subsets in Guillain-Barre syndrome. J Neuroimmunol 1985, 8(2–3):93–101.
10. Cui LY, Pu CQ, Hu XQ: The diagnosis and treatment guidelines of Guillain-Barre syndrome in China. Chin J Neurol 2010, 43(8):583–586.
11. Asbury AK, Cornblath DR: Assessment of current diagnostic criteria for Guillain-Barre syndrome. Ann Neurol 1990, 27(Suppl):S21–S24.
12. Van den Bergh PY, Pieret F: Electrodiagnostic criteria for acute and chronic inflammatory demyelinating polyradiculoneuropathy. Muscle Nerve 2004, 29(4):565–574.
13. Van der Meche FG, Van Doorn PA, Meulstee J, Jennekens FG: Diagnostic and classification criteria for the Guillain-Barre syndrome. Eur Neurol 2001, 45(3):133–139.
14. Puri KS, Suresh KR, Gogtay NJ, Thatte UM: Declaration of Helsinki, 2008: implications for stakeholders in research. J Postgrad Med 2009, 55(2):131–134.
15. Hughes RA, Newsom-Davis JM, Perkin GD, Pierce JM: Controlled trial prednisolone in acute polyneuropathy. Lancet 1978, 2(8093):750–753.
16. Peng M, Jia JP: Predictors at nadir of severity on patients with Guillain-Barre syndrome. Chin J Neurol 2004, 37(2):154–157.
17. Asbury AK, Arnason BG, Adams RD: The inflammatory lesion in idiopathic polyneuritis. Its role in pathogenesis. Medicine (Baltimore) 1969, 48(3):173–215.
18. Hafer-Macko CE, Sheikh KA, Li CY, Ho TW, Cornblath DR, McKhann GM, Asbury AK, Griffin JW: Immune attack on the Schwann cell surface in acute inflammatory demyelinating polyneuropathy. Ann Neurol 1996, 39(5):625–635.
19. Feasby TE, Gilbert JJ, Brown WF, Bolton CF, Hahn AF, Koopman WF, Zochodne DW: An acute axonal form of Guillain-Barre polyneuropathy. Brain 1986, 109(Pt 6):1115–1126.
20. Feasby TE, Hahn AF, Brown WF, Bolton CF, Gilbert JJ, Koopman WJ: Severe axonal degeneration in acute Guillain-Barre syndrome: evidence of two different mechanisms? J Neurol Sci 1993, 116(2):185–192.
21. Greene SK, Rett MD, Vellozzi C, Li L, Kulldorff M, Marcy SM, Daley MF, Belongia EA, Baxter R, Fireman BH, Jackson ML, Omer SB, Nordin JD, Jin R, Weintraub ES, Vijayadeva V, Lee GM: Guillain-Barre syndrome, influenza vaccination, and antecedent respiratory and gastrointestinal infections: a case-centered analysis in the vaccine safety datalink, 2009–2011. PLoS ONE 2013, 8(6):e67185.
22. Souayah N, Yacoub HA, Khan HM, Farhad K, Mehyar LS, Maybodi L, Menkes DL, Qureshi AI: Guillain-Barre syndrome after influenza vaccination in the United States, a report from the CDC/FDA vaccine adverse event reporting system (1990–2009). J Clin Neuromuscul Dis 2012, 14(2):66–71.
23. Dieleman J, Romio S, Johansen K, Weibel D, Bonhoeffer J, Sturkenboom M: Guillain-Barre syndrome and adjuvanted pandemic influenza A (H1N1) 2009 vaccine: multinational case–control study in Europe. BMJ 2011, 343:d3908.
24. van Doorn PA, Ruts L, Jacobs BC: Clinical features, pathogenesis, and treatment of Guillain-Barre syndrome. Lancet Neurol 2008, 7(10):939–950.
25. Lunn MP, Willison HJ: Diagnosis and treatment in inflammatory neuropathies. J Neurol Neurosurg Psychiatry 2009, 80(3):249–258.
26. Drenthen J, Yuki N, Meulstee J, Maathuis EM, van Doorn PA, Visser GH, Blok JH, Jacobs BC: Guillain-Barre syndrome subtypes related to Campylobacter infection. J Neurol Neurosurg Psychiatry 2011, 82(3):300–305.
27. Magira EE, Papaioakim M, Nachamkin I, Asbury AK, Li CY, Ho TW, Griffin JW, McKhann GM, Monos DS: Differential distribution of HLA-DQ beta/DR beta epitopes in the two forms of Guillain-Barre syndrome, acute motor axonal neuropathy and acute inflammatory demyelinating polyneuropathy (AIDP): identification of DQ beta epitopes associated with susceptibility to and protection from AIDP. J Immunol 2003, 170(6):3074–3080.

28. McBreen S, Imlach S, Shirafuji T, Scott GR, Leen C, Bell JE, Simmonds P: Infection of the CD45RA+ (naive) subset of peripheral CD8+ lymphocytes by human immunodeficiency virus type 1 in vivo. *J Virol* 2001, **75**(9):4091–4102.

29. Clement LT, Vink PE, Bradley GE: Novel immunoregulatory functions of phenotypically distinct subpopulations of CD4+ cells in the human neonate. *J Immunol* 1990, **145**(1):102–108.

30. McNeill L, Cassady RL, Sarkardei S, Cooper JC, Morgan G, Alexander DR: CD45 isoforms in T cell signalling and development. *Immunol Lett* 2004, **92**(1–2):125–134.

31. Matto M, Nuutinen UM, Ropponen A, Myllykangas K, Pelkonen J: CD45RA and RO isoforms have distinct effects on cytokine- and B-cell-receptor-mediated signalling in human B cells. *Scand J Immunol* 2005, **61**(6):520–528.

32. Booth NJ, McQuaid AJ, Sobande T, Kissane S, Agius E, Jackson SE, Salmon M, Falciani F, Yong K, Rustin MH, Akbar AN, Vukmanovic-Stejic M: Different proliferative potential and migratory characteristics of human CD4+ regulatory T cells that express either CD45RA or CD45RO. *J Immunol* 2010, **184**(8):4317–4326.

33. Hughes RA, Cornblath DR: Guillain-Barre syndrome. *Lancet* 2005, **366**(9497):1653–1666.

34. Douglas MR, Winer JB: Guillain-Barre syndrome and its treatment. *Expert Rev Neurother* 2006, **6**(10):1569–1574.

4

An unusual case of recurrent Guillain-Barré syndrome with normal cerebrospinal fluid protein levels

Sonali Sihindi Chapa Gunatilake*⑩, Rohitha Gamlath and Harith Wimalaratna

Abstract

Background: Guillain-Barré syndrome is an acquired polyradiculo-neuropathy, often preceded by an antecedent event. It is a monophasic disease but a recurrence rate of 1–6 % is documented in a subset group of patients. Patients with Guillain-Barré syndrome show cerebrospinal fluid albuminocytologic dissociation. Normal cerebrospinal fluid protein levels during both initial and recurrent episodes of Guillain-Barré syndrome is a rare occurrence and has not been described earlier in the literature.

Case presentation: Twenty-five-year-old Sri Lankan female with past history of complete recovery following an acute inflammatory demyelinating polyneuropathy (AIDP) variant of Guillain-Barré syndrome 12 years back presented with acute, ascending symmetrical flaccid quadriparasis extending to bulbar muscles, bilateral VII cranial nerves and respiratory compromise needing mechanical ventilation. Nerve conduction study revealed AIDP variant of Guillain-Barré syndrome. Cerebrospinal fluid analysis done after 2 weeks were normal during both episodes without albuminocytologic dissociation. She was treated with intravenous immunoglobulin resulting in a remarkable recovery. Both episodes had a complete clinical recovery in three and four months' time respectively, rather a faster recovery than usually expected.

Conclusion: Recurrence of Guillain-Barré syndrome can occur in a subset of patients with Guillain-Barré syndrome even after many years of asymptomatic period. Normal cerebrospinal fluid profile does not exclude Guillain-Barré syndrome and may occur in subsequent recurrences of Guillain-Barré syndrome arising the need for further studies to identify the pathophysiology and the possibility of a different subtype of Guillain-Barré syndrome.

Keywords: Guillain-Barré syndrome, Albuminocytologic dissociation, Acute inflammatory demyelinating polyneuropathy, Cerebrospinal fluid, Case report

Abbreviations: AIDP, Acute inflammatory demyelinating polyneuropathy; CIDP, Chronic inflammatory demyelinating polyneuropathy; CSF, Cerebrospinal fluid; GBS, Guillain-Barré syndrome; GBS-TRF, Guillain-Barré syndrome with treatment related fluctuations; RGBS, Recurrent Guillain-Barré syndrome

Background

Guillain-Barré syndrome (GBS) is an acquired heterogeneous group of disorders due to an immune-mediated inflammation and demyelination of the peripheral nervous system, following an antecedent illness in two thirds of the patients, commonly an infection [1–3]. It is a medical emergency which usually presents with acute onset, rapidly progressive symmetrical ascending flaccid paralysis of the limbs with accompanying absent or diminished deep tendon reflexes. It is often associated with sensory symptoms, cranial nerve involvement, less commonly autonomic dysfunction and respiratory compromise.

GBS is a monophasic illness. Although rare, recurrence has been described following an asymptomatic period of few months to years (4 months – 10 years) in 1–6 % of patients [3–6]. Recurrent GBS (RGBS) is characterized by 2 or more attacks of acute inflammatory demyelinating neuropathy with an onset to peak time of 4 weeks or less, and having complete or near complete recovery [3, 5]. It is suggested by Kuitwaard et al. that there is a

* Correspondence: sonaligunatilake@gmail.com
Teaching Hospital, Kandy, Sri Lanka

subset of patients with GBS who are susceptible for recurrence, characterized by younger age, milder course of disease and having Miller-Fisher variant of GBS [3]. Literature revealed that the patients with recurrence had similar but more severe symptoms and signs in subsequent episodes while having similar or different antecedent event [3, 6]. It is important to distinguish recurrent GBS from GBS with treatment related fluctuations (GBS-TRF) and chronic inflammatory demyelinating polyradiculo-neuropathy (CIDP) as the treatment regimens are different. Cerebrospinal fluid (CSF) shows albuminocytologic dissociation in 82–90 % of the patients with GBS after 10–14 days from onset of the illness [7]. Electrophysiological studies and CSF analysis are taken to aid clinical diagnosis of GBS but normal CSF profile can be found in 10 % of GBS patients throughout the disease [8]. Therefore normal values cannot rule out GBS. Grand'maison et al. reported 12 cases of recurrent GBS (total of 32 episodes), where it was observed that all patients who were in the symptomatic phase of GBS and after 1 week of onset of disease showed CSF albuminocytologic dissociation. They observed normal CSF protein levels which was tested at the onset of disease (within 1 week) in two patients but had not identified a variant of RGBS with normal CSF protein levels during the symptomatic episodes, tested atleast 1 week after the onset of symptoms.

We present a rare case of RGBS presenting after 12 years, adding to the limited number of cases with a long asymptomatic interval. Such reported cases from South-Asia are rare. Apart from the young age at initial episode, she did not have other risk factors for recurrence and had a rare findings of normal CSF protein concentrations on both presentations. Extensive literature survey including published case reports and case series did not reveal a similar case report of RGBS or occurrence with normal CSF protein concentrations during both initial and recurrent presentations of GBS.

Case presentation
A 25-year-old Sri Lankan female presented with weakness of all four limbs in January 2014. She had a similar illness 12 years back.

First episode
In 2002, at the age of 13 years, patient had noticed tingling sensation of distal upper and lower limbs followed by weakness of lower limbs, involving both distal and proximal muscle groups. Weakness was progressive and ascending, involving both upper limbs and neck muscles by day 6 of the illness. There was no dysphagia, dysphonia, respiratory difficulty or bladder/bowel involvement. There was no significant medical history suggestive of preceding infection, toxin ingestion or similar disease in the past. On

examination, there was flaccid quadriparesis (muscle power grade - 3/5) with areflexia in all 4 limbs. There were no cranial nerve palsies or features suggestive of autonomic involvement. Sensory system examination was normal. Full blood count, blood picture, serum electrolytes, blood urea and liver enzymes profile were normal. Her erythrocyte sedimentation rate was 13mm during 1st hour. Nerve conduction studies performed on day 4 of the illness showed focal segmental demyelinating type sensory and motor neuropathy with conduction blocks (Table 1), suggestive of acute inflammatory demyelinating polyneuropathy (AIDP). EMG studies were not performed during this episode. CSF analysis on day 14 of the illness revealed normal results with proteins – 30 g/dl (normal 15–40 g/dl), white cells 2 with 100 % lymphocytes and normal CSF glucose levels compared to plasma values. She was treated with intravenous immunoglobulin for 5 consecutive days in addition to physiotherapy and discharged on day 18. She made a complete recovery in 3 months based on normal tone, power and deep tendon reflexes on neurological examination. Follow-up NCS was not performed after clinical recovery.

Second episode
In 2014, patient readmitted with numbness and progressive ascending weakness of all four limbs for 3 days duration and had developed poor cough response, dysphagia and difficulty in breathing during the following 2 days. This episode was preceded by an upper respiratory tract infection two weeks back. There was no similar illness noted in any of her family members. On examination, flaccid quadriparesis with generalized areflexia was noted with a muscle power of 1/5 in lower limbs, 2/5 in upper limbs and 2/5 in neck muscles. Weakness progressed to involve bilateral seventh cranial nerves and bulbar muscle without ophthalmoplegia. Rest of the neurological examination including sensory system and other organ system examination were normal except for a resting tachycardia of 130 beats/min without any significant blood pressure fluctuations. Respiratory rate was 30 cycles/min with oxygen saturation of 92 % on air. Nerve conduction studies done on day 10 of the illness revealed focal segmental demyelinating type sensory and motor neuropathy with prolonged distal motor latency, delayed F-wave and conduction blocks, concluding as AIDP variant of GBS (Table 1). Electromyogram done on day 10 of the illness did not show any evidence of denervation but noted fibrillation potentials of positive sharp waves. CSF analysis on day 10 and a repeat study on day 24 showed normal results without cyto-protein dissociation or pleocytosis (Table 2) Full blood count, blood picture, serum electrolytes, erythrocyte sedimentation rate, blood urea and liver enzymes profile were normal. Serology for *Mycoplasma*, *Campylobacter jejuni*, cytomegalovirus, Epstein-Barr virus,

Table 1 Nerve conduction study during the initial presentation in 2002 (1st episode) and recurrence (2nd episode) of Guillain-Barre syndrome in 2014

Nerve	Episode	Distal latency (ms)	Conduction velocity (m/s)	Amplitude (mV)	F wave (m/s)	Conduction block
Motor						
Median (Right/left)	1st	6.7/6.2	40/45	7.5/11	33/35	Yes
	2nd	9.1/8.9	38/40	5.6/ 6	38/40	Yes
	Recovery (4 months after 2nd Episode)	4.4/4.5	51	6.0	29	No
	Normal Referrence Value	<4.4	>49	>4.2	<31	
Ulnar (Right/left)	1st	4.6/5.0	42/44	6.0/ 6.2	27/32	Yes
	2nd	8.9/9.4	37/41	8.2/ 1.5	36/29	Yes
	Normal Referrence Value	<3.5	>49	>5.6	<31	
Peroneal @ EDB (Right/left)	1st	11.5/13	38/45	2.5/ 2.4	43/49	NP
	2nd	Absent	Absent	1.6/2.0	Absent	Yes
	Recovery (4 months after 2nd Episode)	5.5	50	2.5	33	No
	Normal Referrence Value	<5.7	>50	>2.2		
Tibial (Right/left)	1st	18.8/18.9		3.0/3.2	52/49	NP
	2nd	NP	NP	NP	NP	NP
	Normal Referrence Value			>2.8		
Sensory						
Radial (Right/left)	1st	2.8/ 3.1	38/37	24/23	-	-
	2nd	2.9/ 3.0	28/33	18/20		
	Normal Referrence Value	<2.6	>43	>20		
Sural (Right/left)	1st	2.5/3.0	41/40	34/28		
	2nd	2.6/2.5	46/48	25/27	-	-
	Normal Referrence Value	<2.6	>52	>24		

NP not performed
EDB Extensor digitorum brevis

Table 2 Laboratory findings of Cerebrospinal fluid during the initial presentation in 2002 and recurrence of Guillain-Barré syndrome in 2014

Cerebrospinal fluid profile	2002 episode: 1 – Day 14	2014 recurrence – Day 10	2014 recurrence – Day 24
CSF Glucose (mg/dL)	86	78	80
Proteins (g/dL) (normal: 15 – 40 g/dL)	30	20	26
White blood cells/HPF (normal: 0 – 5 cells/HPF)	2	4	2
Neutrophils %	-	-	-
Lymphocytes %	100	100	100
Red blood cells/HPF	5	-	10
Random blood glucose tested at the time of lumba puncture (mg/dL)	102	110	94

CSF study was performed twice during the episode of recurrence (2014) to clarify the persistence of normal CSF findings during the course of the illness

hepatitis B & C and retroviral studies were negative. Autoimmune panel including anti-nuclear factor was normal. Due to the rapid progressive nature of weakness and respiratory distress, patient was mechanically ventilated for 12 days. Diagnosis of GBS was made and intravenous immunoglobulin 0.4 g/kg/day was administered for 5 days. In addition, she received physiotherapy to support her recover in motor function of limbs and speech therapy following extubation. She made a good clinical recovery assessed subjectively as well as objectively and was discharged home on day 28 with a muscle power of 4/5 and deep tendon reflexes of +1.

On follow-up, patient had normal neurological examination findings and subsequent nerve conduction study after 4 months revealed normal results (Table 1).

Conclusions

GBS is an acute, immune mediated inflammatory polyradiculo-neuropathy involving the peripheral nervous system. Onset is preceded by an antecedent event in two thirds of the patients, usually an upper respiratory tract infection or a diarrheal illness [1–3], where the causative agent is assumed to trigger an immune response against the gangliosides and glycolipids distributed along the myelin sheaths and peripheral nervous system. This results in marked inflammation of the peripheral nerves, resulting in demyelination and defective impulse propagation. It is a heterogeneous group of disorders which involves motor, sensory and autonomic nervous systems to varying degrees depending on the sub type; (1) Acute inflammatory demyelinating polyneuropathy, (2) Acute motor axonal neuropathy, (3) Acute motor sensory axonal neuropathy, (4) Miller Fisher syndrome, (5) Acute pan-autonomic neuropathy and (6) Pure sensory GBS.

GBS is a monophasic illness, with an annual incidence rate of 1.2–3 per 100 000 population [9]. Yet, recurrence of GBS is observed in 1–6 % of patients, where it is defined as 2 or more attacks of acute inflammatory demyelinating neuropathy with an onset to peak time of 4 weeks or less having complete or near complete recovery [3–6]. The time lag between two episodes of GBS was 4 months to 10 years in a study done by Das et al. and a mean of 7 years with a range from 2 months to 37 years was described by Kuitwaard et al. [3, 5]. Patients tend to get similar clinical presentations and shorter intervals in between subsequent episodes of GBS [3]. Results of the study by Kuitwaard also found that RGBS patients were younger, with milder disease and had Miller-Fisher variant of GBS at the initial episode. Patients with above characteristics on initial presentation of GBS are more prone for recurrences [3]. They also identified that there are similar presentations but more severe clinical deficit and residual effects with each recurrence [3, 6]. Yet, there is limited literature addressing why only a certain subset of patients with GBS get recurrences of the disease. The indexed case, although young at presentation, patient had a more alarming disease initially with poor neck muscle power and limb power and did not have Miller-Fisher variant. This shows a deviation from the classically identified features favoring a recurrence of GBS. The time gap between the episodes was 12 years. During the episode of recurrence, she had rapid development of more severe disabling illness involving cranial nerves and respiratory compromise needing mechanical ventilation. Both episodes had AIDP variant of GBS with similar initial presentations.

The RGBS patients with similar presentations during the subsequent episodes had different antecedent infections and this may point towards immunogenic and host factors as major determinants of the disease [3, 5, 6]. Yet, exact mechanism by which similar clinical manifestations occur during recurrence is not established. Our patient also had an upper respiratory tract infection preceding the recurrence of GBS but did not have an event during the initial episode.

It is important to distinguish RGBS from two clinical entities; (1) GBS with treatment related fluctuations (GBS-TRF), (2) Chronic inflammatory demyelinating polyneuropathy (CIDP). GBS-TRF which occurs in 6–16 % of patients with GBS is defined as significant deterioration within 2 months after disease onset following post treatment improvement or stabilization [3]. Repeating immunoglobulin or plasmaparesis in such patients will improve the outcome [10]. Since our patient had a long asymptomatic period, GBS-TRF is less likely but CIDP comes as a differential diagnosis. CIDP is suspected when progression of weakness lasts more than 8 weeks followed by a chronic course but it can be of steadily progressive, relapsing remitting or monophasic. The treatment differs as CIDP can be treated with either immunoglobulin or immunosuppressive therapy with a subsequent maintenance immunosuppressive drug treatment whereas GBS and GBS-TRF do not show a response to immunosuppressant therapy but has good response to immunoglobulin or plasmaparesis. GBS is a more likely diagnosis in our patient as there was a rapid onset of symptoms, subsequent complete or near complete recovery, high incidence of an antecedent illness, normal CSF protein levels at the onset of a recurrence.

Diagnosis of GBS is mainly clinical and supported by evidence from electrophysiological studies and CSF analysis. Characteristically CSF has high protein levels with normal cell counts and sugar levels. Nerve roots that exit from the spinal cord traverse through CSF and when nerve roots are inflamed in GBS, proteins leak in to the CSF. Since the inflammation is confined to the nerve roots, significant numbers of inflammatory cells are not seen. Although normal CSF findings are seen during the first week of disease, albuminocytologic dissociation is seen in 82–90 % of the patients with GBS by the end of second week of the illness [7]. Grand'maison et al. had also observed normal CSF proteins at the onset of recurrent GBS episodes but also noted that it was elevated when measured after 1 week and when the patient is symptomatic [4]. 10 % of patients with typical GBS may have normal CSF findings though out the course of illness [7, 8, 11] but the pathophysiological mechanism leading to normal values is not well understood. Medical literature on above area is not extensive. The index case also had normal levels of CSF total proteins (performed after 2 weeks of onset of illness) during both episodes of GBS, which is uncommon and not described in previously reported cases of RGBS.

Study done by Gonzalez-Quevedo et al. revealed raised CSF total proteins correlated with the degree of inflammation at the nerve roots and higher level of CSF proteins were related to clinical severity [12]. Corston et al. studied amino acids in CSF of GBS patients quantitatively as well as qualitatively. Of the 12 patients studied,

4 had normal CSF protein levels (<40 g/dL) and in 3 of them repeat CSF analysis confirmed normal CSF protein levels. Analysis revealed that 12 amino acids (Eg - ornithine, lysine, arginine, glycine, alanine plus citrulline, leucine, tyrosine and phenylalanine) were raised in patients with high CSF proteins while 6 of the amino acids (alanine plus citrulline, 2 amino-butyric acid, leucin, ornithine and lycine) were raised above normal reference range in patients who had normal CSF total proteins [13]. Three amino acids (phosphoethanolamine, serine and glutamic acid) in the CSF of GBS patients showed reduced concentrations. This study highlights the fact that even when the total protein content in CSF is normal, patients with GBS have alteration of specific amino acids in CSF. Our patient had a severe disease with respiratory compromise during the recurrence but in contrast to the study by Gonzalez-Quevedo et al. she had normal CSF protein levels. Due to the unavailability of the laboratory facilities, we could not perform the CSF amino acid analysis in our patient.

Index patient had a recurrence of GBS after a long asymptomatic period of 12 years as supported by acute onset, rapid progression, disability peaked within 2 weeks followed by complete subsequent recovery following treatment, presence of antecedent infection and supportive electrophysiological evidence. She also had more severe disease during the recurrence. CSF findings were not characteristic and were normal during both episodes occurring 12 years apart, which is a rare finding and not described earlier in patients with RGBS. Mechanism behind normal level of CSF proteins during recurrent episodes remains unclear.

Recurrence of GBS is rare but can occur after many years of asymptomatic period and is associated with more severe clinical manifestations. In such a presentation, it is important to distinguish GBS from CIDP as the treatment modalities are different. Normal CSF total protein levels tested after 1 week after the onset of disease can occur in initial and recurrent episodes of GBS, where the mechanism is not fully understood. Research on recurrent GBS is needed to evaluate the higher probability of certain subgroup of patients with GBS for recurrences, to identify the occurrence and pathophysiology of normal CSF profile and the possibility of a different subtype in recurrent GBS patients.

Acknowledgement

The authors acknowledge the contribution of Dr. W. Dharmakeerthi, Consultant Neuro-electrophysiologist, Teaching Hospital, Kandy, Sri Lanka, staff of biochemistry laboratory, medical intensive care unit and medical ward in Teaching Hospital, Kandy, Sri Lanka for the support provided in the process of diagnosis and management of this patient.

Funding

None of the authors have received any financial assistance for this manuscript.

Authors' contributions

HW made the clinical diagnosis, made clinical decisions in management and supervised the manuscript drafting. SSCG drafted the first manuscript and reviewed the literature. HW, RG and SSCG were involved in direct management of the patient. All authors read and approved the final manuscript.

Authors' information

HW (MBBS, MD, FRCP(Edin), FRCP(Lond), FCCP) is a Consultant Physician. RG (MBBS, MD) is a Senior Registrar in Medicine. SSCG (MBBS) is a Registrar in Medicine. All authors are attached to Teaching Hospital, Kandy, Sri Lanka.

Competing interests

The authors declare that they have no competing interests.

References

1. Winer JB, Hughes RAC, Anderson MJ, et al. A prospective study of acute idiopathic neuropathy. II Antecedent events. J Neurol Neurosurg Psychiatry. 1988;51:613–8.
2. Seneviratne U. Guillain-Barré syndrome. Postgrad Med J. 2000;76:774–82.
3. Kuitwaard K, Koningsveld RV, Ruts L, Jacobs BC, Doorn PAV. Recurrent Guillain–Barré syndrome. J Neurol Neurosurg Psychiatry. 2009;80:56–9.
4. Grand'Maison F, Feasby TE, Hahn AF, Koopman WJ. Recurrent guillain-barre syndrome. Clinical and laboratory features. Brain. 1992;115(4):1093–106.
5. Das A, Kalita J, Misra UK. Recurrent Guillain Barré syndrome. Electromyogr Clin Neurophysiol. 2004;44(2):95–102.
6. Hadden RDM. Deterioration after Guillain-Barré syndrome: recurrence, treatment-related fluctuation or CIDP. J Neurol Neurosurg Psychiatry. 2009;80(1):3.
7. Acute immune polyneuropathies: Neuromuscular. Washington University, 10 Mar 2016. http://neuromuscular.wustl.edu/antibody/gbs.htm. Accessed 20 Mar 2016.
8. Sharma M, Kes P, et al. Guillain-Barré syndrome in a patient suffering acute myocardial infarction. Acta clin Croat. 2002;41(3):255–7.
9. Andary M, et al. Guillain-Barré syndrome: Medscape, 2016. http://emedicine.medscape.com/article/315632-overview#a0156. Accessed 02 Mar 2016.
10. Thivakaran T, Gamage R, Gooneratne IK. Treatment-related fluctuation in Guillain-Barre syndrome. J Neurosci Rural Practice. 2011;2(2):168–70.
11. Kharbanda PS, Prabhakar S, Lal V, Das CP. Visual loss with papilledema in Guillain-Barre syndrome. Neurol India. 2002;50:528.
12. Gonzalez-Quevedo A, Carriera RF, O'Farrill ZL, Luis IS, Becquer RM, Luis Gonzalez RS. An appraisal of blood-cerebrospinal fluid barrier dysfunction during the course of Guillain Barré syndrome. Neurol India. 2009;57:288–94.
13. Corston RN, McGale EH, Stonier C, et al. Abnormalities of cerebrospinal fluid amino acids in patients with Guillain-Barré syndrome. J Neurol Neurosurg Psychiatry. 1981;44:86–9.

5

Capsaicin 8% patch repeat treatment plus standard of care (SOC) versus SOC alone in painful diabetic peripheral neuropathy: a randomised, 52-week, open-label, safety study

Aaron I. Vinik[1*], Serge Perrot[2], Etta J. Vinik[1], Ladislav Pazdera[3], Hélène Jacobs[4], Malcolm Stoker[4], Stephen K. Long[4,8], Robert J. Snijder[4], Marjolijne van der Stoep[4], Enrique Ortega[5] and Nathaniel Katz[6,7]

Abstract

Background: This 52-week study evaluated the long-term safety and tolerability of capsaicin 8% w/w (179 mg) patch repeat treatment plus standard of care (SOC) versus SOC alone in painful diabetic peripheral neuropathy (PDPN).

Methods: Phase 3, multinational, open-label, randomised, controlled, 52-week safety study, conducted in Europe. Patients were randomised to capsaicin 8% patch repeat treatment (30 or 60 min; 1–7 treatments with ≥ 8-week intervals) to painful areas of the feet plus SOC, or SOC alone. The primary objective was the safety of capsaicin 8% patch repeat treatment (30 min and 60 min applications) plus SOC versus SOC alone over 52 weeks, assessed by changes in Norfolk Quality of Life-Diabetic Neuropathy (QOL-DN) total score from baseline to end of study (EOS). Secondary safety endpoints included Utah Early Neuropathy Scale (UENS) assessments and standardised testing of sensory perception and reflex function.

Results: Overall, 468 patients were randomised (30 min plus SOC, $n = 156$; 60 min plus SOC, $n = 157$; SOC alone, $n = 155$). By EoS, mean changes in Norfolk QOL-DN total score from baseline [estimated mean difference versus SOC alone; 90% CI for difference] were: 30 min plus SOC, −27.6% [−20.9; −31.7, −10.1]; 60 min plus SOC, −32.8% [−26.1; −36.8, −15.4]; SOC alone, −6.7%. Mean changes [difference versus SOC alone] in UENS total score by EoS versus baseline were: 30 min plus SOC, −2.1 [−0.9; −1.8, 0.1]; 60 min plus SOC, −3.0 [−1.7; −2.7, −0.8]; SOC alone, −1.2. No detrimental deterioration was observed in any of the Norfolk or UENS subscales by EoS with capsaicin. Also, no worsening in sensory perception testing of sharp, warm, cold and vibration stimuli was found with capsaicin by EoS. Capsaicin treatment was well tolerated and the most frequent treatment-emergent adverse events were application site pain (30 min, 28.2%; 60 min, 29.3%), burning sensation (30 min, 9.0%; 60 min, 9.6%) and application site erythema (30 min, 7.7%; 60 min, 8.9%).

Conclusion: In patients with PDPN, capsaicin 8% patch repeat treatment plus SOC over 52 weeks was well tolerated with no negative functional or neurological effects compared with SOC alone.

Keywords: Capsaicin 8% patch, Norfolk QOL-DN, UENS, TPRV1, Painful diabetic peripheral neuropathy

* Correspondence: vinikai@evms.edu
[1]Eastern Virginia Medical School, Strelitz Diabetes Center, 855 W Brambleton Avenue, Room 2018, Norfolk, VA 23510, USA
Full list of author information is available at the end of the article

Background

Peripheral neuropathic pain (PNP) is widely recognised to have a significant impact on quality of life (QOL) [1]. Painful diabetic peripheral neuropathy (PDPN) has been shown to affect many dimensions of patient QOL, including mood, sleep, work, self-esteem and social relationships, and has a particular impact on individuals with suboptimally managed pain [2, 3]. Approximately one in four people with type 2 diabetes will experience some level of PDPN [4], which often presents as numbness, tingling, burning, aching, electric shocks, or lancinating pains [5].

Many patients with PDPN remain undiagnosed or undertreated and few experience complete resolution of pain. There is a clear unmet need for new therapeutic options to improve current standard of care (SOC); available treatments such as antidepressants, antiepileptic drugs and opioids are often limited by contraindications and safety issues, and frequently have insufficient efficacy to achieve adequate pain relief [6–8]. One alternative to these treatments is the capsaicin 8% patch, which contains 179 mg or 8% weight for weight capsaicin and is optimised for rapid delivery of a high concentration of capsaicin directly into the skin [9]. Defunctionalisation of hyperactive nociceptors in the skin induced by the rapid delivery of capsaicin provides fast, targeted, and sustained pain relief after a single treatment. Furthermore, local application of the capsaicin 8% patch provides minimal systemic absorption, without the potential for drug-drug interactions or requirement for dose adjustment in elderly patients or patients with renal or hepatic impairment [10].

The capsaicin 8% patch is well tolerated and provides effective relief of pain for a variety of types of PNP [11–16]. A single capsaicin 8% patch treatment has demonstrated significant improvements in pain relief versus a placebo patch over 12 weeks, and was well tolerated with no sensory deterioration in patients with PDPN [16]. The present study in patients with PDPN (PACE) was the first evaluation of the long-term safety and tolerability of capsaicin 8% patch repeat treatment plus SOC, compared with SOC alone, over 52 weeks. The study had an open-label design; it primarily assessed the safety of capsaicin 8% patch repeat treatment, with efficacy of the capsaicin 8% patch in PDPN assessed in the double-blind STEP study [16]. In this study, the Norfolk Quality of Life-Diabetic Neuropathy (QOL-DN) questionnaire was chosen as the primary endpoint to assess the safety of capsaicin treatment. The Norfolk scale is a validated patient-reported outcome questionnaire, which captures the entire impact of nerve fibre dysfunction on QOL in diabetic neuropathy [17]. The Norfolk tool includes the concentration of symptoms in the extremities and subtle loss of function, such as fine motor impairments, slight sensory changes, unique problems with proprioception and balance and autonomic symptoms. The Norfolk QOL-DN scale was therefore used to assess any functional consequences associated with potentially deleterious effects of capsaicin treatment on peripheral nerve endings in patients with PDPN.

Methods

Study design

PACE was a Phase 3, multinational, open-label, randomised, controlled, 52-week safety study, conducted in Europe between November 2011 and February 2014 (ClinicalTrials.gov Identifier: NCT01478607). The primary objective assessed the safety of repeat treatment with the capsaicin 8% patch (QUTENZA™ 179 mg capsaicin patch, obtained from Astellas Pharma Europe B.V., Leiden, The Netherlands) in patients with PDPN.

Following a screening visit, patients were assigned a six-digit subject number allocated sequentially according to site and randomised to capsaicin 8% patch (30 min) plus SOC or capsaicin 8% patch (60 min) plus SOC or SOC alone in a ratio of 1:1:1 by chronological order of enrolment to receive treatment with the capsaicin 8% patch to painful areas of the feet for either 30 min plus SOC, 60 min plus SOC, or SOC alone. All patients were pretreated with a eutectic mixture of local anaesthetics (EMLA) containing lidocaine 2.5% and prilocaine 2.5%, to limit pain or discomfort during the application period. The 30-min application time was chosen to align with the approved Summary of Product Characteristics [18]. A 60-min application time was also evaluated in order to ensure that the safety objectives of the study were fully covered with respect to possible exposure periods. SOC was optimised for each patient at the discretion of each investigator and was assessed at clinic visits and on days 1 to 5 post-treatment, by completion of a rescue pain medication diary. The treatment area was mapped at screening and baseline visits, and re-mapped before treatment if the treatment area changed. Treatment borders were defined by the most painful areas of the feet, up to a total combined surface area of 1120 cm^2 (four patches) for both feet. Assessments were scheduled every two months; clinic visits were scheduled for Month 2, 4, 6, 8, 10, and 12, and telephone contact was scheduled at Month 1, 3, 5, 7, 9, and 11. Capsaicin 8% patch retreatment could occur at both scheduled and unscheduled clinic visits at the investigator's discretion, but only after at least 8 weeks had elapsed since the last treatment (Fig. 1).

Patients could not receive more than seven capsaicin 8% patch treatments during the study. Although patients and investigators were unblinded throughout the study, physicians assessing neurological function were blinded to treatment and not involved in the study in any other manner.

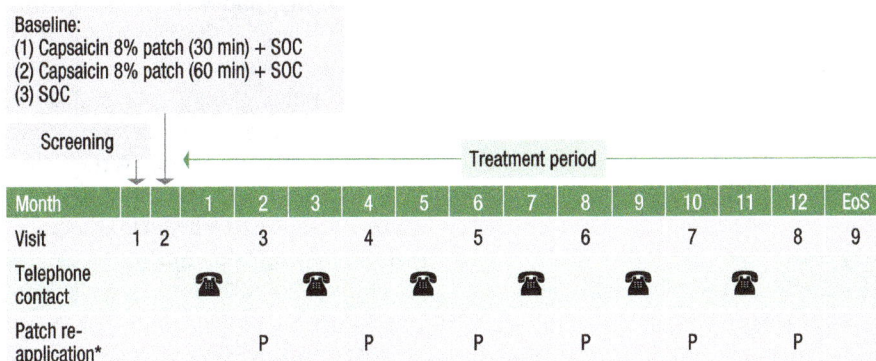

Fig. 1 Study design
*Capsaicin 8% patch treatment (Groups 1 and 2) took place at scheduled bi-monthly visits (P) or unscheduled visit at intervals of at least 8 weeks. EoS visit for Groups 1 and 2 took place between 8 and 12 weeks after last patch application if patch was applied at Visit 8 (Month 12) and between Week 52 and 56 for patients without a patch application at Visit 8 (Month 12). EoS visit for Group 3 took place between Week 52 and 56. *EoS* end of study, *SOC* standard of care, *UENS* Utah Early Neuropathy Scale

Patients

Patients were aged ≥18 years with a diagnosis of PDPN due to type 1 or type 2 diabetes mellitus for ≥1 year prior to the screening visit. Key criteria for inclusion and exclusion are presented in Table 1.

Safety endpoints

Primary endpoint

Norfolk QOL-DN Scale

The primary objective was to evaluate the safety of repeat treatment with the capsaicin 8% patch, assessed by the percentage change from baseline to end of study (EoS) in the Norfolk QOL-DN total score. The scale has been shown to correlate with clinical Total Neuropathy Score along with the different features of diabetic neuropathy such as small fibre function (including loss of pain and thermal sensation), large fibre function (including motor function and touch/pressure discrimination) and autonomic nerve function [19]. The Norfolk QOL-DN scale was specifically developed to reliably measure changes in nerve function that translate into changes in QOL, activities of daily living, and health of the individual, where a reduction in score is associated with improved function [17]. In this study, it was used to assess any functional consequences of potential small nerve fibre dysfunction that may have been associated with capsaicin 8% patch repeat treatment and adversely affected QOL.

Secondary endpoints

Secondary safety variables evaluated to support the primary endpoint included Norfolk QOL-DN subscale scores, Utah Early Neuropathy Scale (UENS) [20] assessments and standardised testing of sensory perception and reflex function. Average pain score, pain severity index, pain interference index, obtained from the Brief Pain Inventory-Diabetic Neuropathy (question 5),

response rates and Patient Global Impression of Change were recorded as other secondary endpoints in this study and will be reported separately.

Secondary Norfolk QOL-DN endpoints

Secondary safety variables related to Norfolk QOL-DN included: percentage change from baseline in

Table 1 Key inclusion and exclusion criteria

Inclusion criteria

- Aged ≥ 18 years with a diagnosis of PDPN confirmed by a score ≥ 3 on the MNSI
- HbA1c ≤ 9% (74.9 mmol/mol) at 3–6 months prior to screening and at screening
- Stable glycaemic control for ≥ 6 months prior to screening visit
- Average daily pain score over the last 24 h ≥ 4 (question 5 of BPI-DN) at the screening and the baseline visit

Exclusion criteria

- Primary pain associated with PDPN in the ankles or above
- Significant pain (moderate or above) due to an aetiology other than PDPN
- Any amputation of lower extremity
- Clinically significant cardiovascular disease within 6 months prior to screening visit
- Any active signs of skin inflammation around onychomycosis sites such as tenderness, redness, swelling or drainage
- Body mass index ≥ 40 kg/m²
- Hypersensitivity to capsaicin any capsaicin 8% patch excipients, EMLA ingredients, or adhesives
- Use of oral or transdermal opioids within 7 days preceding patch application at baseline

- Pain that could not be clearly differentiated from, or conditions that might have interfered with, the assessment of PDPN, e.g., claudication, fasciitis tendinitis and arthritis
- Current or previous foot ulcer
- Severe renal disease as defined by a creatinine clearance < 30 mL/min
- Significant peripheral vascular disease[a]
- Impaired glucose tolerance only – without diabetes mellitus
- Previous treatment with capsaicin 8% patch
- Use of any topical pain medication on the painful areas within 7 days preceding patch application at baseline

BPI-DN Brief pain inventory-diabetic neuropathy version, EMLA eutectic mixture of local anaesthetics, HbA1c glycosylated haemoglobin of A1c, MNSI Michigan neuropathy screening instrument, PDPN painful diabetic peripheral neuropathy
[a]Intermittent claudication or lack of pulsation of either the dorsal pedis of posterior tibias artery, or ankle-brachial systolic BP index of 0.80

Norfolk QOL-DN total score by number of capsaicin treatments; percentage change from baseline in Norfolk QOL-DN subscale scores ('small fibre', 'symptoms', 'autonomic', 'physical functioning', 'activities of daily living'); and absolute Norfolk QOL-DN total score. A reduction in subscale score was associated with improved function.

Utah early neuropathy scale

The UENS, a validated clinical tool developed to detect and quantify signs of early neuropathy and identify modest changes in the severity and spatial distribution of sensation, was used to assess any functional consequences of capsaicin treatment. A reduction in score indicates improvement in sensory function over time. Endpoints related to the UENS included: change from baseline in UENS total score; change from baseline in UENS total score by number of capsaicin treatments; change from baseline in UENS subscale scores ('pinprick sensation', 'motor', 'allodynia/hyperaesthesia', 'large fibre', 'deep tendon reflex'); clinically significant change in UENS total score (defined as a decrease of > 4 points from baseline); and absolute UENS total score.

Sensory perception, reflex function and tolerability

Sensory examination was performed by neurologists as well as by non-neurologist physician-investigators given study training, and were ideally performed by the same person (Additional file 1). Physicians conducting sensory examinations were blinded to treatment. 'Bedside' sensory and reflex testing was performed on both feet at baseline and EoS to identify any clinically relevant deficits in sensory function. Ratings of evoked sensation were compared with an asymptomatic site and recorded using standardised categorical reporting scales: assessment of warm, cold, and sharp sensations were rated as 'absent', 'diminished', 'normal', or 'painful'. Sensation of vibration on the dorsal surface of the great toe was rated as 'absent', 'markedly diminished', 'mild loss', or 'normal' sensation. Testing areas on the dorsal surface included the great toe, midpoint and medial malleolus and on the plantar surface included the ball and midpoint. Achilles tendon reflex assessment was rated as 'absent', 'diminished', 'normal', 'hyperactive', or 'clonus'. To assess the proportion of patients with changes in sensory perception or reflex category, patients were judged to have improved, stayed the same, or worsened depending on the change in reported category at EoS versus baseline (Fig. 2).

A post-hoc analysis in patients who received the maximum of seven capsaicin 8% patch treatments was performed to determine within-group changes of sensory perception testing over time.

Adverse events (AEs) observed after randomisation (post-randomisation AEs [PRAEs]) were collected for all

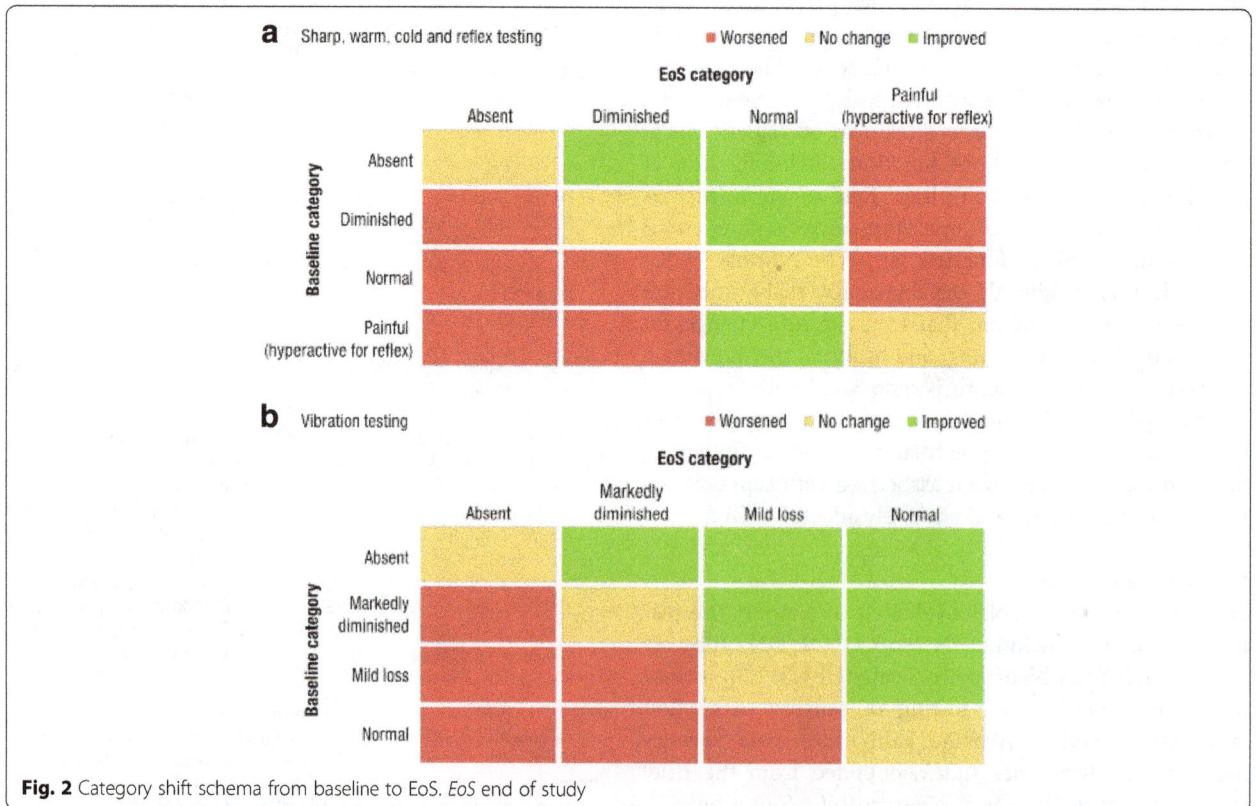

Fig. 2 Category shift schema from baseline to EoS. *EoS* end of study

groups, allowing for comparison of the capsaicin 8% patch arms with the SOC arm. Treatment-emergent AEs (TEAEs) were observed following administration of the capsaicin 8% patch, therefore no TEAEs are reported for the SOC alone group. 'Pain now' Numeric Pain Rating Scale (NPRS) scores, within 15 min and after 60 min following patch removal, were also assessed during the study.

The change in use of concomitant medication was assessed throughout the study; classes of interest were antidepressants, antiepileptic drugs, and opioids.

Statistical methods

Regarding sample size, the number of patients planned for the trial were such that safety concerns related to the Norfolk questionnaire would have been picked up. The power calculation for this study used the principle of a non-inferiority study with 90% power and a 95% one sided confidence interval [CI]. The non-inferiority limit was 20%. A clinically meaningful difference in the percentage reduction from baseline on the Norfolk scale was chosen using data from a clinical trial in diabetic peripheral neuropathy with ruboxistaurin [21], which showed a drug effect of 37.2%, and selecting 20% as the lower margin for clinically meaningful effect. A number of statistical measures were used to describe the data: descriptive statistics for absolute and change from baseline values at each visit and at EoS; 90 or 95% CI for the estimated mean difference between each of the active treatment groups against SOC control for change from baseline; percentage change from baseline at each post-baseline analysis visit and EoS. As the objective of the trial was to assess the safety and tolerability of long-term capsaicin 8% patch treatment, no formal statistical testing was performed to calculate p-values for the difference between both capsaicin groups and SOC alone. At EoS, for each subject, the last available observation was used with the last observation carried forward (LOCF) imputation method. The results were also analysed using the baseline observation carried forward method.

The safety analysis set (SAS) included all patients who received study treatment and was used for all analyses of safety and analgesic effectiveness.

Results

Patient disposition

Of the 555 patients screened, a total of 468 patients were randomised at 71 centres across 11 European countries (30 min plus SOC, $n = 156$; 60 min plus SOC, $n = 157$; SOC alone, $n = 155$). A total of 388 patients completed the study (30 min plus SOC, $n = 132$; 60 min plus SOC, $n = 128$; SOC alone, $n = 128$); 80 patients (17.1%) discontinued the study post baseline, most commonly due to withdrawal of consent ($n = 44$) and adverse events ($n = 18$; Fig. 3).

Baseline characteristics were similar across treatment groups and specifically, were comparable for age, glycosylated haemoglobin of A1c (HbA1c), average daily pain, Norfolk QOL-DN total score, UENS total score, duration of PDPN and use of prior treatments for PDPN (including pain medications and SOC) (Table 2).

The most commonly prescribed categories of pain medications during the study were analgesics and antiepileptics; the most commonly prescribed drugs for pain during the study were gabapentin and pregabalin (Table 3).

The average interval between each capsaicin retreatment was 68.4 days in the capsaicin 30-min group and 68.3 days in the 60-min group. The mean number of

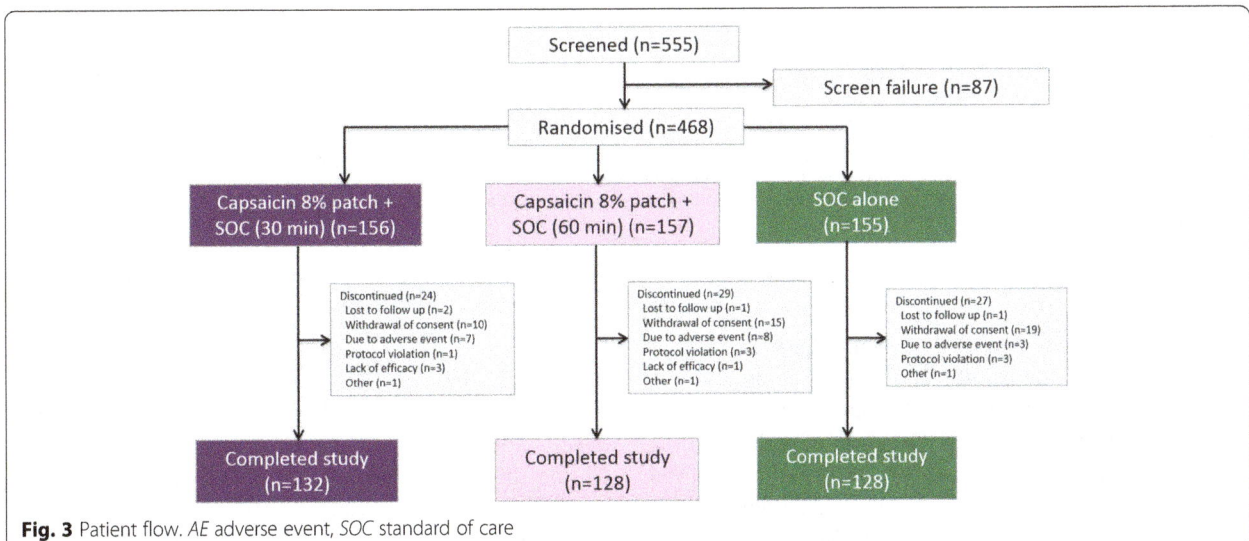

Fig. 3 Patient flow. *AE* adverse event, *SOC* standard of care

Table 2 Summary of demographics and baseline characteristics (safety analysis set)

Parameter	Capsaicin 8% patch (30 min) + SOC (n = 156)	Capsaicin 8% patch (60 min) + SOC (n = 157)	SOC (n = 155)
Sex, n (%)			
Male	74 (47.4)	79 (50.3)	71 (45.8)
Female	82 (52.6)	78 (49.7)	84 (54.2)
Ethnicity, n (%)			
Caucasian	154 (98.7)	155 (98.7)	154 (99.4)
Other	2 (1.3)	2 (1.3)	1 (0.6)
Age, years			
Mean [SD]	60.9 [10.9]	61.0 [10.3]	59.1 [10.3]
Weight, kg			
Mean [SD]	86.6 [14.5]	86.7 [16.4]	89.6 [17.6]
Height, cm			
Mean [SD]	169.7 [8.9]	169.7 [9.0]	169.3 [10.9]
Body mass index, kg/m^2			
Mean [SD]	30.1 [4.6]	30.1 [5.0]	31.2 [5.0]
Duration of PDPN, years			
Mean [SD]	4.1 [3.7]	4.4 [3.9]	4.4 [3.6]
Pain medications before baseline, n (%)			
Overall	70 (44.9)	71 (45.2)	79 (51.0)
Analgesics[a]	56 (35.9)	54 (34.4)	59 (38.1)
Antiepileptics	44 (28.2)	49 (31.2)	52 (33.5)
Psycholeptics	22 (14.1)	19 (12.1)	24 (15.5)
Anti-inflammatory/antirheumatic products	14 (9.0)	12 (7.6)	17 (11.0)
Topical joint/muscular pain products[b]	14 (9.0)	11 (7.0)	15 (9.7)
Baseline average pain score (BPI-DN question 5)			
Mean [SD]	5.6 [1.3]	5.6 [1.4]	5.5 [1.3]
Baseline Norfolk QOL-DN score			
Mean [SD]	42.8 [19.5]	40.6 [18.3]	41.0 [18.5]
Baseline UENS total score			
Mean [SD]	17.0 [7.4]	16.5 [7.0]	15.6 [6.2]
HbA1c at screening			
Mean, % [SD]	7.3 [1.0]	7.4 [1.0]	7.4 [1.0]
Mean, mmol/mol [SD]	56.6 [10.8]	57.5 [10.8]	57.6 [11.4]

BPI-DN Brief pain inventory diabetic neuropathy, *HbA1c* glycosylated haemoglobin of A1c, *PDPN* painful diabetic peripheral neuropathy, *QOL-DN* Quality-of-life questionnaire for diabetic neuropathy, *SD* standard deviation, *SOC* standard of care
[a]Analgesics were categorised by analgesics, anilides, natural opium alkaloids, other analgesics and antipyretics, other opioids, pyrazolones and salicylic acid and derivatives
[b]Anti-inflammatory preparations, non-steroidals for topical use, preparations with salicylic acid derivatives

patches used was similar between capsaicin groups (30 min, 1.53; 60 min, 1.42) and the mean duration of patch application was 30.2 min in the 30-min group and 60.2 min in the 60-min group. Over half of patients in the capsaicin 8% patch groups received the maximum seven capsaicin treatments (167/313 [53.4%]) (Additional file 2: Figure S1 and Additional file 3: Figure S2).

Safety

Norfolk QOL-DN

No deterioration (denoted by a reduction in score) in mean (estimated mean difference versus SOC alone; 90% CI for difference) Norfolk QOL-DN total score from baseline to EoS was observed in the capsaicin 8% patch plus SOC groups (30 min, −27.6% [−20.9; −31.7, −10.1];

Table 3 Pain medication during the study (safety analysis set)

Pain medication[a]	Capsaicin 8% patch (30 min) + SOC (n = 156)	Capsaicin 8% patch (60 min) + SOC (n = 157)	SOC (n = 155)
Overall, n (%)	98 (62.8)	105 (66.9)	107 (69.0)
Most commonly used category (>10 % patients in either group), n (%)			
Analgesics[b]	79 (50.6)	84 (53.5)	81 (52.3)
Antiepileptics	54 (34.6)	57 (36.3)	73 (47.1)
Topical products for joint and muscular pain	30 (19.2)	35 (22.3)	29 (18.1)
Anti-inflammatory/antirheumatic products	29 (18.6)	35 (22.3)	30 (19.4)
Psycholeptics	24 (15.4)	22 (14.0)	40 (25.8)
Stomatological preparations	18 (11.5)	22 (14.0)	18 (11.6)
Psychoanaleptics	16 (10.3)	6 (3.8)	21 (13.5)
Ophthalmologicals[c]	15 (9.6)	20 (12.7)	16 (10.3)
Most commonly used drugs (>5% patients in any group), n (%)			
Gabapentin	26 (16.7)	26 (16.6)	35 (22.6)
Pregabalin	24 (15.4)	22 (14.0)	39 (25.2)
Paracetamol	23 (14.7)	36 (22.9)	6 (3.9)
Tramadol	16 (10.3)	14 (8.9)	6 (3.9)
Diclofenac	12 (7.7)	13 (8.3)	12 (7.7)
Ibuprofen	11 (7.1)	15 (9.6)	14 (9.0)
Metamizole	10 (6.4)	10 (6.4)	5 (3.2)
Duloxetine	9 (5.8)	3 (1.9)	10 (6.5)
Carbamazepine	7 (4.5)	14 (8.9)	10 (6.5)
Alpha lipoic acid	3 (1.9)	1 (0.6)	8 (5.2)

SOC standard of care

[a]Medication used for pain (check box of 'pain medication' is YES on electronic case report form [eCRF])

[b]Analgesics were categorised by class: anilides, natural opium alkaloids, other analgesics and antipyretics, other opioids, pyrazolones, and salicylic acid and derivatives

[c]Ophthalmologicals (eye treatments) were categorised by anti-inflammatory agents and nonsteroids, local anaesthetics, corticosteroids (plain) and other ophthalmologicals

60 min, −32.8% [−26.1; −36.8, −15.4]) compared with SOC alone (−6.7%) (Fig. 4). By EoS, patients who received the maximum seven capsaicin treatments plus SOC also had no deterioration in Norfolk QOL-DN when compared with the overall SAS population (Fig. 4).

The mean difference [90% CI] from baseline in Norfolk QOL-DN total score between groups increased throughout the study (Fig. 5).

In addition, no deterioration in any of the Norfolk QOL-DN subscale scores from baseline to EoS was observed in both capsaicin plus SOC groups versus SOC alone (Fig. 4).

Utah early neuropathy scale

The mean change [SD] from baseline to EoS in absolute UENS total score was −2.1 [5.0] with capsaicin 30 min and −3.0 [5.1] with capsaicin 60 min, compared with −1.2 [4.2] in SOC alone group (least squares mean difference [90% CI]: 30 min, −0.9 [−1.8, 0.1]; 60 min: −1.7 [−2.7, −0.8]) (Fig. 6).

No deterioration in UENS total score was noted in patients who received the maximum seven capsaicin treatments plus SOC compared with the overall SAS population (Fig. 6). A clinically significant improvement in UENS total score (defined as a decrease of > 4 points from baseline) was observed in 35.6 and 37.9% of patients in the capsaicin 30-min and capsaicin 60-min groups, respectively, compared with 22.5% of patients in the SOC alone group.

Regarding UENS subscales, no deterioration in mean [SD] 'pinprick sensation' score was observed in the capsaicin plus SOC groups compared with SOC alone (30 min, −1.4 [3.84]; 60 min, −2.2 [3.99]; SOC, −0.7 [3.14]). There were no noticeable differences or only minimal changes across treatment groups in the other UENS subscale scores (Fig. 6).

No differences were observed between treatment groups (data not show) using the baseline observation carried forward method.

Sensory perception and reflex testing

The capsaicin 8% patch had no negative impact on sensory perception and reflex testing and the majority of patients had no change from baseline to EoS (Fig. 7, Additional file 4: Table S1). In patients who received the

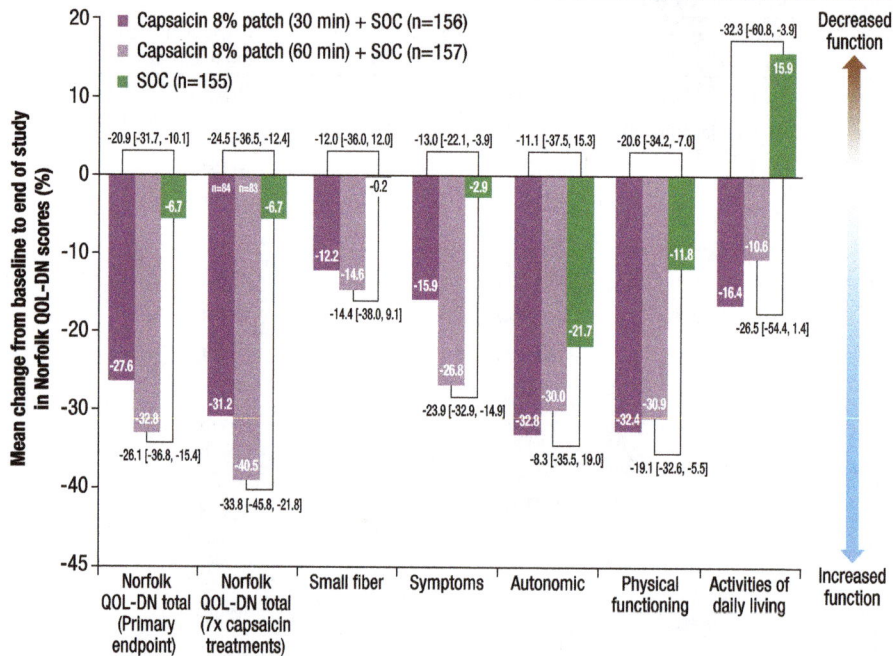

Fig. 4 Mean percentage change from baseline to end of study in Norfolk QOL-DN scores (LOCF) (SAS)
Treatment group comparisons are least squares mean difference [90% CI]. *CI* confidence interval, *LOCF* last observation carried forward, *SAS* safety analysis set, *SOC* standard of care

maximum seven capsaicin treatments, there was also no negative impact from baseline to EoS (Additional file 5: Figure S3). A shift to worsened sensation was reported by a lower proportion of patients in both the overall population and the capsaicin 8% patch seven treatment cohort (Fig. 7, Additional file 5: Figure S3).

By EoS, the proportion of patients reporting 'normal' sensation increased for the majority of tests in all three groups; however, reporting of 'normal' sharp (on ball of foot), warm, and cold sensation was greater for capsaicin groups plus SOC versus SOC alone (Fig. 8a). The proportion of patients reporting 'absent' sharp (on

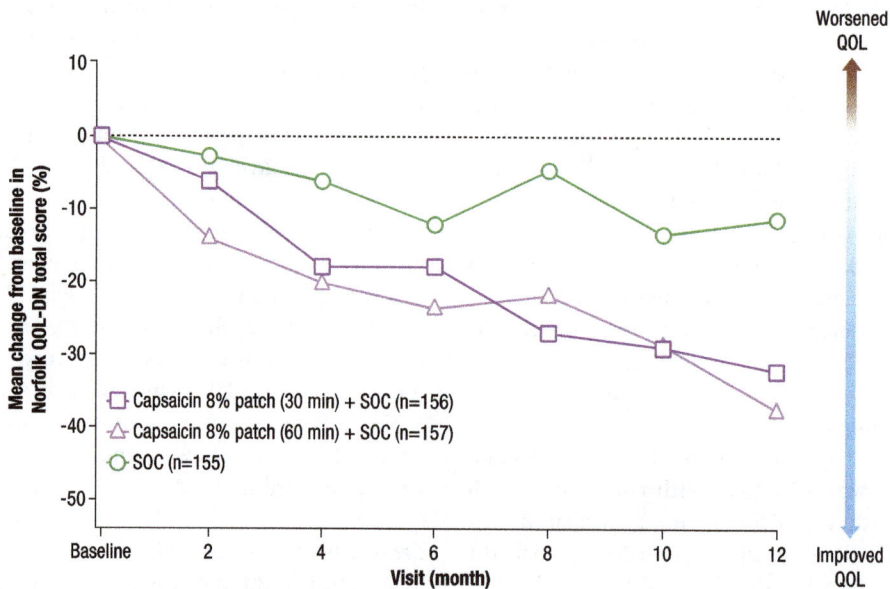

Fig. 5 Mean percentage change in Norfolk QOL-DN total score from baseline during the study (SAS)
In patients who received a capsaicin treatment at Month 12 and had an end of study visit at Month 14, mean [SD] change in Norfolk total score by Month 14 was: 30 min, −36.1% [51.6] (*n* = 79); 60 min, −40.2% [39.4] (*n* = 76). *SAS* safety analysis set, *SOC* standard of care

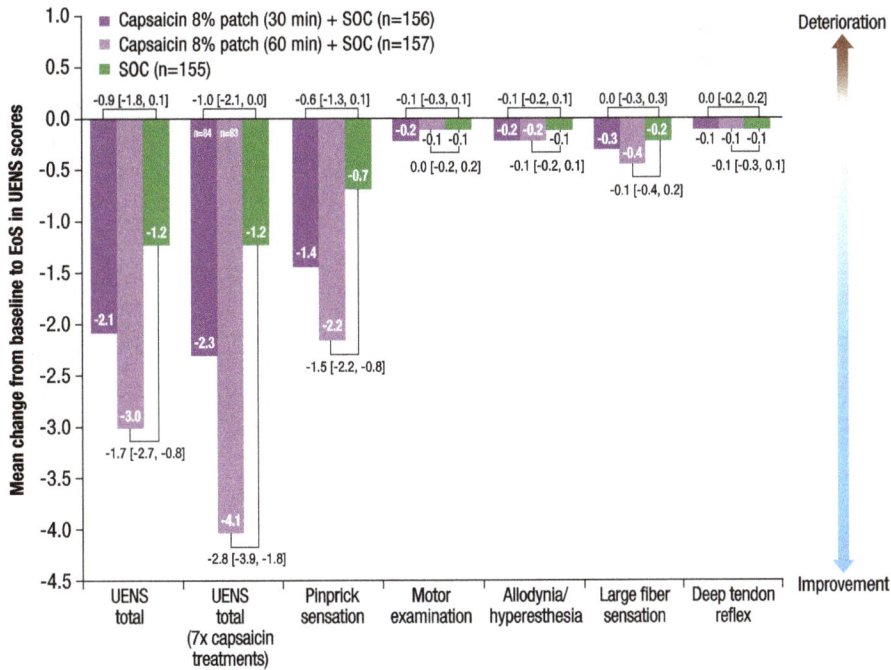

Fig. 6 Mean change in UENS total and subscale scores from baseline to EoS (LOCF) (SAS)
Treatment group comparisons are least squares mean difference [90% CI]. *CI* confidence interval, *EoS* end of study, *LOCF* last observation carried forward, *SAS* safety analysis set, *SOC* standard of care

plantar midpoint), warm, cold and vibration sensation decreased in all groups by EoS, with the greatest change in warm, cold and vibration seen in the capsaicin 60 min plus SOC group (Fig. 8b). There was also a decrease in the proportion of patients, in all groups, reporting 'absent' or 'markedly diminished' vibration sensation by EoS, and this was accompanied by a corresponding increase in 'mild loss' vibration in all groups (Fig. 8b). These findings were mirrored in the subset of patients who received the maximum seven capsaicin treatments plus SOC, with more patients in the capsaicin groups reporting 'normal' sensation for sharp,

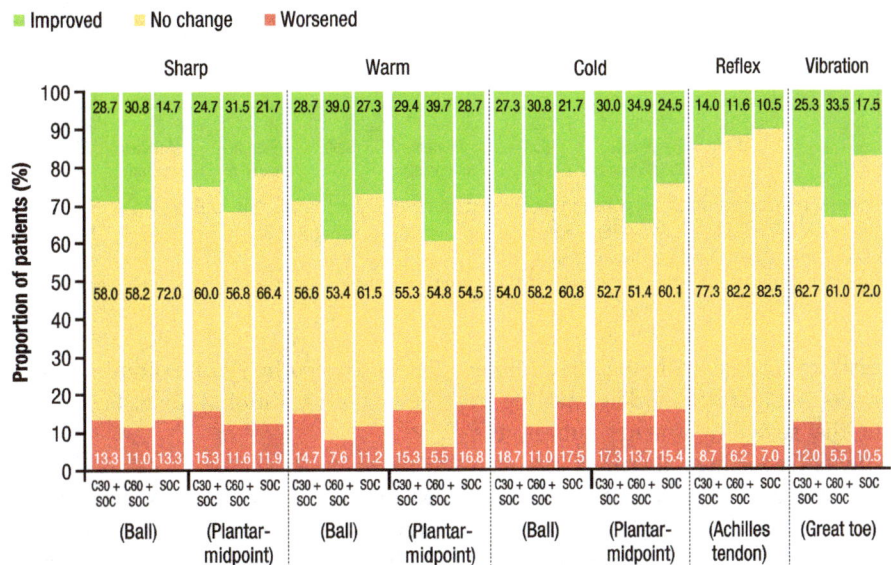

Fig. 7 Proportion of patients reporting improved, unchanged, or worsened sensory or reflex function by EoS (SAS)
C30 + SOC, capsaicin 8% patch (30 min) + SOC (*n* = 150); C60 + SOC, capsaicin 8% patch (60 min) + SOC (*n* = 146)
EoS end of study, *SAS* safety analysis set, *SOC* standard of care (*n* = 143); *n* is number of patients with non-missing data

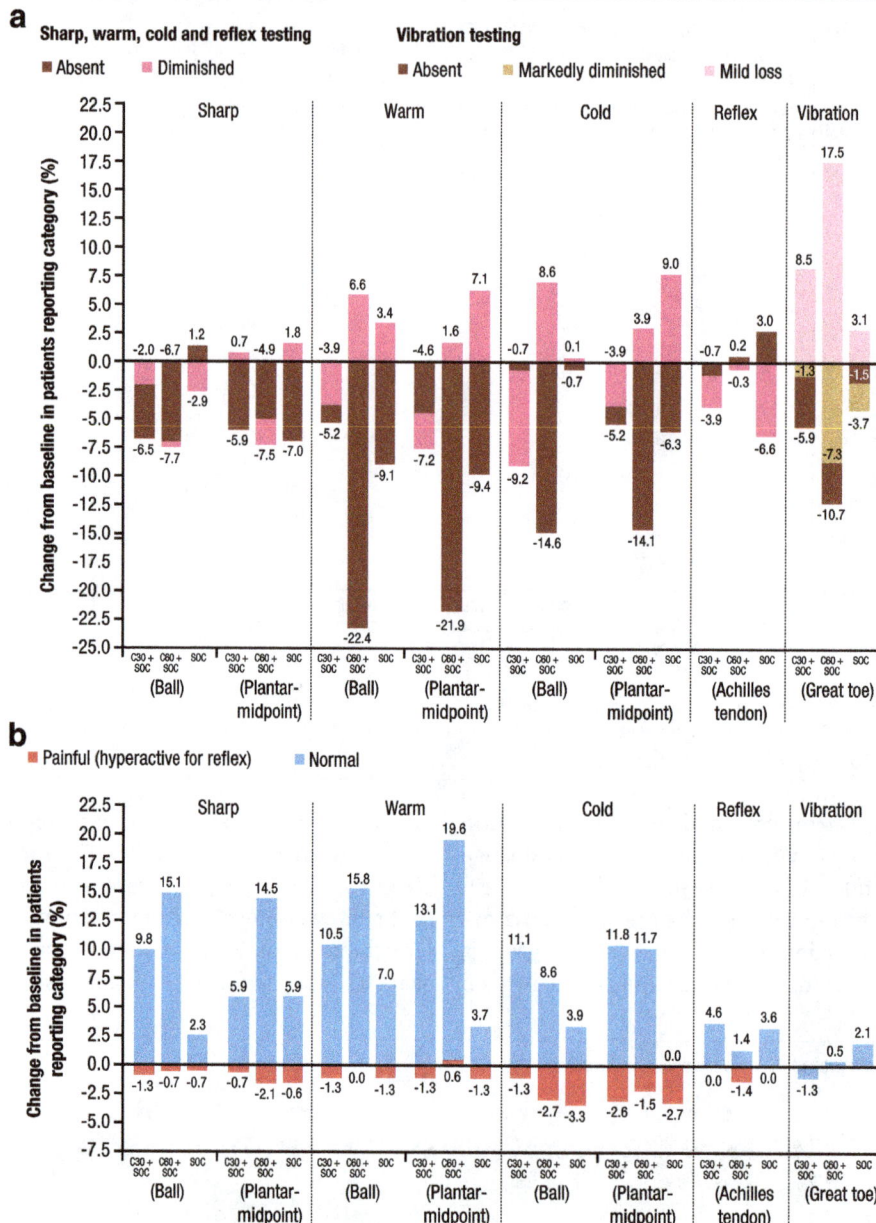

Fig. 8 a and **b** Change in proportion of patients reporting sensory and reflex testing from baseline to EoS (SAS)
C30 + SOC, capsaicin 8% patch (30 min) + SOC (*n* = 156); C60 + SOC, capsaicin 8% patch (60 min) + SOC (*n* = 157)
EoS end of study, *SAS* safety analysis set, *SOC* standard of care (*n* = 155)

warm, and cold tests compared with the SOC alone group (Additional file 6: Figure S4, Additional file 7: Table S2). Also in the seven treatments subset, the proportion of patients reporting 'absent' sharp (on plantar midpoint), warm, cold and vibration sensation decreased in all groups by EoS, with the greatest change in warm and cold seen in the capsaicin 60 min plus SOC group (Additional file 8: Figure S5). In addition, fewer patients in the seven treatment subset reported 'absent' vibration sensation by EoS,

accompanied by a corresponding increase in 'mild loss' vibration (Additional file 8: Figure S5).

Tolerability
Mean 'pain now' NPRS scores after patch application were low (≤3.5); peak mean pain scores were observed within 15 min after the first patch removal (3.5; median 3.0, interquartile range 2.0–5.0) to 60 min after the first patch removal (3.3; median 3.0, interquartile range 1.0–5.0). However, 'pain now' NPRS scores decreased after

the second patch removal and were stable from the fifth to the last patch removal. More patients in the capsaicin 8% patch 60-min group used concomitant analgesics for application site-related pain (29.9%) compared with the 30-min group (22.4%).

The proportion of patients reporting any PRAE was 67.3% (30 min plus SOC), 69.4% (60 min plus SOC) and 48.4% (SOC alone) (Table 4), and the majority of PRAEs were of mild or moderate severity.

Severe PRAEs were reported by 12.2, 7.6 and 6.5% in the patients in the capsaicin 30 min, capsaicin 60 min, and SOC alone, groups, respectively; overall, these severe PRAEs were most commonly categorised as cardiac disorders, infections and infestations, and musculoskeletal and connective tissue disorders. The difference in PRAEs between the capsaicin plus SOC groups and SOC alone was primarily due to the reporting of application site pain or erythema in the capsaicin groups, which were predominately mild or moderate in severity (Table 4).

TEAEs were similar in the capsaicin 8% patch 30-min and 60-min plus SOC treatment groups (66.7 and 67.5%, respectively) and were generally mild or moderate in severity (Table 4). Over one-third of TEAEs in the capsaicin groups were application site reactions; the type and frequency of these reactions were comparable between both capsaicin groups. The proportion of patients with application site reactions decreased throughout the study, from between the first and second to between the sixth and seventh treatments (application site pain: 30 min, −6.9%; 60 min, −7.9%, burning sensation: 30 min, −2.8%; 60 min −2.2%). Four patients in the 60-min group discontinued due to drug-related TEAEs (four events: muscle spasms, rectal adenocarcinoma, neuralgia, and psoriasis); no drug-related discontinuations were reported in the 30-min group. Severe TEAEs were reported by 12.2% in the 30-min group and 7.6% in the 60-min group; severe TEAEs considered as drug related were reported by 2.6% in the 30-min group and 1.9% in the 60-min group. Serious TEAEs considered as drug related were reported by two patients in the 60-min group (three events: angina pectoris, rectal adenocarcinoma and accelerated hypertension), and by no patients in the 30-min group. These events were officially classified as drug-related by the investigator because causation could not be excluded; however, the sponsor considered it unlikely that repeat treatment with capsaicin 8% patch was the cause of these events. Four deaths were reported during the study: capsaicin 30 min, multiple injuries and brain death ($n = 1$); capsaicin 60 min, hypotension ($n = 1$); SOC alone, pneumonia ($n = 1$), atrial fibrillation ($n = 1$). None of the deaths were considered to be drug related by the investigator. The only finding of note from vital sign and laboratory analyses was that the change in HbA1c from screening to EoS was marginally greater in the SOC alone arm (0.24%), compared with the capsaicin 30 min (0.06%) and 60 min (0.06%) arms, although HbA1c levels were generally controlled throughout the study.

Concomitant medications
Overall, there was no decrease in the use of concomitant medications in any of the treatment groups throughout the study; use of concomitant medications was comparable from baseline to EoS in both capsaicin groups (Additional file 9: Table S3). The proportion of patients using antiepileptics at the end of the study was comparable with the proportion reported at baseline for both capsaicin groups. However, the proportion of patients using antiepileptic drugs had increased by > 10% in the SOC alone group at the end of the study. Small increases were also observed in antidepressant and opioid use in the SOC alone group from baseline to the EoS.

Discussion
In patients with PDPN, capsaicin 8% patch repeat treatment plus SOC over 52 weeks was well tolerated, had no negative functional or neurological effects and raised no new safety concerns compared with SOC therapy.

While the efficacy and safety of a single capsaicin 8% treatment has been previously characterised in patients with PDPN in the double-blind STEP study [16], the open-label PACE study was the first to assess the long-term safety and tolerability of repeated treatment over 52 weeks in PDPN. Capsaicin 8% patch repeat treatment plus SOC was not associated with any deterioration in Norfolk QOL-DN total or subscale scores compared with SOC alone. For the safety endpoints, few differences were observed in results between the 30-min and 60-min capsaicin groups.

Regarding the UENS total score and 'pinprick sensation' subscale, and sharp, cold, warm and vibration sensation on standardised neurological tests, no deterioration was observed with capsaicin 8% patch repeat treatment. By EoS, the majority of patients showed no change in sensation category, indicating that the changes observed in Figs. 8a and b and Additional file 6: Figure S4 and Additional file 8: Figure S5 were predominantly in patients who transitioned from 'absent' to 'diminished' or to 'normal' during the study. Taken together, these findings indicate that there was no small fibre mediated sensory loss with capsaicin 8% patch repeat treatment. The sensory testing observations in the subset of patients who received seven consecutive capsaicin treatments demonstrated that regular, repeat treatment with the capsaicin 8% patch was also not associated with deterioration in sensory function.

Alongside the double-blind STEP study, the PACE study formed part of a successful regulatory submission to remove the restriction of treatment with capsaicin 8% patch

Table 4 Summary of PRAEs, TEAEs, and drug-related TEAEs (safety analysis set)

Event, n (%)	Capsaicin 8% patch (30 min) + SOC (n = 156)	Capsaicin 8% patch (60 min) + SOC (n = 157)	SOC (n = 155)
PRAEs	105 (67.3)	109 (69.4)	75 (48.4)
Mild PRAEs	83 (53.2)	89 (56.7)	55 (35.5)
Moderate PRAEs	50 (32.1)	54 (34.4)	34 (21.9)
Severe PRAEs	19 (12.2)	12 (7.6)	10 (6.5)
PRAEs identified as general disorders or administration site conditions	54 (34.6)	53 (33.8)	10 (6.5)
Application site pain	44 (28.2)	46 (29.3)	0 (0)
Mild	23 (14.7)	28 (17.8)	0 (0)
Moderate	19 (12.2)	16 (10.2)	0 (0)
Severe	2 (1.3)	2 (1.3)	0 (0)
Application site erythema	12 (7.7)	14 (8.9)	0 (0)
Mild	12 (7.7)	13 (8.3)	0 (0)
Moderate	0 (0)	1 (0.6)	0 (0)
Severe	0 (0)	0 (0)	0 (0)
PRAEs leading to permanent discontinuation	7 (4.5)	8 (5.1)	3 (1.9)
TEAEs	104 (66.7)	106 (67.5)	N/A
Application site reactions	60 (38.5)	69 (43.9)	
TEAEs most commonly reported (>5% of each group)			N/A
Application site pain	44 (28.2)	46 (29.3)	
Burning sensation	14 (9.0)	15 (9.6)	
Application site erythema	12 (7.7)	14 (8.9)	
Pain in extremity	6 (3.8)	13 (8.3)	
TEAEs leading to permanent discontinuation	7 (4.5)	8 (5.1)	N/A
Drug-related[a] TEAEs	62 (39.7)	71 (45.2)	N/A
Drug-related[a] TEAEs leading to permanent discontinuation	0 (0)	4 (2.5)	N/A
Muscle spasms[b]	0 (0)	1 (0.6)	
Rectal adenocarcinoma[c]	0 (0)	1 (0.6)	
Neuralgia[d]	0 (0)	1 (0.6)	
Plantar psoriasis[e]	0 (0)	1 (0.6)	
Severe TEAEs	19 (12.2)	12 (7.6)	N/A
Drug-related[a] severe TEAEs	4 (2.6)	3 (1.9)	N/A

Table 4 Summary of PRAEs, TEAEs, and drug-related TEAEs (safety analysis set) *(Continued)*

Application site pain	2 (1.3)	2 (1.3)	
Rectal adenocarcinoma[c]	0 (0)	1 (0.6)	
Burning sensation	1 (0.6)	0 (0)	
Hypoaesthesia	1 (0.6)	0 (0)	
Serious TEAEs	20 (12.8)	13 (8.3)	N/A
Drug-related[a] serious TEAEs	0 (0)	2 (1.3)	N/A
Angina pectoris[f]	0 (0)	1 (0.6)	
Accelerated hypertension[g]	0 (0)	1 (0.6)	
Rectal adenocarcinoma[c]	0 (0)	1 (0.6)	
Deaths	1 (0.6)	1 (0.6)	2 (1.3)

N/A not applicable in SOC alone group, *PRAE* post-randomisation adverse event, *SOC* standard of care, *TEAE* treatment-emergent adverse event
[a]Possible or probable, as assessed by the investigator, or records where relationship is missing
[b]Muscle spasms in both legs of one patient were considered unlikely to have been caused by the capsaicin 8% patch, but a causal association could not be excluded. The same patient also previously reported cramps in the toes
[c]Rectal adenocarcinoma was considered unlikely to have started during the study and reach grade T3 within 129 days; however, a causal association with the capsaicin 8% patch could not be excluded
[d]One case of neuralgia was considered probably related to the study drug in view of the close temporal association with dosing and the known ability of the capsaicin 8% patch to cause application site pain
[e]Although the capsaicin 8% patch could not be excluded as a cause of one event of plantar psoriasis, the mechanism by which it could cause an autoimmune condition such as psoriasis is unclear and a causal association was considered unlikely
[f, g]Angina pectoris and accelerated hypertension were likely related to the patient's co-existing ischemic heart disease and hypertension but a causal association with the capsaicin 8% patch could not be excluded

in patients with diabetes in Europe. The capsaicin 8% patch is now indicated for the treatment of peripheral neuropathic pain in adults either alone or in combination with other medicinal products for pain in Europe [18].

Although the open-label design of this study may be perceived as more representative of capsaicin 8% patch repeat treatment in clinical practice than in a double-blind design, the observed safety evaluations may have been biased by the open-label design. Although the physicians assessing neurological function were blinded to treatment, patients and investigators were unblinded, which may have impacted on the findings. As the primary objective of this open-label study was to assess the safety and tolerability of capsaicin 8% patch repeat treatment, *p*-values were not calculated to supplement the 90% CIs for the between-group differences each month. Furthermore, differences between treatment groups in an open-label study may be caused by the fact that patients know which treatment they are receiving. The LOCF imputation method is a conservative method to estimate the treatment effect. The underlying assumption is that subjects that withdraw have worse efficacy than those that stay in the trial. The LOCF imputation method did use the data of withdrawn subjects and therefore, theoretically, gave worse results in this study than from a non-imputed analysis. As the limitations of the LOCF for missing data methodology are recognised, the results were also analysed using the baseline observation carried forward method, and no differences in the results were observed. Quantitative Sensory Testing (QST) was not performed in this multicenter study and instead, 'bedside' sensory testing was used. Although it was not feasible in this multicenter study to provide adequate QST training across all centres, or standardise all assessments in all study centres, potential advantages of QST such as quantification of sensory deficits and allodynia/hyperalgesia, and standardisations of values for several painful sites [22, 23] may have provided greater sensitivity in detecting small variations of thermal or mechanical deficits, and reduced possible variability in testing within and between centres. Other limitations include the impact of concomitant opioid use on the results and that the patient population was 99% Caucasian, and therefore the findings may not be widely applicable to patients of other ethnicity.

Conclusion

Repeat treatment with the capsaicin 8% patch plus SOC versus SOC alone over 52 weeks in patients with PDPN was well tolerated and consistent with the established safety profile of the capsaicin 8% patch. Capsaicin plus SOC had no negative functional or neurologic effects compared with SOC alone.

Additional files

Additional file 1: Sensory examination. Details of how sensory examination conducted.

Additional file 2: Figure S1. Exposure to capsaicin 8% patch (SAS). Bar chart of number of patients by number of capsaicin treatments.

Additional file 3: Figure S2. Maximum number of treatments with capsaicin 8% patch (SAS). Bar chart of number of patients by maximum number of capsaicin treatments.

Additional file 4: Table S1. Sensory and reflex testing categories at baseline and end of study (SAS). Table of absolute mean values.

Additional file 5: Figure S3. Proportion of patients who reported improved, unchanged, or worsened sensory reflex function by EoS (capsaicin seven treatment cohort). Bar char of proportion of patients by sensory or reflex function.

Additional file 6: Figure S4. Change in proportion of patients reporting sensory and reflex testing categories from baseline to EoS (capsaicin seven treatment cohort). Bar chart of change from baseline in patients reporting category by sensory or reflex function.

Additional file 7: Table S2. Sensory and reflex testing categories at baseline and end of study (capsaicin seven treatment cohort). Table of absolute mean values.

Additional file 8: Figure S5. Change in proportion of patients reporting sensory and reflex testing categories from baseline to EoS (capsaicin seven treatment cohort). Bar chart of change from baseline in patients reporting category by sensory or reflex function.

Additional file 9: Table S3. Use of concomitant medications at baseline and at end of study. Table of number of antidepressants, antiepileptic drugs and opioids.

Abbreviations

AE: Adverse event; BPI-DN: Brief pain inventory diabetic neuropathy; CI: Confidence interval; eCRF: Electronic case report form; EMLA: Eutectic mixture of local anaesthetics; EoS: End of study; HbA1c: Glycated haemoglobin of A1c; LOCF: Last observation carried forward; MNSI: Michigan neuropathy screening instrument; N/A: Not applicable; NPRS: Numeric pain rating scale; PDPN: Painful diabetic peripheral neuropathy; PNP: Peripheral neuropathic pain; PRAE: Post randomisation adverse event; QOL: Quality of life; QOL-DN: Quality-of-life questionnaire for diabetic neuropathy; QST: Quantitative sensory testing; SAS: Safety analysis set; SOC: Standard of care; TEAE: Treatment emergent adverse event; UENS: Utah early neuropathy scale

Acknowledgments

The Coordinating Investigator of this study was Dr. Ladislav Pazdera. The authors would like to thank all study investigators (for full list see Additional file 4: Table S1) and Faysal Riaz of Astellas Pharma Europe Ltd., Chertsey, UK for critical review and his valuable comments.

Funding

This study was funded by Astellas Pharma Europe B.V., Leiden, The Netherlands. Astellas Pharma Europe B.V. developed the study design and protocol in conjunction with the clinical investigators, were responsible for collection and statistical analysis of the data and provided the study drug. The authors received editorial support for manuscript preparation from Sarah Reynolds of NexGen Healthcare Communications, London, UK, and this assistance was supported by Astellas Pharma Europe Ltd.

Authors' contributions

The authors directed and are fully responsible for all interpretation of the data and editorial decisions for this manuscript. All authors listed have contributed sufficiently to the manuscript to be included as authors, and all those who are qualified to be authors are listed in the author by line in line with ICMJE requirements. HJ, MS, SL, RS and MvS contributed to study design and data collection, analysis and interpretation. AV and NK contributed to study design and data analysis and interpretation. EV contributed to data analysis and interpretation. SP, LP and EO contributed to data collection, analysis and interpretation. All authors listed were involved in drafting the manuscript and have read and approved the final version.

Competing interests

A.V. has received research funding from Astellas Pharma, Pfizer, and Daiichi Sankyo; Astellas Pharma has licensed the Norfolk QOL-DN from Eastern Virginia Medical School; A.V. and E.V. have received royalties from the licensing. N.K. was a paid consultant for Astellas Pharma to support the design of this study and received a research grant from Astellas Pharma. M.S., H.J., R.S., and M.v.d.S. are employed by Astellas Pharma Europe B.V. Stephen Long was employed by Astellas Pharma Europe B.V. at the time of the study. Serge Perrot, Ladislav Pazdera and Enrique Ortega have no disclosures.

Author details

[1]Eastern Virginia Medical School, Strelitz Diabetes Center, 855 W Brambleton Avenue, Room 2018, Norfolk, VA 23510, USA. [2]Hôpital Hôtel Dieu, Paris Descartes University, Paris, France. [3]Vestra Clinics - Dedicated Research Clinics, Rychnov nad Kneznou, Czech Republic. [4]Astellas Pharma Europe B. V, Leiden, The Netherlands. [5]Hospital Rio Hortega, Valladolid, Spain. [6]Analgesic Solutions, Natick, MA, USA. [7]Tufts University School of Medicine, Boston, MA, USA. [8]INC Research, Camberley, UK.

References

1.   Jensen MP, Chodroff MJ, Dworkin RH, et al. The impact of neuropathic pain on health-related quality of life: review and implications. Neurology. 2007; 68:1178–82.

2.   Tölle T, Xu X, Sadosky AB. Painful diabetic neuropathy: a cross-sectional survey of health state impairment and treatment patterns. J Diabetes Complicat. 2006;20:26–33.

3.   Schmader KE. Epidemiology and impact on quality of life of postherpetic neuralgia and painful diabetic neuropathy. Clin J Pain. 2002;18:350–4.

4.   Davies M, Brophy S, Williams R, Taylor A. The prevalence, severity, and impact of painful diabetic peripheral neuropathy in type 2 diabetes. Diabetes Care. 2006;29:1518–22.

5.   Huizinga MM, Peltier A. Painful diabetic neuropathy: a management-centered review. Clin Diabetes. 2007;25:6–15.

6.   Jensen TS, Backonja MM, Hernández Jiménez S, et al. New perspectives on the management of diabetic peripheral neuropathic pain. Diab Vasc Dis Res. 2006;3:108–19.

7.   Rudroju N, Bansal D, Talakokkula ST, et al. Comparative efficacy and safety of six antidepressants and anticonvulsants in painful diabetic neuropathy: a network meta-analysis. Pain Physician. 2013;16:E705–14.

8.   Vinik AI, Tuchman M, Safirstein B, et al. Lamotrigine for treatment of pain associated with diabetic neuropathy: results of two randomized, double-blind, placebo-controlled studies. Pain. 2007;128:169–79.

9.   Finnerup NB, Attal N, Haroutounian S, et al. Pharmacotherapy for neuropathic pain in adults: a systematic review and meta-analysis. Lancet Neurol. 2015;14:162–73.

10. Anand P, Bley K. Topical capsaicin for pain management: therapeutic potential and mechanisms of action of the new high-concentration capsaicin 8% patch. Br J Anaesth. 2011;107:490–502.

11. Backonja M, Wallace MS, Blonsky ER, et al. NGX-4010, a high-concentration capsaicin patch, for the treatment of postherpetic neuralgia: a randomised, double-blind study. Lancet Neurol. 2008;7:1106–12.

12. Brown S, Simpson DM, Moyle G, et al. NGX-4010, a capsaicin 8% patch, for the treatment of painful HIV-associated distal sensory polyneuropathy: integrated analysis of two phase III, randomized, controlled trials. AIDS Res Ther. 2013;10:5.

13. Haanpää M, Cruccu G, Nurmikko T, et al. Capsaicin 8% patch versus oral pregabalin in patients with peripheral neuropathic pain. Eur J Pain. 2016;20: 316–28.

14. Irving GA, Backonja MM, Dunteman E, et al. A multicenter, randomized, double-blind, controlled study of NGX-4010, a high-concentration capsaicin patch, for the treatment of postherpetic neuralgia. Pain Med. 2011;12:99–101.

15. Simpson DM, Brown S, Tobias J, for the NGX-4010 C107 Study Group. Controlled trial of high-concentration capsaicin patch for treatment of painful HIV neuropathy. Neurology. 2008;70:2305–13.

16. Simpson DM, Robinson-Papp J, Van J, Stoker M, et al. Capsaicin 8% Patch in Painful Diabetic Peripheral Neuropathy: A Randomized, Double-Blind, Placebo-Controlled Study. J Pain. 2016. [Epub ahead of print].

17. Vinik EJ, Hayes RP, Oglesby A, et al. The development and validation of the Norfolk QOL-DN, a new measure of patients' perception of the effects of diabetes and diabetic neuropathy. Diabetes Technol Ther. 2005;7:497–508.

18. Astellas Pharma Ltd. QUTENZA™ 179 mg cutaneous patch SPC (2015). Available at https://www.medicines.org.uk/emc/medicine/23156. Accessed 4 Apr 2016.

19. Boyd A, Casselini C, Vinik E, Vinik A. Quality of life and objective measures of diabetic neuropathy in a prospective placebo-controlled trial of ruboxistaurin and topiramate. J Diabetes Sci Technol. 2011;5:714–22.

20. Singleton J, Bixby B, Russel JW, et al. The Utah early neuropathy scale: a sensitive clinical scale for early sensory predominant neuropathy. J Peripher Nerv Syst. 2008;13:218–27.

21. Casellini CM, Barlow PM, Rice AL, Casey M, Simmons K, Pittenger G, et al. A 6-month, randomized, double-masked, placebo-controlled study evaluating the effects of the protein kinase C-beta inhibitor ruboxistaurin on skin microvascular blood flow and other measures of diabetic peripheral neuropathy. Diabetes Care. 2007;30:896–902.

22. Maier C, Baron R, Tölle TR, et al. Quantitative sensory testing in the German research network on neuropathic pain (DFNS): somatosensory abnormalities in 1236 patients with different neuropathic pain syndromes. Pain. 2010;150: 439–50.

23. Backonja MM, Attal N, Baron R, et al. Value of quantitative sensory testing in neurological and pain disorders: NeuPSIG consensus. Pain. 2013;154:1807–19.

6

Guillain-Barré syndrome as a cause of acute flaccid paralysis in Iraqi children: a result of 15 years of nation-wide study

Jagar Jasem[1,2*], Kawa Marof[3], Adnan Nawar[4], Yosra Khalaf[5], Sirwan Aswad[3], Faisal Hamdani[5], Monirul Islam[6] and Andre Kalil[7]

Abstract

Background: Guillain-Barré syndrome (GBS) is the most common cause of acute flaccid paralysis (AFP) in the post-poliomyelitis eradication era. This is the first study done to identify the epidemiology, clinical features, and outcome of GBS in Iraqi children over 15 years.

Methods: The surveillance database about AFP cases < 15 years reported during January 1997-December 2011 was used.

Results: GBS represented 52.5% of AFP cases, with an incidence of 1.33 case/100,000 population < 15 years/year. There was a higher incidence in the Southern provinces, age group 1–4 years, males, and outside the capital city of province, with no significant seasonal variations (p = .22). Survival probability after the 1 year of onset for those with respiratory muscle involvement was .76 (95% CI: .60-.86), versus .97 (95% CI: .96-.98) for those who did not develop it (*p* < .001); and .97 (95% CI: .96-.98) for those living inside the capital city, versus .94 (.93-.95) for those living outside (*p* = .001). Cumulative incidence of residual paralysis for patients living inside the capital city was .21 (95% CI: .18-.24), versus .27 (95% CI: .25-.29) for those living outside (*p* < .001).

Conclusions: The incidence, age and gender distribution, and seasonality of GBS among Iraqi children is similar to those reported from other previous studies. It is the most important cause of AFP, especially in those between the age of 1 to 4 years living in rural areas.

Background

Guillain-Barré syndrome (GBS) is mostly an acute inflammatory demyelinating ascending polyradiculoneuropathy [1-3]. Flu-like illness or gastroenteritis precedes the onset of paralysis by 6 weeks in about two-thirds of patients [3]. The culprit infectious agent often remains unrecognized, but *Compylobacter jejuni Mycoplasma pneumonia*, and cytomegalovirus are commonly reported triggering pathogens. Molecular mimicry between structural components of both pathogens and myelin sheath of peripheral nerves, with subsequent cross-reaction of antibodies with the lat-

ter, is a commonly proposed hypothesis for the pathogenesis of disease [3-6].

Worldwide, GBS is considered the most common cause of acute flaccid paralysis in the post-poliomyelitis eradication era [5-14]. It affects people in various geographical locations and virtually all age groups [15]. Similar studies about the epidemiology and clinical features of GBS yield a wide range of minor to major differences [4,10,15-18]. Information about the epidemiology of the disease can give insights into the changing patterns of the disease incidence following exposure to new potential provoking factors [16]. Measuring the outcome of the disease in terms of mortality and morbidity can help direct attention towards modifying the risk factors of adverse disease outcomes. This is the first study done to identify the epidemiology, clinical features, and outcome of GBS in Iraqi children over 15 years of study.

---

* Correspondence: jagar.jasem@osumc.edu
[1]School of Medicine/ Faculty of Medical Sciences/ University of Duhok, Nakhoshkhana Street, Duhok, Kurdistan Region, Iraq
[2]Internal Medicine, Ohio State University, Columbus, Ohio, USA
Full list of author information is available at the end of the article

Methods

The surveillance database about acute flaccid paralysis (AFP) cases under the age of 15 reported from Iraq during January 1997 to December 2011 was used in the current study. AFP surveillance is an essential strategy of the Polio Eradication Initiative adopted by the World Health Organization (WHO) in 1988. AFP is defined as "any child under 15 years of age with acute flaccid paralysis (including GBS) or any person of any age with paralytic illness if polio is suspected". AFP information is routinely included in the weekly and monthly reporting system from the Preventive Health Department (PHD) in the Directorate General of Health (DGoH) of every Iraqi province, even if there is no reported case (routine surveillance "zero-reporting"). Notifications are done via mailing the standard communicable notification forms designed by the Iraqi Ministry of Health to the Communicable Disease Control Unit (CDCU) of the regional PHD. Active surveillance for the suspected cases of AFP is ideally done within 48 hours via a designed investigating team from the CDCU visiting the reporting sources (hospitals, rehabilitation centers, or private clinics). Case investigation is done using a WHO-standardized form [19].

Two stool specimens are collected from each suspected case with an interval of 24–48 hours between collections, given that no more than two months have elapsed since the onset of paralysis. Following collection, the specimens are kept in a cold box to be sent for the National Polio Laboratory in Baghdad. At least 60 days after the onset of paralysis, all surviving patients are re-examined by an expert committee for residual paralysis. The diagnosis of GBS was made based on clinical evaluation and cytochemical analysis of the cerebrospinal fluid retrieved via conducting a lumbar puncture test of the suspected cases.

There is no clear classification for "urban" and "rural" areas in Iraq. Hence, the most approximate encounter for that fact is via dividing each Province into areas inside and outside the Capital City of each; referring to more urban and more rural areas, respectively.

The study was approved by the Ethical Committee of the Faculty of Medical Sciences/University of Duhok, Duhok, Iraq and the Institutional Review Board (IRB) of the University of Nebraska Medical Center, Omaha, Nebraska, USA. The statistical analysis was done using SPSS 18 for Windows/MAC, (PASW® Statistics Grad-Pack 18). Statistical analyses included: Chi-square test, univariate Kaplan-Meier survival analysis and stratified log-rank tests. All tests were two sided with .05 level of significance.

Results

A total number of 5027 cases were reported from Iraq between January 1997 and December 2011. Out of these, 53 cases were excluded as they were not AFP (nutritional deficiencies and skeletal diseases). A total of 4974 cases of AFP were used in the final analysis. GBS represented more than half of the reported cases (N = 2611, 52.5%) (Table 1), corresponding to an annual incidence of 1.33 case/100,000 population under the age of 15 years (95% CI: .97-1.68). There was a higher incidence in the Southern provinces compared to the Central and Northern ones (Figure 1). The vast majority of cases belonged to the age group 1–4 years old (Figure 2). Male–female ratio was 1.35:1. About 65% of cases occurred outside the capital city of province of more rural social characteristics. Cases were reported throughout the year with the highest number being in January (261) and the lowest in August (173) (Figure 3). This monthly variation was not statistically significant ($p = .22$).

Fever was observed in 1358 (55.4%) of cases, and progression of paralysis to the maximum within 4 days of onset occurred in 2450 (97.1%) of cases. At least 60 days from the onset of paralysis, 619 (24.6%) of cases had residual paralysis and 118 (4.8%) others died (Table 2).

The probability of survival after the 1 year of onset for those with respiratory muscle involvement was .76 (95% CI: .60-.86), versus .97 (95% CI: .96-.98) for those who did not develop respiratory muscle weakness ($p < .001$) (Figure 4). Kaplan-Meier analysis of household location, gender, and age showed that only household location was significantly associated with the decreased probability of survival. The cumulative survival for patients living inside the capital city of province was .97 (95% CI: .96-.98), versus .94 (.93-.95) for those living outside the capital city of province ($p = .001$) (Figure 5). This effect was eliminated when stratified log-rank test was performed for both respiratory muscle paralysis and household location ($p = .21$). Likewise, Kaplan-Meier analysis of household location, gender, and age showed that both household location and age were significantly associated with increased cumulative incidence of residual paralysis. The cumulative incidence of residual weakness

Table 1 Causes of acute flaccid paralysis in Iraqi children, 1997-2011

Cause	Number (%)
Guillain-Barré syndrome	2611 (52.5)
Traumatic neuritis	715 (14.4)
Meningitis/Encephalitis	292 (5.9)
Poliomyelitis	166 (3.3)
Myopathy	89 (1.8)
Hypokalemia	74 (1.5)
Unknown	568 (11.4)
Others	459 (9.4)
Total	4974 (100)

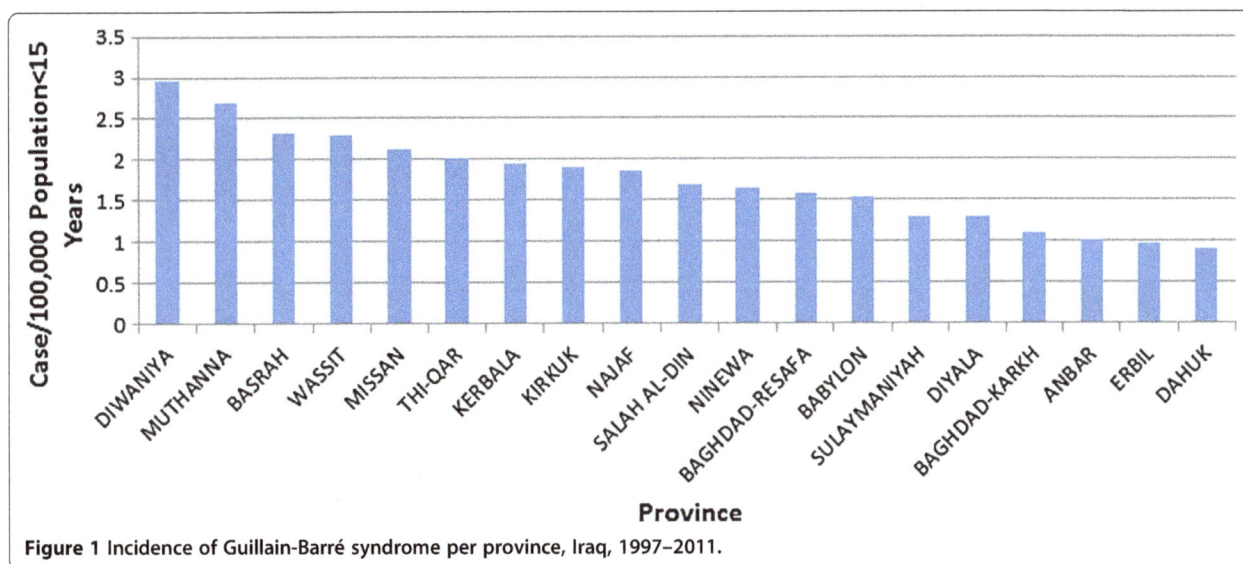

Figure 1 Incidence of Guillain-Barré syndrome per province, Iraq, 1997–2011.

increased with age was: .22 (95% CI: -.20-.24) for those below the age of 5 years and .35 (.29-.41) for those above the age of 5 years (*p* = .001) (Figure 6). The cumulative incidence of residual paralysis for patients living inside the capital city of province was .21 (95% CI: .18-.24), versus .27 (95% CI: .25-.29) for those living outside the capital city of province (*p* < .001) (Figure 7). This effect was maintained when stratified log-rank test was performed for both age and household location (*p* = .001).

Discussion

The annual incidence among Iraqi children was 1.33/100,000 population under the age of 15 years. This rate is at the upper limit of the reported international range of .34-1.34 cases/100,000/year among children aged <15 years [16]. Figures as high as 5 cases/100,000/year have been reported from some districts in Bangladesh [7].

Unlike other autoimmune diseases, males are typically affected more than females [10,16,20,21]. However, male predilection is found in other immune-mediated peripheral neuropathies like chronic inflammatory demyelinating polyneuropathy, multifocal motor neuropathy and Miller-Fisher syndrome [4]. Our study showed a male–female ratio of 1.3:1. Individual studies report ratios of 1.5 to 2.7 males to 1 female [20]. However, estimated 662 children reported in different studies have shown a male–female ratio of 1.3:1. Likewise, a total of 1607 patients of all ages reported in different studies have shown a similar ratio of 1.3:1 [20]. Pooled data about the cases of GBS in Latin America showed the exact same ratio [21]. This indicates that the higher preponderance of males in individual studies is likely to be the product of the confounding effect of sample size (Simpson's paradox) [20].

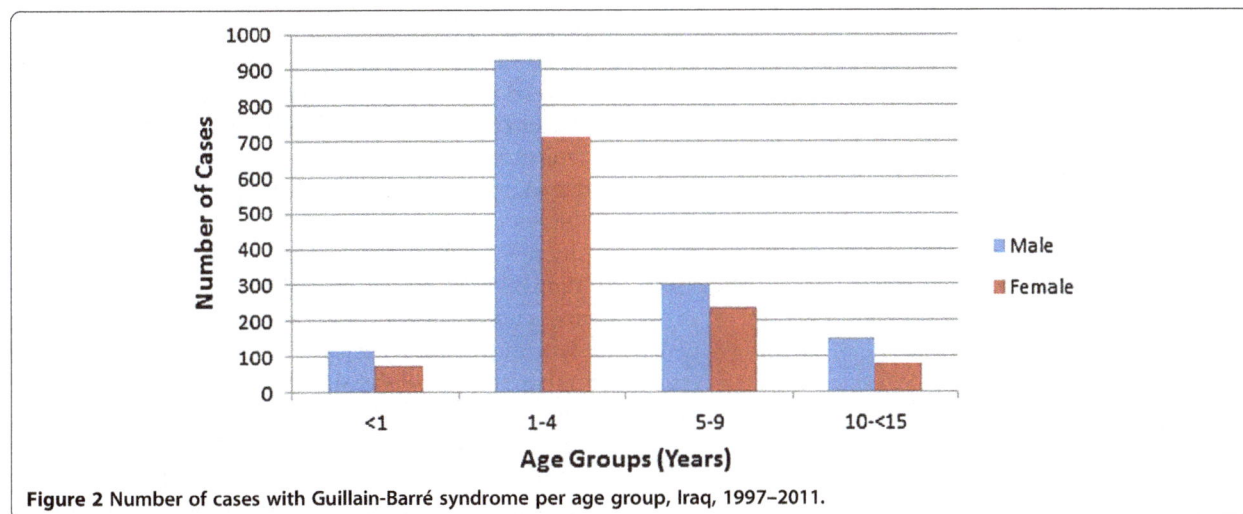

Figure 2 Number of cases with Guillain-Barré syndrome per age group, Iraq, 1997–2011.

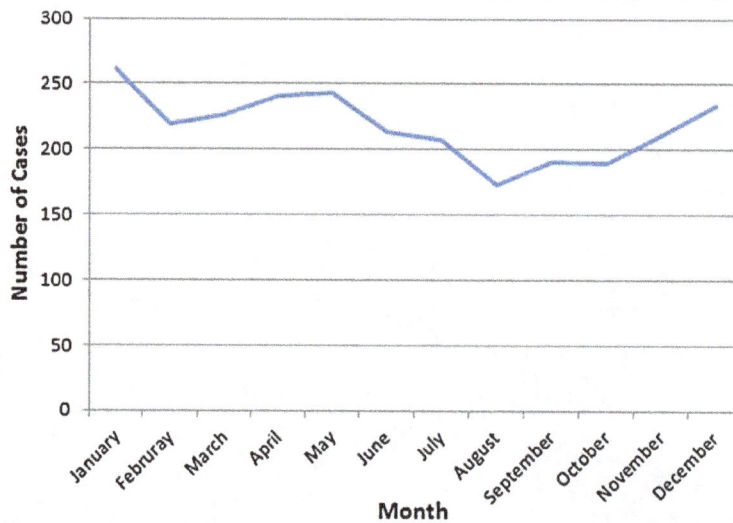

Figure 3 Number of cases with Guillain-Barré syndrome per month, Iraq, 1997–2011.

In accordance with other reports, children 1–4 years old were the most commonly affected age group with GBS in our study [9,10,22,23]. This is believed to be due to their relatively high susceptibility to infections in this age group and the increased susceptibility to the young myelinated peripheral nerves to demyelination [22,23]. Southern provinces have a statistically significant higher incidence of GBS compared to both Central and Northern ones. Although no specific reason was found, geographic variation in the incidence of disease in Iraq may be due to differences in the infection rates and climate among the different regions [7,9].

Table 2 Selected clinical characteristics of cases with Guillain-Barré syndrome, Iraq, 1997-2011

Features	Cases (%)
Fever at the onset of paralysis	2449 (93.8)
Yes	1358 (55.4)
No	1091 (44.5)
Progression to the maximum paralysis within 4 days of onset	2523 (96.6)
Yes	2450 (97.1)
No	73 (2.9)
Residual paralysis at least 60 days from onset	2343 (89.7)
Yes	619 (26.4)
No	1724 (73.6)
Survival at least 60 days from onset	2461 (94.2)
Alive	2343 (95.2)
Dead	118 (4.8)

Many studies have addressed the seasonality in the incidence of GBS, [9,15,16,24,25] only a few demonstrated a significant seasonal trend [18,24,26,27]. The lack of clear seasonal association may be due to the fact that the respiratory and enteric infections that precede GBS have opposite seasonal patterns [17]. The higher number of cases reported in winter and spring in our study is similar to reports from Southern Iran and Kuwait [18,28]. In general, different countries have different clustering patterns of cases, which might reflect the heterogeneity of the infectious agents that trigger the disease. The same reason may explain the higher number of cases reported outside the capital city of provinces, dominated by rural areas.

Although not classically attributed to the disease process of GBS [9,29], fever at the onset of paralysis is reported from previous studies and may be attributed to the effect of the triggering infectious disease [9,21,30]. Our study revealed that 55.4% of cases had fever at the onset of paralysis. As it might be expected from a study that is primarily concerned about AFP surveillance as a sensitive measure to detect cases of poliomyelitis, specific details about the progression pattern of weakness, sensory involvement, and dysautonomia in patients with GBS were not recorded in the study.

Although information about respiratory muscle involvement were only recorded for 1166 (44.7%) of patients, cumulative survival was significantly lower in those with respiratory muscle involvement. Likewise, the cumulative survival was significantly lower among those living outside the capital city of province. However, the latter association was insignificant when stratified by respiratory muscle involvement. This indicates that household location is not an independent cause of death per

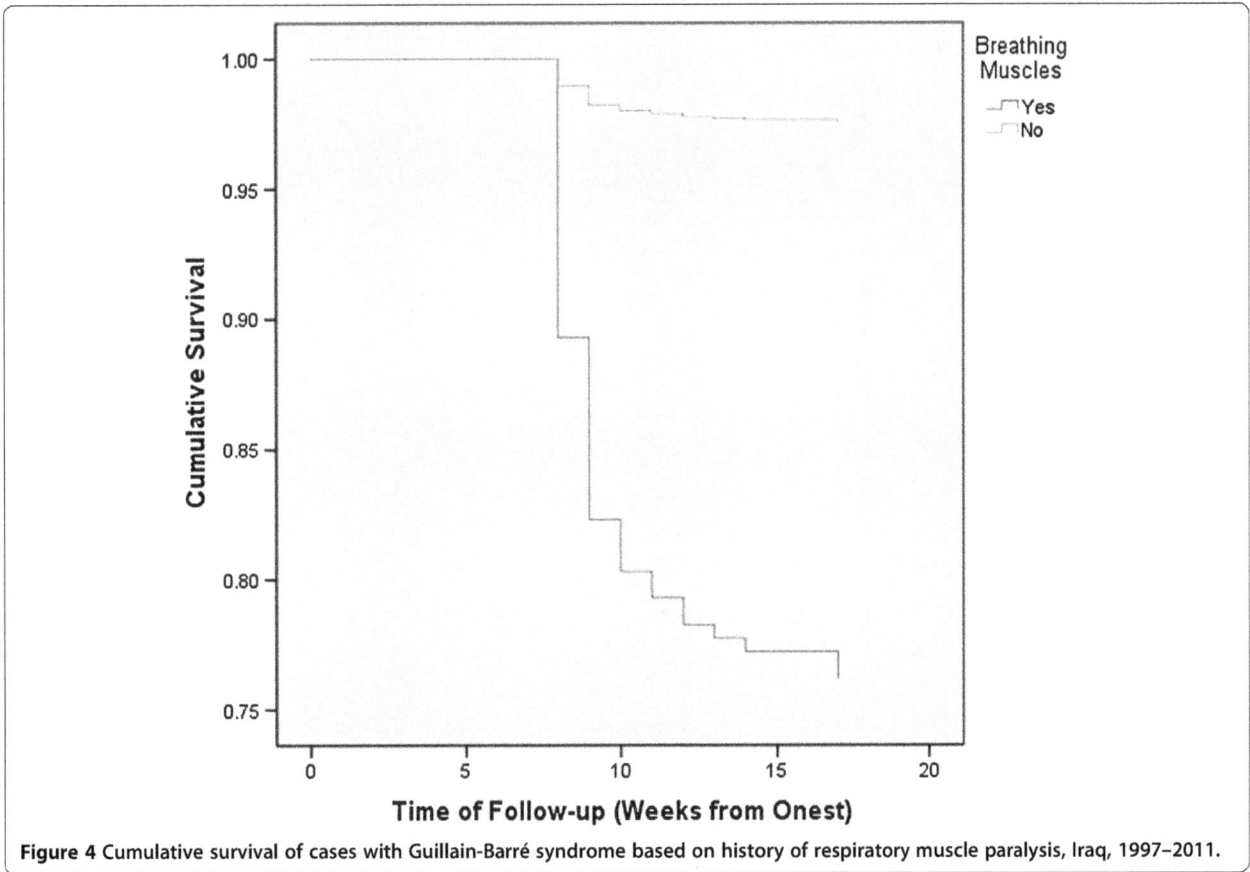

Figure 4 Cumulative survival of cases with Guillain-Barré syndrome based on history of respiratory muscle paralysis, Iraq, 1997–2011.

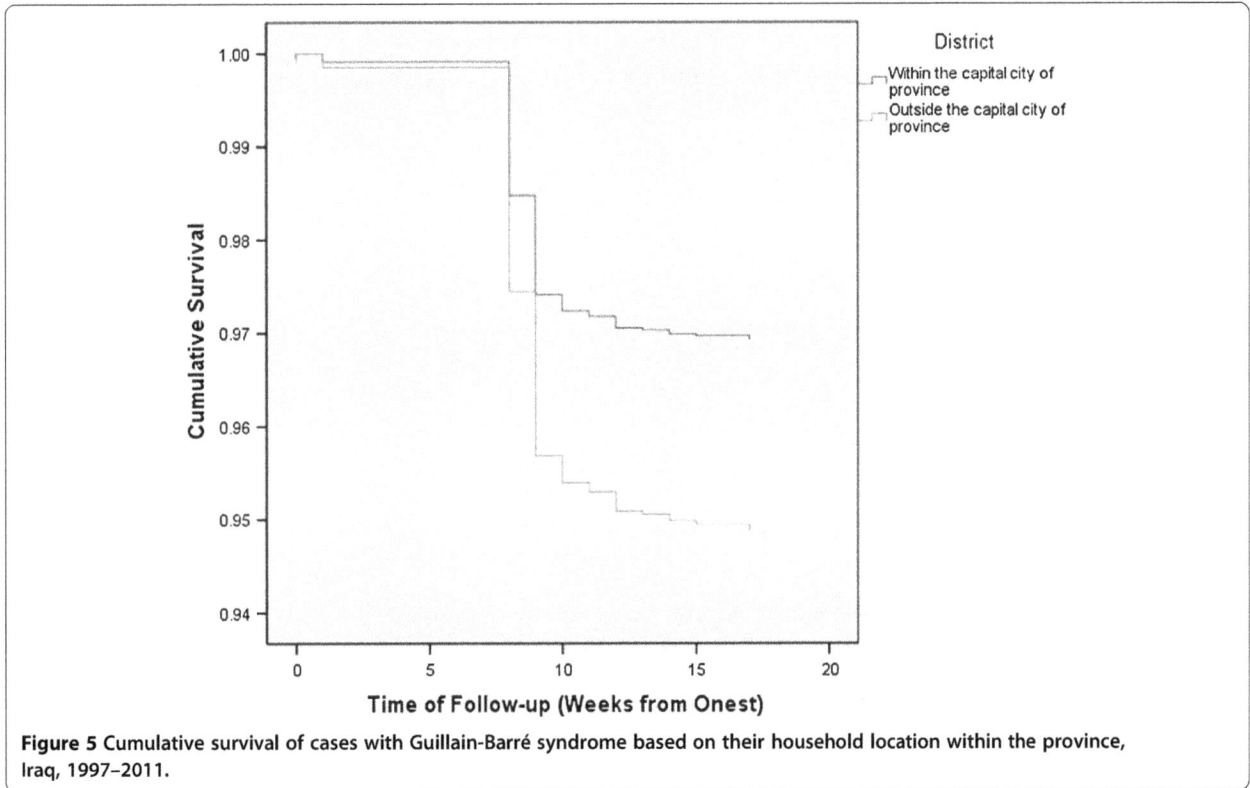

Figure 5 Cumulative survival of cases with Guillain-Barré syndrome based on their household location within the province, Iraq, 1997–2011.

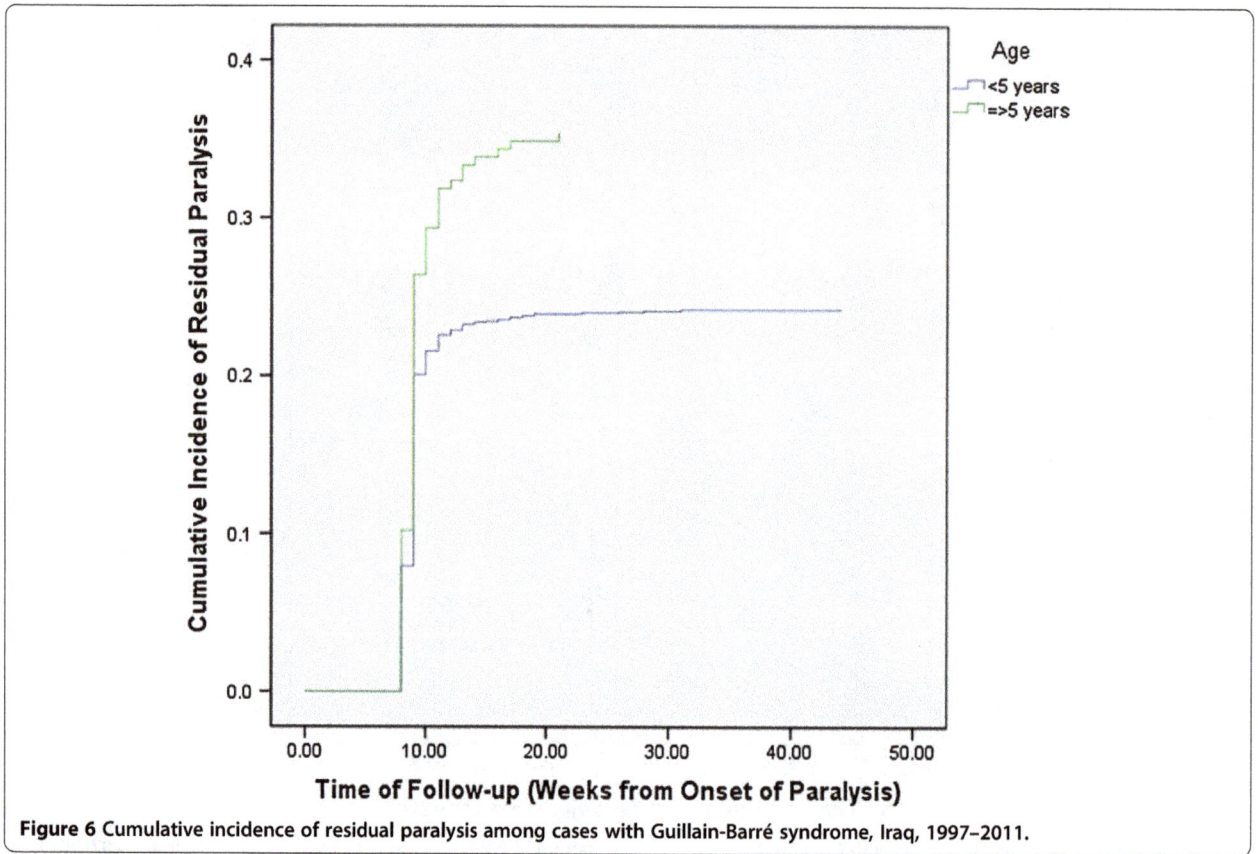

Figure 6 Cumulative incidence of residual paralysis among cases with Guillain-Barré syndrome, Iraq, 1997–2011.

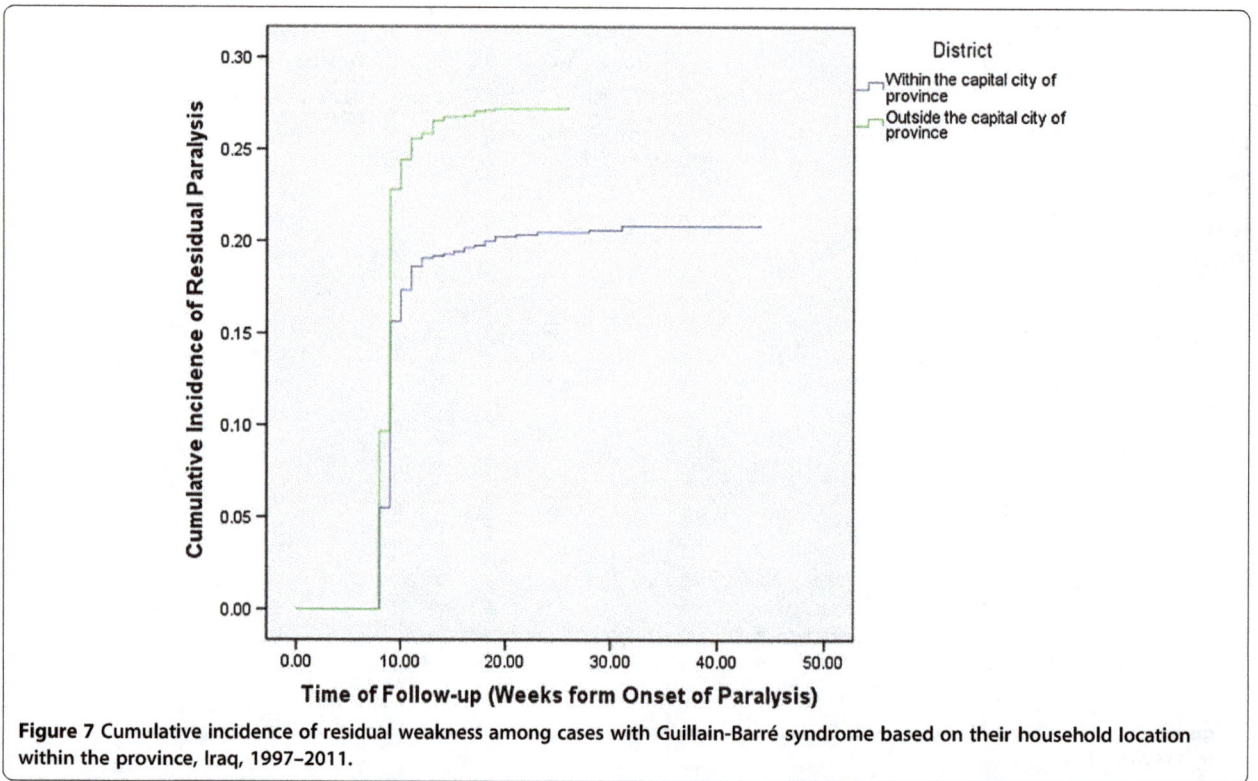

Figure 7 Cumulative incidence of residual weakness among cases with Guillain-Barré syndrome based on their household location within the province, Iraq, 1997–2011.

se, but rather causes death via respiratory paralysis, which plays a "mediating" effect. Furthermore, the association between household location and respiratory paralysis was insignificant too ($p = .12$), indicating that although respiratory paralysis occurs equally among those living inside and outside the capital city of province; the latter group are more likely die from it. This finding may be due to one or more of: differences of the inciting factors, delayed diagnosis in the rural areas, and inaccessibility to the required intensive care in those areas. Respiratory intensive care units do not exist in the vast majority of hospitals serving the rural communities in Iraq.

The risk of residual paralysis was higher among children above the age of 5 years. In general, the prognosis of GBS is shown to be better among younger age groups, although comparisons were generally made with adults [31-33]. In the largest prospective study by Korinthenberg et al., 96% of children were either asymptomatic or had minor symptoms at the end of the 288-day observation period [34]. This might reflect poorer axonal outgrowth and regeneration and less effective remyelinization process with increasing age [32]. Again, lower quality of and access to health care might underlie the increased risk of residual paralysis among cases residing outside the capital city of province.

The current study is the first to be done in Iraq involving analysis of nation-wide data over 15 years of study. It presents information about the overall incidence of disease, as well as the differences in disease incidence with time, age, gender, season, province of residence, and household location within the province of residence. It also provides information about the case-fatality rate of the disease and the likelihood of developing residual weakness following the resolution of acute disease, with emphasis on gender, age, and household location differences in those adverse outcomes. The sensitivity of AFP investigation was 2.5 cases/100,000 population below the age of 15 (above the WHO-recommended cut-off level of 1/100,000) and completeness of reporting was 96% (above the above the WHO-recommended cut-off level of 80%). These two performance indicators imply that the vast majority of GBS cases among children below15 years were effectively detected and recorded in the current database. However, since the data were collected for the purpose of acute flaccid surveillance as a strategy for detecting cases of poliomyelitis, the study provides limited information about the clinical features and subtypes of disease. Future studies are needed to at least identify the main 4 main subtypes of GBS, including: acute inflammatory demyelinating polyradiculoneuropathy (AIDP), acute motor axonal neuropathy (AMAN) and acute motor and sensory axonal neuropathy (AMSAN), and Miller Fisher syndrome [16]. Likewise, no data were available about the treatment modalities used for treating GBS cases. However, IVIG therapy remains largely unavailable in Iraq. Information about the history of preceding respiratory and gastrointestinal infection needs to be documented in future studies.

Conclusions

The incidence, age and gender distribution, and seasonality of GBS among Iraqi children is similar to those reported from other previous studies. It is the most important cause of AFP, especially in those between the age of 1 to 4 years living in rural areas.

Competing interests
The authors declare that they have no competing interests.

Authors' contributions
JJ has made substantial contributions to design of the study, data analysis, and writing and submitting the manuscript. KM, AN, YK, SA, and FH have contributed in data acquisition and manuscript revision. MI and AK have supervised study design and data analysis, as well as critically revised the manuscript. All authors have read and approved the final manuscript.

Author details
[1]School of Medicine/ Faculty of Medical Sciences/ University of Duhok, Nakhoshkhana Street, Duhok, Kurdistan Region, Iraq. [2]Internal Medicine, Ohio State University, Columbus, Ohio, USA. [3]Directorate of Preventive Health Affairs, Directorate General of Health, Mazi Street, Duhok, Kurdistan Region, Iraq. [4]National Communicable Disease Control, Ministry of Health, Bab Al Mudam Area, Baghdad, Iraq. [5]AFP Surveillance Laboratory, Ministry of Health, Bab Al Mudam Area, Baghdad, Iraq. [6]College of Public Health, University of Nebraska Medical Center, Omaha, Nebraska, USA. [7]Division of Infectious Diseases/Department of Internal Medicine, University of Nebraska Medical Center, Omaha, Nebraska, USA.

References
1. Beherman R, Kliegman R, Jenson H: *Nelson's Textbook of Pediatrics*. Philadelphia: Saunders; 2003.
2. Kasper D, Braunwals E, Hauser S, Longo D, Jameson L, Antony F: *Harrison's principles of internal medicine*. New York: McGraw-Hill Professional; 2005.
3. Hughes RA, Cornblath DR: **Guillain-Barre syndrome.** *Lancet* 2005, **366**(9497):1653–1666.
4. Kuwabara S: **Guillain-Barre syndrome: epidemiology, pathophysiology and management.** *Drugs* 2004, **64**(6):597–610.
5. Oomes PG, Jacobs BC, Hazenberg MP, Banffer JR, van der Meche FG: **Anti-GM1 IgG antibodies and Campylobacter bacteria in Guillain-Barre syndrome: evidence of molecular mimicry.** *Ann Neurol* 1995, **38**(2):170–175.
6. Sladky JT: **Guillain-Barre syndrome in children.** *J Child Neurol* 2004, **19**(3):191–200.
7. Islam Z, Jacobs BC, van Belkum A, Mohammad QD, Islam MB, Herbrink P, Diorditsa S, Luby SP, Talukder KA, Endtz HP: **Axonal variant of Guillain-Barre syndrome associated with Campylobacter infection in Bangladesh.** *Neurology* 2010, **74**(7):581–587.
8. Lam RM, Tsang TH, Chan KY, Lau YL, Lim WL, Lam TH, Leung NK, National Committee for the Certification of Wild Poliovirus Eradication: **Surveillance of acute flaccid paralysis in Hong Kong: 1997 to 2002.** *Hong Kong Med J* 2005, **11**(3):164–173.
9. Landaverde JM, Danovaro-Holliday MC, Trumbo SP, Pacis-Tirso CL, Ruiz-Matus C: **Guillain-Barre syndrome in children aged <15 years in Latin America and the Caribbean: baseline rates in the context of the influenza A (H1N1) pandemic.** *J Infect Dis* 2010, **201**(5):746–750.
10. Molinero MR, Varon D, Holden KR, Sladky JT, Molina IB, Cleaves F: **Epidemiology of childhood Guillain-Barre syndrome as a cause of acute flaccid paralysis in Honduras: 1989–1999.** *J Child Neurol* 2003, **18**(11):741–747.

11. Morris AM, Elliott EJ, D'Souza RM, Antony J, Kennett M, Longbottom H: **Acute flaccid paralysis in Australian children.** *J Paediatr Child Health* 2003, **39**(1):22–26.

12. Oostvogel PM, Spaendonck MA, Hirasing RA, van Loon AM: **Surveillance of acute flaccid paralysis in The Netherlands, 1992–94.** *Bull World Health Organ* 1998, **76**(1):55–62.

13. Poorolajal J, Ghasemi S, Farahani LN, Hosseini AS, Bathaei SJ, Zahiri A: **Evaluation of acute flaccid paralysis in hamadan, iran from 2002 to 2009.** *Epidemiol Health* 2011, **33**:e2011011.

14. Saraswathy TS, Zahrin HN, Apandi MY, Kurup D, Rohani J, Zainah S, Khairullah NS: **Acute flaccid paralysis surveillance: looking beyond the global poliomyelitis eradication initiative.** *Southeast Asian J Trop Med Public Health* 2008, **39**(6):1033–1039.

15. Chroni E, Papapetropoulos S, Gioldasis G, Ellul J, Diamadopoulos N, Papapetropoulos T: **Guillain-Barre syndrome in Greece: seasonality and other clinico-epidemiological features.** *Eur J Neurol* 2004, **11**(6):383–388.

16. McGrogan A, Madle GC, Seaman HE, de Vries CS: **The epidemiology of Guillain-Barre syndrome worldwide. A systematic literature review.** *Neuroepidemiology* 2009, **32**(2):150–163.

17. Hughes RA, Rees JH: **Clinical and epidemiologic features of Guillain-Barre syndrome.** *J Infect Dis* 1997, **176**(Suppl 2):S92–S98.

18. Borhani Haghighi A, Banihashemi MA, Zamiri N, Sabayan B, Heydari ST, Safari A, Lankarani KB: **Seasonal variation of Guillain-Barre syndrome admission in a large tertiary referral center in southern Iran: a 10 year analysis.** *Acta Neurol Taiwan* 2012, **21**(2):60–63.

19. World Health Organization, Iraqi Ministry of Health: *Acute Flaccid Paralysis Field Manual.* Baghdad: WHO & Iraqi MOH; 2009.

20. Ammache Z, Afifi AK, Brown CK, Kimura J: **Childhood Guillain-Barre syndrome: clinical and electrophysiologic features predictive of outcome.** *J Child Neurol* 2001, **16**(7):477–483.

21. Olive JM, Castillo C, Castro RG, de Quadros CA: **Epidemiologic study of Guillain-Barre syndrome in children <15 years of age in Latin America.** *J Infect Dis* 1997, **175**(Suppl 1):S160–S164.

22. Koul R, Al-Futaisi A, Chacko A, Fazalullah M, Nabhani SA, Al-Awaidy S, Al-Busaidy S, Al-Mahrooqi S: **Clinical characteristics of childhood guillain-barre syndrome.** *Oman Med J* 2008, **23**(3):158–161.

23. Rantala H, Cherry JD, Shields WD, Uhari M: **Epidemiology of Guillain-Barre syndrome in children: relationship of oral polio vaccine administration to occurrence.** *J Pediatr* 1994, **124**(2):220–223.

24. Nachamkin I, Arzarte Barbosa P, Ung H, Lobato C, Gonzalez Rivera A, Rodriguez P, Garcia Briseno A, Cordero LM, Garcia Perea L, Perez JC, Ribera M, Aldama PC, Guiterrez GD, Sarnat LF, Garcia MR, Veitch J, Fitzgerald C, Cornblath DR, Rodriguez Pinto M, Griffin JW, Willison HJ, Asbury AK, McKhann GM: **Patterns of Guillain-Barre syndrome in children: results from a Mexican population.** *Neurology* 2007, **69**(17):1665–1671.

25. Van Koningsveld R, Van Doorn PA, Schmitz PI, Ang CW, Van der Meche FG: **Mild forms of Guillain-Barre syndrome in an epidemiologic survey in The Netherlands.** *Neurology* 2000, **54**(3):620–625.

26. Jiang GX, Cheng Q, Link H, de Pedro-Cuesta J: **Epidemiological features of Guillain-Barre syndrome in Sweden, 1978–93.** *J Neurol Neurosurg Psychiatry* 1997, **62**(5):447–453.

27. Lyu RK, Tang LM, Cheng SY, Hsu WC, Chen ST: **Guillain-Barre syndrome in Taiwan: a clinical study of 167 patients.** *J Neurol Neurosurg Psychiatry* 1997, **63**(4):494–500.

28. Ismail EA, Shabani IS, Badawi M, Sanaa H, Madi S, Al-Tawari A, Nadi H, Zaki M, Al-saleh Q: **An epidemiologic, clinical, and therapeutic study of childhood Guillain-Barre syndrome in Kuwait: is it related to the oral polio vaccine?** *J Child Neurol* 1998, **13**(10):488–492.

29. van Doorn PA, Ruts L, Jacobs BC: **Clinical features, pathogenesis, and treatment of Guillain-Barre syndrome.** *Lancet Neurol* 2008, **7**(10):939–950.

30. Koga M, Yuki N, Hirata K: **Antecedent symptoms in Guillain-Barre syndrome: an important indicator for clinical and serological subgroups.** *Acta Neurol Scand* 2001, **103**(5):278–287.

31. Kalra V, Sankhyan N, Sharma S, Gulati S, Choudhry R, Dhawan B: **Outcome in childhood Guillain-Barre syndrome.** *Indian J Pediatr* 2009, **76**(8):795–799.

32. Anonymous: **The prognosis and main prognostic indicators of guillain-barre syndrome. A multicentre prospective study of 297 patients. The Italian guillain-barre study group.** *Brain* 1996, **119**(Pt 6):2053–2061. Pt 6.

33. Walgaard C, Lingsma HF, Ruts L, van Doorn PA, Steyerberg EW, Jacobs BC: **Early recognition of poor prognosis in Guillain-Barre syndrome.** *Neurology* 2011, **76**(11):968–975.

34. Korinthenberg R, Schessl J, Kirschner J: **Clinical presentation and course of childhood Guillain-Barre syndrome: a prospective multicentre study.** *Neuropediatrics* 2007, **38**(1):10.

7

Utility of somatosensory evoked potentials in the assessment of response to IVIG in a long-lasting case of chronic immune sensory polyradiculopathy

Angelo Maurizio Clerici[1*], Eduardo Nobile-Orazio[2], Marco Mauri[1], Federico Sergio Squellati[1] and Giorgio Giovanni Bono[1]

Abstract

Background: Chronic immune sensory polyradiculopathy (CISP) identifies a progressive acquired peripheral dysimmune neuropathy recognized as a chronic inflammatory demyelinating polyradiculoneuropathy (CIDP) variant. We describe a young woman with a thirteen-year history of CISP with a belated variable response to intravenous immunoglobulin (IVIG) and an almost erratic anticipation of symptoms between IVIG cycles. The association of IVIG and corticosteroids, immunosuppressants, plasmapheresis, did not lead to clinical improvement and was characterized by significant side effects. We evaluated a combined clinical and somatosensory evoked potentials (SSEPs) approach aimed to identify possible predictive parameters concerning the effect and duration of each IVIG administration. Neurologic disability was evaluated using INCAT - Overall Disability Sum Score (INCAT-ODSS).

Case presentation: A 30-year-old woman presented on 2004 for the subacute onset of asymmetric paresthesias in the lower limbs over the previous six months. The symptoms had been relapsing-remitting during the first four months, followed by a slow progression, resulting in limbs ataxia and a progressive gait disturbance requiring Canadian crutches. Motor and sensory nerve conduction studies and electromyographic evaluation were into normal limits. Median SSEPs were normal, while tibial SSEPs were characterised by the bilateral absence of both lumbar and cortical responses. Cerebrospinal fluid detected an increased protein concentration, while spinal MRI showed a pronounced thickening of the sacral nerve roots, together with a tube-shaped enlargement. These findings led to the diagnosis of CISP and the patient was treated with IVIG reaching a stable remission over the following 9 years. In early 2014, the patient began to show a variable response to treatment with erratic anticipation of sensory disturbances, and a more pronounced walking disability: corticosteroids, plasmapheresis, mycophenolate mofetil and cyclophosphamide were uneffective and burdened by relevant side effects. To better assess the response to IVIG in terms of time-effect, consistency and duration, we have combined a scheduled clinical and SSEPs evaluation during and after each IVIG cycle.

Conclusions: The correlation between the neurophysiological data and the INCAT-ODSS scores has allowed the modulation of IVIG cycles with a significant reduction of the clinical fluctuations and disability. SSEPs may therefore represent an useful and recommended additional aid for the treatment schedule of this rare clinical form.

Keywords: Chronic immune sensory polyradiculopathy, Somatosensory evoked potentials, Chronic inflammatory demyelinating polyneuropathy, Intravenous immunoglobulin, INCAT - Overall disability sum score

* Correspondence: angelomaurizio.clerici@asst-settelaghi.it
[1]Neurology Unit, Circolo & Macchi Foundation Hospital - Insubria University – DBSV, Viale L. Borri 57, 21100 Varese, Italy
Full list of author information is available at the end of the article

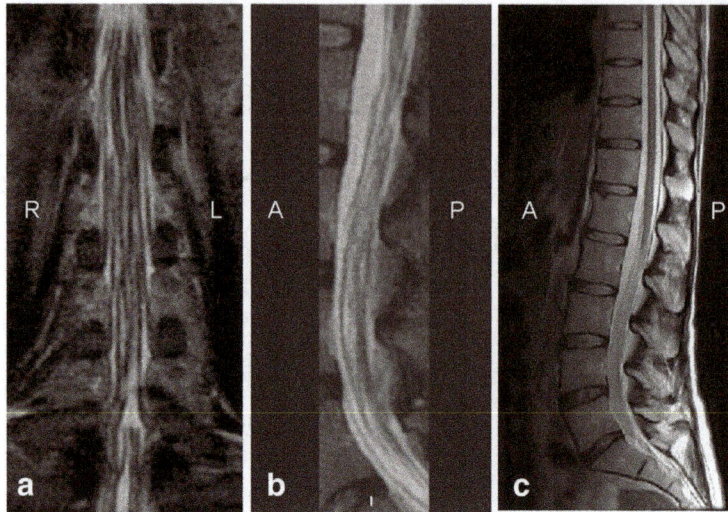

Fig. 1 Spinal MRI study. MR coronal STIR (**a**), sagittal STIR (**b**) and T2-weighted sagittal (**c**) images of the cauda equina showing marked thickening of the nerve roots together with a tube-shaped enlargement. (R = right; L = left; A = anterior; P = posterior)

Background

The term chronic inflammatory demyelinating polyradiculoneuropathy (CIDP) identifies a chronic-progressive acquired peripheral neuropathy. The clinical picture is characterised by sensorimotor signs and symptoms due to an inflammatory demyelinating process that is dysimmune in nature [1, 2].

The symptoms usually develop over a period of at least 8 weeks and are usually characterised by muscle weakness associated with sensory disturbances (paresthesia, dysesthesia, and hypoesthesia in some cases), moderate muscle wasting and areflexia. The weakness, distal and symmetric at onset, gradually tends to involve the proximal limb's segments, resulting in a progressive disability in walking, climbing stairs and in all movements against gravity, while the cranial district is usually spared. Occasionally, a postural tremor may be present, usually due to muscle weakness [1, 2].

Several CIDP variants have been described and classified as "atypical forms" in the diagnostic criteria of the European Federation of Neurological Societies/Peripheral Nerve Society (EFNS/PNS) [3]. Chronic immune sensory polyradiculopathy (CISP) is an almost rare form: paresthesia, pain, numbness, and ataxia represent the main symptoms with an asymmetric distribution at onset and progression to a distal symmetric pattern [4]. Nerve conduction studies are normal and the diagnosis of a demyelinating process is revealed by prolonged somatosensory evoked potentials (SSEPs) [5–7]. We describe the results of a combined clinical (INCAT - Overall Disability Sum Score - ODSS) and neurophysiological (SSEPs) approach we adopted to assess the effect and duration of response to intravenous immunoglobulin (IVIG) treatment in a long-lasting case of CISP with belated variable response to treatment and erratic anticipation of sensory symptoms [8].

Case presentation

An otherwise healthy 30-year-old woman presented on 2004 for the subacute onset of asymmetric paresthesias in the lower limbs over the previous six months. The symptoms had been relapsing-remitting during the first four months, followed by a slow progression that resulted in limbs ataxia and a progressive gait disturbance requiring Canadian crutches (ODSS: 4). Routine blood examinations, vitamins E and B12, folate, lipid profile, serum protein electrophoresis with immunofixation,

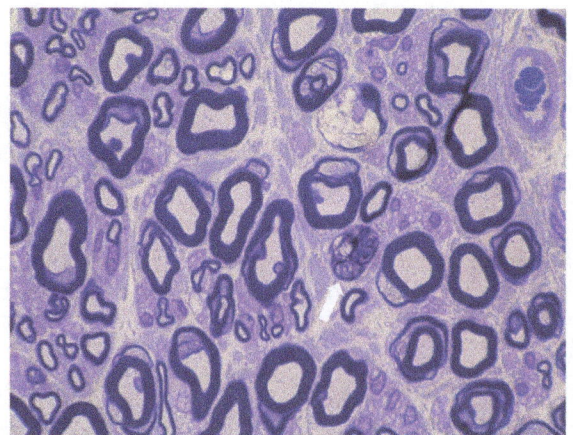

Fig. 2 Sural nerve biopsy. Cross section of plastic embedded left sural nerve stained with Toluidin blue showing slight axonal impairment without inflammatory infiltrate, a minimal reduction in myelinated fibers density with some isolated aspects of chronic (cluster) reinnervation (white arrow) and sporadic fibers in Wallerian

ceruloplasmin, angiotensin-1-converting enzyme, thyroid function including anti-thyroid antibodies were normal. Laboratory research for neoplastic, rheumatic, celiac and venereal disease, as well as myelin associated glycoprotein, sulfatide and anti-peripheral nerve antibodies showed normal values.

Motor and sensory nerve conduction studies (median, ulnar, common peroneal, tibial, sural nerves) and electromyographic evaluation (extensor digitorum brevis, tibialis anterior, quadriceps femoris, first dorsal interosseous, extensor digitorum communis, deltoid, L4-L5 and D9 paraspinal muscles) were into normal limits, with the exception of a bilateral mild elongation of the tibial F-waves

latencies (< 15% of the upper normal limit). Median SSEPs were normal, while tibial SSEPs were characterised by the bilateral absence of both lumbar (N22) and cortical (P40) responses.

A lumbar puncture detected clear cerebrospinal fluid (CSF) without cellularity, a normal glucose level (52 mg/dl) and an increased protein concentration of 128 mg/dl (NV < 50 mg/dl).

Spinal MRI showed a pronounced thickening of the sacral nerve roots, together with a tube-shaped enlargement (Fig. 1).

A left sural nerve biopsy was performed, showing slight axonal impairment without inflammatory infiltrate, a

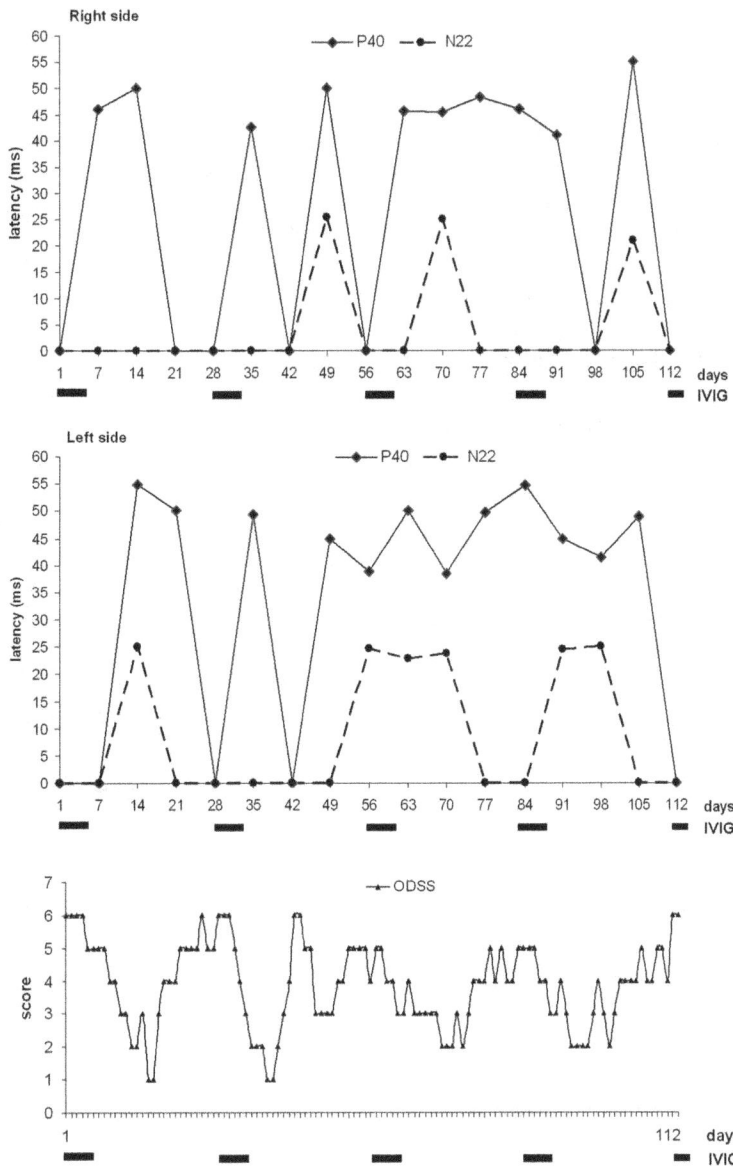

Fig. 3 Superimposed graphs of the daily ODSS and the longitudinal trend of tibial SSEPs (N22 and P40 latencies) recorded every 7 days over a period of 16 consecutive weeks. The bold lines below the horizontal axis refer to each cycle of IVIG scheduled every 28 days. Note the large P40 latencies fluctuations significantly correlated to the highest ODSS values

minimal reduction in myelinated fibre density with some isolated aspects of chronic (cluster) reinnervation, and sporadic fibres in Wallerian degeneration (Fig. 2).

These findings led to the diagnosis of CISP and the patient was treated with a high dose course of methylprednisolone (500 mg/day for 8 consecutive days), without significant effects on ataxia and on walking disability (ODSS: 4–5). As a second step, ten days after high dose steroid course, she was treated with IVIG (0.4 g/kg per day, for 5 consecutive days) every 4 weeks: vibration sense and joint position began to improve after the third IVIG-dose, with a marked reduction of the ataxic pattern, and an almost normal walking ability was achieved on the tenth day (ODSS: 1–2). This regimen has ensured a prolonged and stable remission over the following 9 years with an ODSS of 0–1.

In early 2014, the patient started to have symptom fluctuations, a variable response to treatment with erratic anticipation of sensory disturbances, and a more pronounced walking disability (ODSS: 2–4): she was treated with plasmapheresis (3 a week cycles for 3 weeks without benefit), mycophenolate mofetil (500 mg per day, discontinued after 4 weeks for relevant side effects - diarrhoea and vomiting), and cyclophosphamide (100 mg per day added to IVIG, maintained for 5 months, and then discontinued because of loss of weight and leukopenia). The patient was therefore subsequently kept only on IVIG therapy. To better assess the response to IVIG in terms of time-effect, consistency and duration, we have combined a scheduled clinical (ODSS scale) and SSEPs evaluation during and after each IVIG cycle.

Materials and methods

Basing on the patient's IVIG regimen (5 consecutive days every 4 weeks) we have assessed bilaterally tibial and median SSEPs together with nerve conduction studies (NCS) at the first day of each IVIG administration and after 7, 14 and 21 days for 16 consecutive weeks; the neurologic disability was recorded daily using the INCAT-ODSS [8].

Obtained the informed consent, NCS and SSEPs have been performed at a skin temperature of 32 °C, following the standard guidelines [9–11].

For each registration, we have considered the "peak latency" (ms) and "peak-to-peak amplitude" (µV) for N9, N13, N20, N22, and P40 responses, with any faulty recordings being marked as "0".

All collected data underwent statistical analysis, conducted with Statistical Package for Social Science -Version 19.0 (SPSS Inc), by setting the statistical significance level at 0.05. For descriptive statistics, we presented the data as the percentage distributions for categorical variables and as the means with standard deviations for continuous variables. Frequency distributions were compared by the chi-square test, and means were compared by the Kruskal-Wallis H-test for continuous variables. Correlations were assessed by the Spearman's regression analysis.

Results

The baseline evaluation of the SSEPs data showed a wide fluctuation of P40 latencies, ranging from 0 (41.1% of cases after right-side stimulation; 29.4% after left-side stimulation) to 55 ms for both sides (NV ≤ 44.2 ms); these values were greater than 6 standard deviations (SDs) compared with our normative data. For the N22 component, the absence of the evoked response has been documented in 82.3% of cases after right-side stimulation and in 64.7% after left-side stimulation. At the same time, ODSS values were quantified in the range of major disabilities (4–6) in 61.4% (70/114) of the total recordings, and with scores 5–6 (severe disability) in 35% (40/114) (Fig. 3-4). The amplitudes of the evoked responses (if present) were consistently 2 SDs under the normative values, with marked chronodispersion. The data derived from the upper

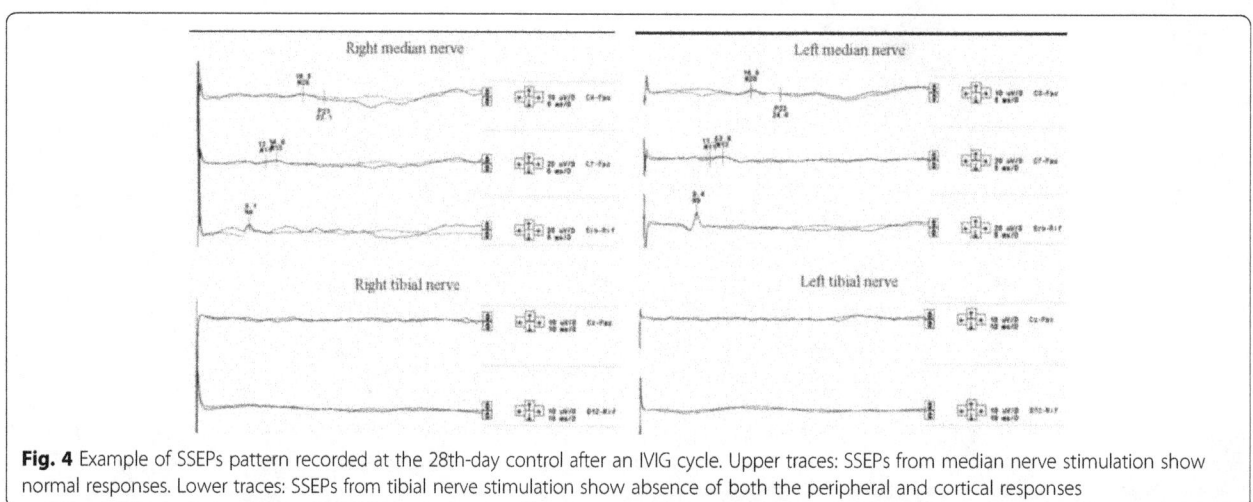

Fig. 4 Example of SSEPs pattern recorded at the 28th-day control after an IVIG cycle. Upper traces: SSEPs from median nerve stimulation show normal responses. Lower traces: SSEPs from tibial nerve stimulation show absence of both the peripheral and cortical responses

limbs stimulation have instead shown stable and normal values for all the evoked components (N9, N13, N20), as for the central conduction time (Fig. 4).

The statistical correlation between neurophysiological data and the daily ODSS scores has shown a mean clinical worsening 16 ± 3.1 days after IVIG treatment, while the longitudinal analysis of ODSS scores, compared to the frequency of IVIG cycles (5 consecutive days every 4 weeks), has shown, for each cycles, a significant clinical worsening (ataxia) respectively at days 17, 12, 19 and 18 (Fig. 3). The isolated record on day 12 has been observed in the context of a minor infectious event of

the upper airways which may contribute to a negative modulation of the dysimmune pattern. Thus excluding this confounding data, the mean clinical deterioration was estimated to occur on the eighteenth day. As a consequence, we have planned 5 consecutive IVIG doses every 18 days, repeating the neurophysiological monitoring at the first day of IVIG infusion, after 7 and 14 days for 13 consecutive registrations, together with a daily evaluation of the ODSS.

The statistical analysis of the new data collection has shown, unlike the baseline assessments, a) an always reliable N22 and P40 responses; b) a significant reduction

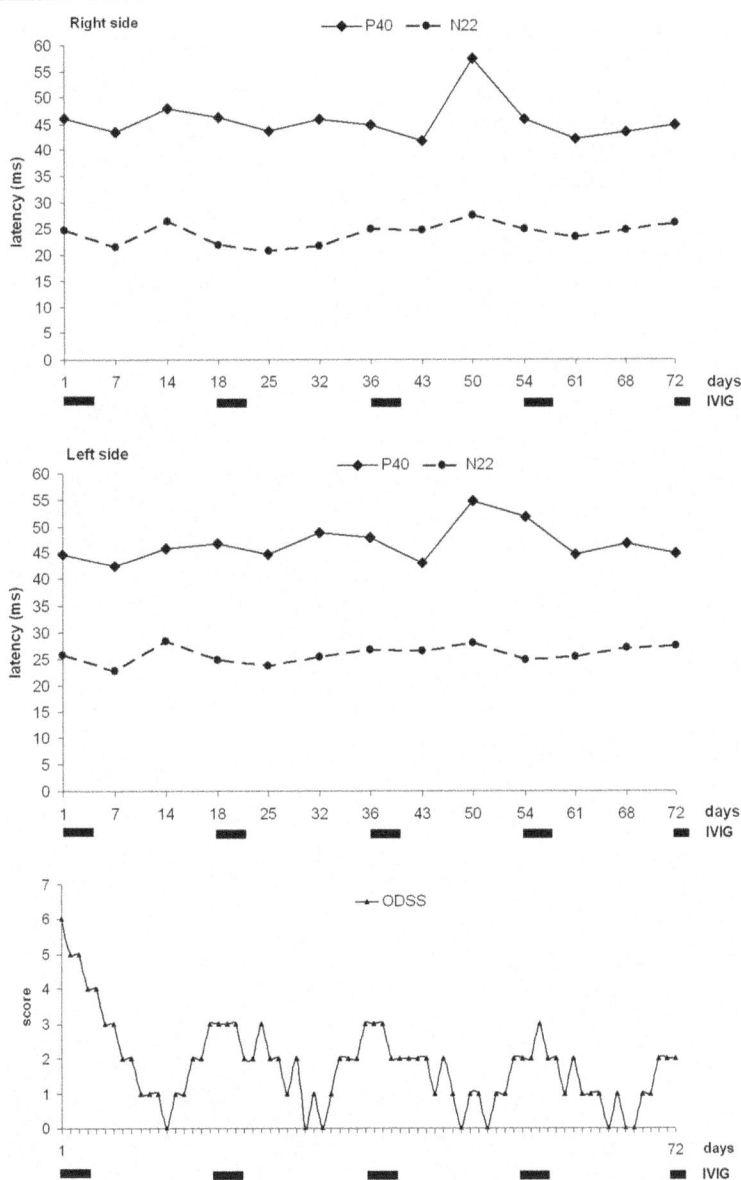

Fig. 5 Superimposed graphs of the daily ODSS and the longitudinal trend of tibial SSEPs (N22 and P40 latencies) recorded the first day of each IVIG administration and after 7–14 days for 13 consecutive recordings. The bold lines below the horizontal axis refer to each cycle of IVIG scheduled every 18 days. Note the relevant stabilization of P40/N22 latencies and the reduction of ODSS values

of P40 and N22 latencies ($p < 0.04$) with a mean values of 45.6 ± 3.9 ms (range: 42.0–57.0) in the right-side, 46.6 ± 3.4 ms (range: 42.4–54.7) in the left side for P40, and 24.0 ± 2.0 ms (range: 20.7–27.4) in the right side, 25.6 ± 1.58 ms (range: 22.8–28.4) in the left side for N22, respectively. Note that the highest scores (57 ms for P40, and 27.4 ms for N22) have been recorded only once during the whole neurophysiological monitoring (Figs. 5 and 6). The ODSS scores were in the range 0–2 (moderate or absent disability) in 77.7% (56/72) of the total recordings, and with score 3 ("requires unilateral support to walk 10 meters - stick, single crutch, one arm") in only 15.2% (11/72) (Fig. 5). When compared to baseline results, the new data are much more homogeneous, as confirmed by the significant reduction of SDs from the average values (1–1.5 SDs).

The time course analysis of P40 latencies (from the first day of IVIG infusion to the beginning of the subsequent cycle) showed an improving trend, for the right side, between the first and the second week (from a mean value of 45.5 ± 0.71 ms to 42.7 ± 0.9 ms), followed by a worsening trend between the second and third week (mean value: 48,65 ± 6,06 ms). These trends were found to be statistically significant ($p = 0.046$ - Kruskal-Wallis H test), and similar results have been detected on the left side, reaching the threshold of statistical significance ($p = 0.051$). The pejorative and ameliorative trend is also confirmed by the changes in ODSS scores, from a mean value of 2.6 in the first week (discrete disability), to 0.8 in the second week (minimal disability), and finally equal to 1.8 in the third week ($p < 0.001$ - Kruskal-Wallis H test). No statistical correlation has been found considering N22 and P40 amplitudes.

Nerve conduction studies were consistently within the normative values, including F-waves, without statistical correlation between clinical exacerbations or improvement after each IVIG protocol.

Discussion and conclusion

An inflammatory radiculoneuropathy with the predominant involvement of the dorsal roots has been originally described by Sinnreich as a cause of sensory ataxia, introducing the term of chronic immune sensory polyradiculopathy (CISP). All the patients had gait ataxia, large-fibre sensory impairment, paraesthesias, an high CSF protein level, a completely normal motor and sensory nerve conduction studies, and abnormal SSEPs as a specific hallmark, as in our case [12–15]. Moreover, the neuropathological findings were also not specific for a peripheral demyelinating process, and ruled out the presence of an inflammatory infiltrate [16].

According to the EFNS/PNS guidelines CISP is clinically classified within the subgroup of atypical-CIDP, but the diagnosis is feasible only by considering several "supportive criteria", and it cannot be further characterised in terms of "definite", "probable" or "possible" since electrodiagnostic criteria do not include SSEPs, which represent the more sensitive diagnostic tool [3, 17]. Several authors have indeed recently underlined the diagnostic properties and utility of SSEPs in evaluating CIDP patients [18–21].

In the present case, considering clinical fluctuations and the erratic response to IVIG treatment, we have planned a neurophysiological approach (SSEPs) together with the daily ODSS record, not only for a diagnostic confirmation, but also to search possible correlations between neurophysiological and clinical data potentially exploitable for therapeutic purposes. Consider also that we often modulate "empirically" the IVIG cycles following the criterion of the clinical worsening, as well as the choice of other

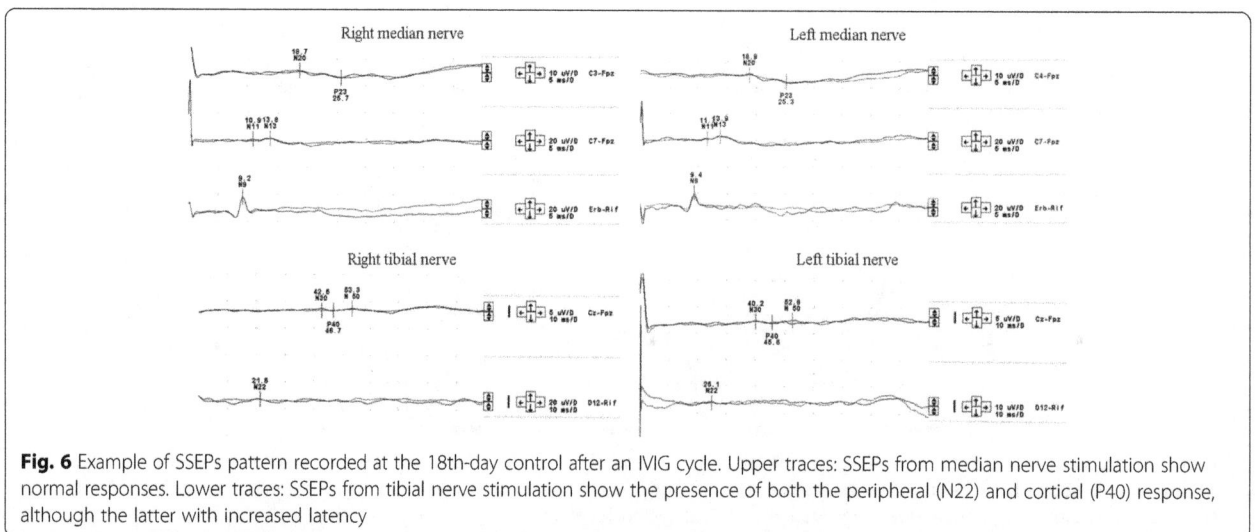

Fig. 6 Example of SSEPs pattern recorded at the 18th-day control after an IVIG cycle. Upper traces: SSEPs from median nerve stimulation show normal responses. Lower traces: SSEPs from tibial nerve stimulation show the presence of both the peripheral (N22) and cortical (P40) response, although the latter with increased latency

therapeutic measures (corticosteroids, immunosuppressants, plasmapheresis) [22–24].

Our data, although derived from a single case, show a close correlation between serial SSEPs and ODSS scores, thus contributing to the assessment of the effect and duration of IVIG administration and, accordingly, into the modulation of the frequency of IVIG intake, allowing the patient to reduce both clinical fluctuations and disability with any further significant relapse. In addition, the new therapeutic regimen, scheduled according to the neurophysiological evidences, has enabled a significant improvement of the ODSS global average score from 3.85 to 1.83.

We agree with some previous evidences about the non-localizing property of tibial SSEPs in the demyelinating process but, as shown in this case, they may be an useful supportive aid to establish the more appropriate therapeutic program faithfully reproducing the evolution of the clinical picture [4, 18, 21]. Undoubtedly, none of the two resources (SSEPs and ODSS) reaches an absolute diagnostic power, but we recommend their execution and integration in such rare and selective clinical forms.

Abbreviations

CIDP: Chronic inflammatory demyelinating polyradiculoneuropathy; CISP: Chronic immune sensory polyradiculopathy; CSF: Cerebrospinal fluid; EFNS/PNS: European Federation of Neurological Societies/Peripheral Nerve Society; INCAT-ODSS: Inflammatory Neuropathy Cause and Treatment - Overall Disability Sum Score; IVIG: Intravenous immunoglobulin; MRI: Magnetic resonance imaging; NV: Normal value; SDs: Standard Deviations; SPSS: Statistical Package for Social Science; SSEPs: Somatosensory evoked potentials

Acknowledgements

We wish to thank Chiara Luoni (MD) for the availability and expertise in statistical analysis, Ms. Emiliana Motta and Mrs. Tiziana Callari for the contribution to the neurophysiological recordings.

Funding

None.

Authors' contributions

AMC contributed to the study design, to the writing and revision of the manuscript; conducted and controlled the whole neurophysiological investigations, as well as the clinical assessments. ENO contributed to the study design, to the writing and revision of the manuscript. MM contributed to the data collection, statistical analysis, and revision of the manuscript. FSS contributed to the neurophysiological investigations and literature review. GGB contributed to the study design, to the writing and revision of the manuscript. All authors read and approved the final manuscript.

Competing interests

The Authors declare that they have no competing interests.

Author details

[1]Neurology Unit, Circolo & Macchi Foundation Hospital - Insubria University – DBSV, Viale L. Borri 57, 21100 Varese, Italy. [2]2nd Neurology, Humanitas Clinical and Research Institute, Department of Medical Biotechnology and Translational Medicine (BIOMETRA), Milan University, Rozzano, Milan, Italy.

References

1. Vallat JM, Sommer C, Magy L. Chronic inflammatory demyelinating polyradiculoneuropathy: diagnostic and therapeutic challenges for a treatable condition. Lancet Neurol. 2010;9(4):402–12. doi:10.1016/S1474-4422(10)70041-7.
2. Reynolds J, Sachs G, Stavros K. Chronic inflammatory demyelinating polyradiculoneuropathy (CIDP): clinical features, diagnosis, and current treatment strategies. R I Med J (2013). 2016;99(12):32–5. Review
3. Van den Bergh PY, Hadden RD, Bouche P, Cornblath DR, Hahn A, Illa I, et al. European Federation of Neurological Societies; Peripheral nerve society. European Federation of Neurological Societies/peripheral nerve society guideline on management of chronic inflammatory demyelinating polyradiculoneuropathy: report of a joint task force of the European Federation of Neurological Societies and the peripheral nerve society - first revision. Eur J Neurol. 2010;17(3):356–63. doi:10.1111/j.1468-1331.2009.02930. x. Erratum in: Eur J Neurol. 2011 May;18(5):796
4. Sinnreich M, Klein CJ, Daube JR, Engelstad J, Spinner RJ, Dyck PJ. Chronic immune sensory polyradiculopathy: a possibly treatable sensory ataxia. Neurology. 2004;63(9):1662–9.
5. Rajabally YA, Wong SL. Chronic inflammatory pure sensory polyradiculoneuropathy: a rare CIDP variant with unusual electrophysiology. J Clin Neuromuscul Dis. 2012;13(3):149–52. doi:10.1097/CND.0b013e31822484fb.
6. Trip SA, Saifee T, Honan W, Chandrashekar H, Lunn MP, Yousry T, et al. Chronic immune sensory polyradiculopathy with cranial and peripheral nerve involvement. J Neurol. 2012;259(6):1238–40. doi:10.1007/s00415-011-6326-0. Epub 2011 Nov 29
7. Salhi H, Corcia P, Remer S, Praline J. Somatosensory evoked potentials in chronic inflammatory demyelinating polyradiculoneuropathy. J Clin Neurophysiol. 2014;31(3):241–5. doi:10.1097/WNP.0000000000000050.
8. Merkies IS, Schmitz PI. Getting closer to patients: the INCAT Overall disability sum score relates better to patients' own clinical judgement in immune-mediated polyneuropathies. J Neurol Neurosurg Psychiatry. 2006;77(8):970–2. Epub 2006 Mar 20
9. Cruccu G, Aminoff MJ, Curio G, Guerit JM, Kakigi R, Mauguiere F, et al. Recommendations for the clinical use of somatosensory-evoked potentials. Clin Neurophysiol. 2008;119(8):1705–19. doi:10.1016/j.clinph.2008.03.016. Epub 2008 May 16. Review
10. Chiappa KH. Evoked potentials in clinical medicine. 3rd ed. Philadelphia, PA: Lippincott-Raven; 1997.
11. Aminoff MJ, Eisen AA. Somatosensory evoked potentials. Muscle Nerve. 1998;21:277–90.
12. Khadilkar SV, Deshmukh SS, Dhonde PD. Chronic dysimmune neuropathies: beyond chronic demyelinating polyradiculoneuropathy. Ann Indian Acad Neurol. 2011;14(2):81–92. doi:10.4103/0972-2327.82789.
13. Sheikh SI, Amato AA. The dorsal root ganglion under attack: the acquired sensory ganglionopathies. Pract Neurol. 2010;10(6):326–34. doi:10.1136/jnnp. 2010.230532.
14. Bril V, Katzberg H, Donofrio P, Banach M, Dalakas MC, Deng C, et al. ICE study group. Electrophysiology in chronic inflammatory polyneuropathy with IGIV. Muscle Nerve. 2009;39(4):448–55. doi:10.1002/mus.21236.
15. Nicolas G, Maisonobe T, Le Forestier N, Leger JM, Bouche P. Proposed revised electrophysiological criteria for chronic inflammatory demyelinating polyradiculoneuropathy. Muscle Nerve. 2002;25:26–30.
16. Kulkarni GB, Mahadevan A, Taly AB, Nalini A, Shankar SK. Sural nerve biopsy in chronic inflammatory demyelinating polyneuropathy: are supportive pathologic criteria useful in diagnosis? Neurol India. 2010;58(4):542–8. doi:10.4103/0028-3886.68673.
17. Sander HW, Latov N. Research criteria for defining patients with CIDP. Neurology. 2003;60(8 Suppl 3):S8–15.
18. Yiannikas C, Vucic S. Utility of somatosensory evoked potentials in chronic acquired demyelinating neuropathy. Muscle Nerve. 2008;38(5):1447–54. doi:10.1002/mus.21078.
19. Ayrignac X, Viala K, Koutlidis RM, Taïeb G, Stojkovic T, Musset L, et al. Sensory chronic inflammatory demyelinating polyneuropathy: an under-recognized entity? Muscle Nerve. 2013;48(5):727–32. doi:10.1002/mus.23821. Epub 2013 Aug 30
20. Devic P, Petiot P, Mauguiere F. Diagnostic utility of somatosensory evoked potentials in chronic polyradiculopathy without electrodiagnostic signs of peripheral demyelination. Muscle Nerve. 2016;53(1):78–83. doi:10.1002/mus. 24693. Epub 2015 Nov 26
21. Koutlidis RM, Ayrignac X, Pradat PF, Le Forestier N, Léger JM, Salachas F, et al. Segmental somatosensory-evoked potentials as a diagnostic tool in

chronic inflammatory demyelinating polyneuropathies and other sensory neuropathies. Neurophysiol Clin. 2014;44(3):267–80. doi:10.1016/j.neucli.2014. 08.006. Epub 2014 Aug 23

22. Chroni E, Veltsista D, Gavanozi E, Vlachou T, Polychronopoulos P, Papathanasopoulos P. Pure sensory chronic inflammatory polyneuropathy: rapid deterioration after steroid treatment. BMC Neurol. 2015;15:27. doi:10.1186/s12883-015-0291-7.

23. Oaklander AL, Lunn MP, Hughes RA, van Schaik IN, Frost C, Chalk CH. Treatments for chronic inflammatory demyelinating polyradiculoneuropathy (CIDP): an overview of systematic reviews. Cochrane Database Syst Rev. 2017;1:CD010369. doi:10.1002/14651858.CD010369.pub2.

24. Bright RJ, Wilkinson J, Coventry BJ. Therapeutic options for chronic inflammatory demyelinating polyradiculoneuropathy: a systematic review. BMC Neurol. 2014;14:26. doi:10.1186/1471-2377-14-26.

Arthropathy-related pain in a patient with congenital impairment of pain sensation due to hereditary sensory and autonomic neuropathy type II with a rare mutation in the *WNK1/HSN2* gene

Keiko Yamada[1,2], Junhui Yuan[3], Tomoo Mano[4], Hiroshi Takashima[3] and Masahiko Shibata[1,5*]

Abstract

Background: Hereditary sensory and autonomic neuropathy (HSAN) type II with *WNK1/HSN2* gene mutation is a rare disease characterized by early-onset demyelination sensory loss and skin ulceration. To the best of our knowledge, no cases of an autonomic disorder have been reported clearly in a patient with *WNK/HSN2* gene mutation and only one case of a Japanese patient with the *WNK/HSN2* gene mutation of HSAN type II was previously reported.

Case presentation: Here we describe a 54-year-old woman who had an early childhood onset of insensitivity to pain; superficial, vibration, and proprioception sensation disturbances; and several symptoms of autonomic failure (e.g., orthostatic hypotension, fluctuation in body temperature, and lack of urge to defecate). Genetic analyses revealed compound homozygous mutations in the *WNK1/HSN2* gene (c.3237_3238insT; p.Asp1080fsX1). The patient demonstrated sensory loss in the "stocking and glove distribution" but could perceive visceral pain, such as menstrual or gastroenteritis pain. She experienced frequent fainting episodes. She had undergone exenteration of the left metatarsal because of metatarsal osteomyelitis at 18 years. Sural nerve biopsy revealed a severe loss of myelinated and unmyelinated nerves. She complained of severe pain in multiple joints, even on having pain impairment. Although non-steroidal anti-inflammatory drugs are generally more effective than acetaminophen for arthritis, in our case, they were ineffective and acetaminophen (2400 mg/day) adequately controlled her pain and improved quality of life. Over 3 months, the numerical rating scale, pain interference scale of the Brief Pain Inventory, and the Pain Catastrophizing Scale decreased from 6/10 to 3/10, from 52/70 to 20/70, and from 22/52 to 3/52 points, respectively.

Conclusions: This is the second reported case of a Japanese patient with *WNK/HSN2* gene mutation of HSAN type II and the first reported case of an autonomic disorder in a patient with the *WNK/HSN2* gene mutation. Acetaminophen adequately controlled arthropathy related pain in a patient with congenital impairment of pain sensation.

Keywords: Hereditary sensory and autonomic neuropathies, Arthropathy, Demyelinating diseases, Acetaminophen, Case report

* Correspondence: mshibata@pain.med.osaka-u.ac.jp
[1]Center for Pain Management, Osaka University Hospital, 2-15 Yamadaoka, Suita-shi, Osaka 565-0871, Japan
[5]Department of Pain Medicine, Osaka University Graduate School of Medicine, 2-2 Yamadaoka, Suita-shi, Osaka 565-0871, Japan
Full list of author information is available at the end of the article

Background

Hereditary sensory and autonomic neuropathies (HSANs) are clinical and genetic disorders of the peripheral nerve [1]. HSANs are linked to 12 genes and have been classified into types I–V on the basis of age at onset, mode of inheritance, and predominant clinical symptoms [1]. Patients with HSAN type II present with loss of pain, temperature, and touch and mutations in the hands and feet [1]. Autonomic disorder is not a dominant feature of HSAN type II, although this disease is called "hereditary sensory and *autonomic* neuropathy" [1]. HSAN type II, with mutation in the nervous system-specific HSN2 exon of the with-no-lysine(K)-1 (*WNK1*) gene (*HSN2/WNK1*), is a very rare autosomal recessive disease. A few cases of *WNK1/HSN2* have been reported among the following ethnic groups: French–Canadian families (c.594delA, c.918_919insA, c.943c > T) [2, 3], a Lebanese family (c.947delC) [4], and two British families (c.60_61delTG + c.1168_1171delACAG and c.1168_1171delACAG + c.1168_1171delACAG) [5] and in Austrian (c.550C > T) [6], Italian (c.255delC, c.1089_1090insT) [6], Belgian (c.1064_1065delTC) [6], Polish (c.539_540delAG, c.2897_2898delAG) [7], Korean (c.1134_1135insT, c.217C > T) [8], and Japanese (c.1134_1135insT) [9] ethnicities. With the exception of dry hands in a Korean case, autonomic complications have not been reported in patients with HSAN type II with *HSN/WNK1* mutation [8].

Charcot arthropathy includes deforming and destructive process in joints and is one of the complications of neurosensory disorders [10]. The lack of protective sensation in patients with sensory neuropathies could cause delayed identification of bone injuries by overload [10]. Because of the lack of sensation experienced by patients with Charcot arthropathy, they are not expected to experience much pain despite severe deformation. However, a previous study reported that among 55 patients with Charcot arthropathy, more than 75 % complained of pain in the foot at the final stage of deformation, although all patients had clinical loss of sensation [11]. The reasons for this remain unclear.

Case presentation

A 54-year-old woman presented with loss of touch, temperature, position, and vibration sense and taste disorder, and she was insensitive to pain at the body surface since infancy. She also suffered from an autonomic disorder, with symptoms, such as orthostatic hypotension, fluctuation in body temperature, and lack of urge to defecate.

She had normal mental growth and development, although she did not walk until 18 months of age. Her family history was unremarkable; she had a healthy younger sister and her parents were not related (Fig. 1). She had repeated injuries during childhood because of insensitivity to pain, and she was diagnosed with Freiberg disease at 6 years. She experienced frequent fainting episodes and was diagnosed with an autonomic nervous system imbalance at 21 years. Even in cold temperatures, she perspired on her back and reported not needing a snowsuit. She did not have high blood pressure.

After repeated jumping from a squatting position in gym class at 14 years, the sole of her left foot developed severe blisters, and the wounds transitioned into metatarsal osteomyelitis after a few weeks. As a result of the refractory osteomyelitis, a left metatarsal was replaced by an autogenous bone graft when she was 18 years. It took approximately 10 years to recover fully from the wounds.

She had migraine since childhood until she was 20 years and took a painkiller (an antipyrine medication) daily during that time. Although she could feel a toothache/headache, she lacked sensation on the surface of her face, except around the jaw. She showed a "stocking and glove distribution", and the detection range of sensation varied along a gradient from the periphery to center. She could perceive visceral pain, such as menstrual or gastroenteritis pain, which she controlled with an antipyrine medication. Since 42 years of age, she started using a cane for walking outside.

Although she had known that she was different from others concerning pain perception since childhood, she and her parents had never consulted a doctor regarding the impaired pain sensation until 48 years of age.

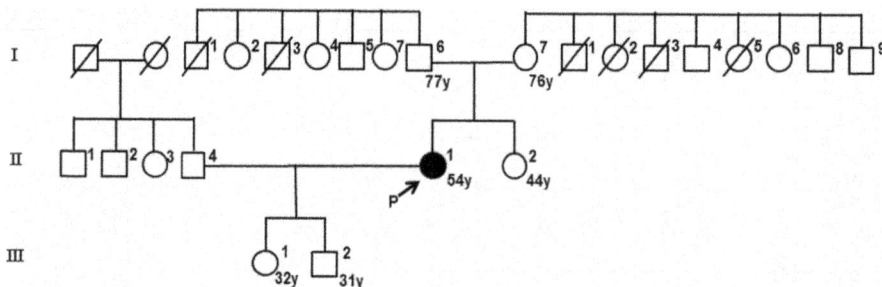

Fig. 1 The family tree of the patient

Arthropathy-related pain in a patient with congenital impairment of pain sensation due to hereditary...

59

At 48 years of age, the patient developed sudden severe pain and swelling in her right joint, and her previous physician diagnosed Charcot arthropathy (X-ray photograms are shown in Fig. 2). At 50 years of age, she was confined to a wheelchair to avoid putting weight on her joints. The pain gradually affected multiple joints over subsequent years. Non-steroidal anti-inflammatory drugs (NSAIDs) improved her joint pain to a limited degree. At 54 years of age, her joint pain became intolerable. NSAIDs were not effective enough for her to resume activities of daily living. Mexiletine hydrochloride treatment was not effective. She experienced side effects of pregabalin and duloxetine. Subsequently, her physician referred her to our multidisciplinary center for pain management. She was diagnosed with HSAN type II using molecular genetic analysis and was prescribed acetaminophen (2400 mg/day), which controlled her pain very well and improved her quality of life.

During our follow-up, she reported: "one day severe 'electric-shock-like or piercing pain' occurred, and which made me suffer few times per hour and keeping for months after this episode, and which was naturally decreased."

Pain-related assessment

Brief Pain Inventory (BPI), including numerical rating scale (NRS) [12, 13], was used to assess pain intensity and interference. Pain-related psychosocial factors were quantitated using the Hospital Anxiety and Depression scale (HADS) [14] and Pain Catastrophizing Scale (PCS) [15]. NRS and pain interference scale of BPI decreased from 6/10 to 3/10 and from 52/70 to 20/70 points, respectively, over 3 months. PCS scores also decreased from 22/52 to 3/52 points. At baseline, HADS indicated normal mental state; both the anxiety and depressive scales of HADS were relatively low (both 5/21 points) despite severe pain. After 3 months, the anxiety and depressive scales of HADS decreased from 5/21 to 3/21 points and from 5/21 to 4/21 points, respectively.

Neurological examination

A neurological examination revealed normal mental status, speech, and comprehension and intact cranial nerve-innervated muscles. Manual muscle testing revealed moderate weakness in the distal parts of the extremities and mild weakness in the proximal parts. Grip strength was significantly reduced (right, 4.0 kg; left, 6.0 kg). Deep tendon reflexes were absent. Plantar responses were flexor on both sides. The sensory examination revealed that the tactile and pinprick sensations were moderately decreased in the face and trunk and severely diminished in the upper and lower distal extremities. Sensations were diminished in a stocking and glove pattern. The vibration sense was reduced till the knees and absent in the ankles. The joint position sense was absent at the hallux. There was no apparent laterality of the sensory disturbance. Pseudoathetosis was observed in the upper limbs, and Romberg's test was not positive in the seated position. With the exception of abnormal sweating, thermoregulatory failure, and lack of urge to defecate, there were no signs of autonomic dysfunction, such as pupillary responses, dry eyes, or dry mouth. Her blood pressure was 138/85 bpm in the supine position and 126/72 bpm while standing. The head-up tilt test did not reveal any orthostatic intolerance. On electrocardiogram, the coefficient of variation of the R-R intervals (CVR-R) measured at rest was normal. The early and delayed heart-to-mediastinum (H/M) ratio was not decreased on 123I-MIBG myocardial scintigraphy (early: 3.14, delay: 2.97).

Nerve conduction and electromyographic evaluation

The nerve conduction study revealed normal compound muscle action potentials (CMAPs) values, except for a slightly reduced motor nerve conduction velocity of 50.0 m/s, 41.0 m/s, and 39.0 m/s in the median, peroneal, and tibial nerves, respectively. The velocity was in the normal range in the ulnar nerve (>50.5 m/s) and in the tibial and peroneal nerves (>48.0 m/s). The sensory nerve action potentials of the median, ulnar, and sural nerves were not evoked. The electromyography revealed a reduction in recruitment in the distal muscles of the upper and lower limbs. The patient was diagnosed with pure sensory neuropathy.

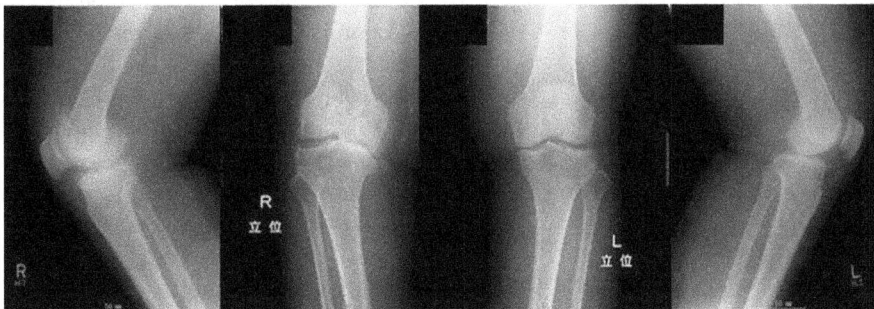

Fig. 2 X-ray photograms of the legs

Pathologic examination

Sural nerve biopsy revealed a severe loss of myelinated and unmyelinated nerve which were observed by light microscopy of the epon section with toluidine blue staining (Fig. 3a, b) and electron microscopy (Fig. 4a, b). Collagen pockets, which were indicative of unmyelinated nerve loss, were observed by electron microscopy (indicated by the arrows in Fig. 4c). Myelinated nerve tissue was completely lost. The density of unmyelinated nerve tissue (7620 per mm^2), calculated by electron microscopy, was significantly decreased. Skin biopsy was not performed.

Molecular genetic analysis

Mutation screening was conducted as previously described [16]. Target sequencing with 16 HSAN disease-related genes were conducted using Illumina MiSeq (Illumina Inc., San Diego, CA, USA). The *WNK1* mutation observed in this patient was validated by Sanger sequencing. A homozygous frame shift mutation was identified in the *WNK1/HSN2* gene c.3237_3238insT (p.Asp1080fsX1; ENST00000537687), which was previously reported as c.1134_1135insT (p.Asp379fsX1; ENST00000574564) [8, 9]. This mutation is absent in 1000

Genomes, ExAC, or HGVD, which comprises exome sequencing of 1208 Japanese individuals (http://www.genome.med.kyoto-u.ac.jp/SnpDB/).

Conclusion

We would like to highlight three important points from this case. First, this is the second case of *WNK/HSN2* gene mutation of HSAN type II reported in a Japanese patient. Second, this is the first reported case of an autonomic disorder in a patient with the *WNK/HSN2* gene mutation. Third, the patient's arthropathy-related pain, despite congenital impairment of pain sensation, was a noteworthy symptom.

The current patient is the second reported case of a patient with *WNK1/HSN2* gene mutation in Japan, both of which resulted from the same homozygous mutation, c.3237_3238insT [9]. *WNK1/HSN2* with homozygous 1134–1135 ins T mutation was reported in a Japanese patient by Takagi et al. [9], and the same mutation was reported in Korea by Cho et al. [8].

Although an autonomic disorder has never been reported in HSAN type II with the WNK1/HSN2 gene mutation, our patient presented with several symptoms of autonomic disturbances. In particular, the lack of urge to defecate through decreased parasympathetic pelvic nerve activity resulted in serious disruptions in her activities of daily living. Although there have been no reports of hyperhidrosis in patients with HSAN type II, fluctuation in body temperature is one of the most common symptoms of autonomic failure. In the presence of partial hyperhidrosis, there may be peripheral autonomic dysfunction. WNK influences transient receptor potential vanilloid 4 (TRPV4) channel function, which controls osmoregulation at the cellular level and regulates water balance. Therefore, there is an association between WNK1 and severe hypertension as reported previously [17]. However, our patient did not present with hypertension. Although our examination did not reveal autonomic dysfunction, we think that the possibility of autonomic failure cannot be excluded. This is the first reported case of an autonomic disorder in a patient with the *WNK/HSN2* gene mutation, and HSAN type II should be carefully considered because symptoms of autonomic dysfunction appeared in our patient.

Recurrent skin ulcers on the tips of the fingers and toes were previously reported [1, 8, 9]. Our patient had a difficult in recovering from injury and an amputated metatarsal due to osteomyelitis, but she did not develop skin ulcers. Except the autonomic disorder, her neurological examination had almost the same clinical features as those of previous patients with HSAN type II with *WNK1/HSN2* gene mutations.

NSAIDs are generally more effective than acetaminophen for arthritis with inflammation. However, in our

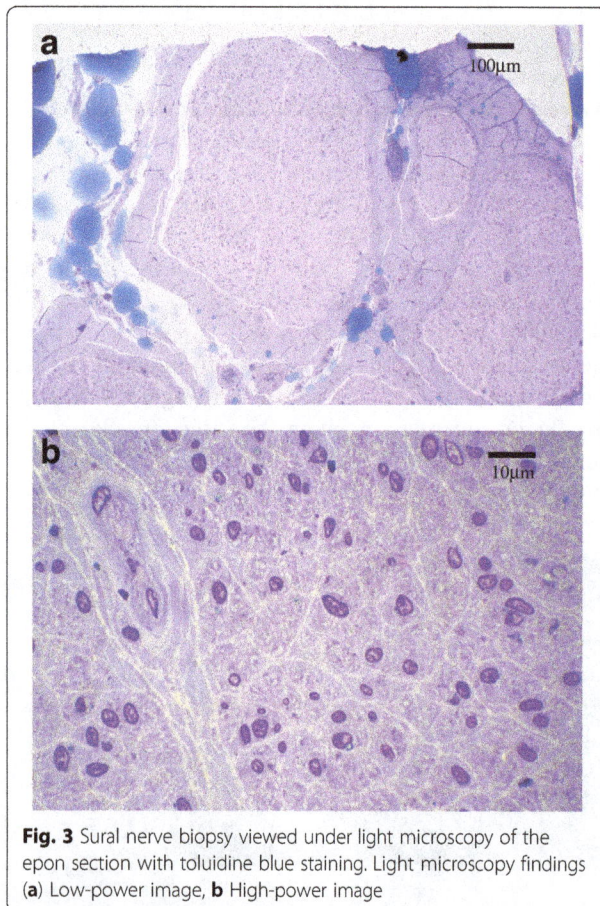

Fig. 3 Sural nerve biopsy viewed under light microscopy of the epon section with toluidine blue staining. Light microscopy findings (**a**) Low-power image, **b** High-power image

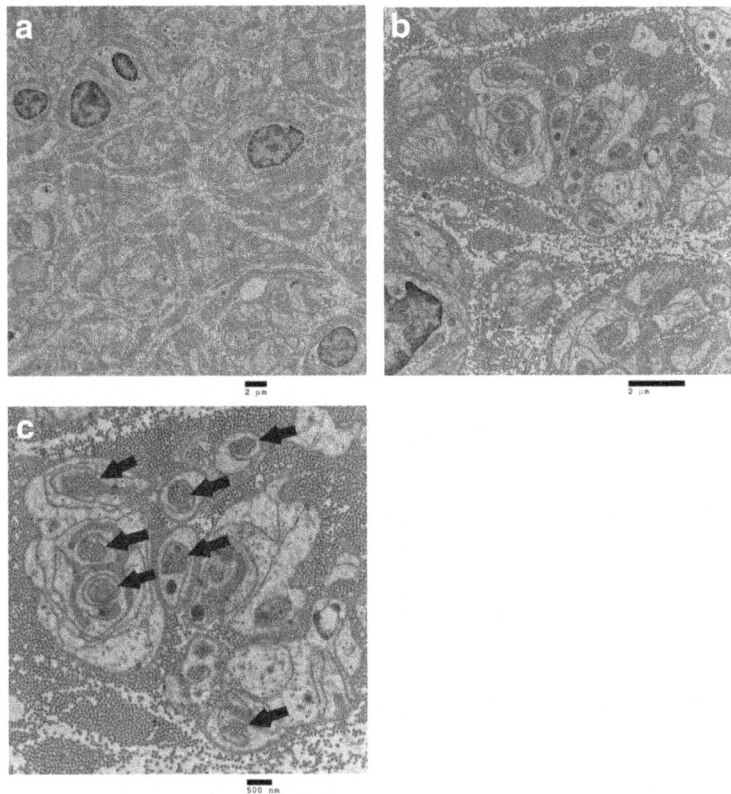

Fig. 4 Sural nerve biopsy viewed under electron microscopy. Electron microscopy findings (**a**) Low-power image, **b** High-power image. Myelinated nerve completely disappeared, and the density of unmyelinated nerves (7620 per mm^2) significantly decreased. **c** Collagen pockets are indicated by the arrows

patient, acetaminophen was more effective than NSAIDs for alleviating multiple joint pain. Theoretically, her arthropathy pain was conducted by unmyelinated nerve fibers (C fibers) and was possibly modified by central pain because acetaminophen was very effective for controlling her pain, although she had a reduction in unmyelinated nerve tissue. The antinociceptive mechanism of acetaminophen is still unclear, but the theory of multiple pathways is supportive. Although acetaminophen inhibits cyclooxygenase (COX), anti-inflammatory effect of acetaminophen is weak. Acetaminophen is lipid-soluble, passes through the blood–brain barrier, and has an effect on the central nerve system [18]. Acetaminophen activates 5-hydroxytryptamine 3 receptors in the serotonergic pathways, which are part of the descending pain system, with resulting pain relief [19]. The gamma-aminobutyric acid receptor is associated with acetaminophen [20]. Cannabinoid is one of the key factors of acetaminophen-induced antinociception [21]. Moreover, TRPV1 has an important role in antinociception induced by acetaminophen in the brain [22].

The patient felt non-specific 'electric shock-like or piercing' pain suddenly, but she was innately unable to feel sharp pain because of complete demyelination. Her non-specific pain might have been phantom pain, derived from the central nervous system because it was correlated with her strong emotional episode. When she complained about non-specific pain, her father was diagnosed of cancer and reported a pins-and-needles sensation in his fingers due to peripheral nerve disorder, which was caused by anti-cancer chemotherapy. He had complained about the pins-and-needles sensation every day, and she was told that she had empathized with and imagined his pain. We suspect that her non-specific pain was central pain from this emotional episode relating to her father. A previous study reported that empathy for pain may effectively activate pain neural circuits in an individual observing another person's pain [23]. Consistent with our findings, Danzier et al. reported a 32-year-old woman with HSAN type V who experienced tension-type headaches shortly after the sudden loss of her brother, despite complete absence of physical pain [24].

Abbreviations
BPI: Brief Pain Inventory; CMAPs: Compound muscle action potentials; HADS: Hospital Anxiety and Depression scale; HSAN: Hereditary sensory and autonomic neuropathy; NRS: Numerical rating scale; NSAIDs: Non-steroidal anti-inflammatory drugs; PCS: Pain Catastrophizing Scale; TRPV4: Transient receptor potential vanilloid 4; WNK1: With-no-lysine(K)-1

Acknowledgments

The authors would like to express their appreciation to Dr. Hiroki Yamazaki, Dr. Masanori Sawamura, and Dr. Kazuhito Nishinaka for providing the patient information. The authors would like to express gratitude to Dr. Daita Kaneda for his professional comment, Dr. Nobuyuki Oka for his contribution to nerve biopsy, Dr. Tamotsu Kubori for his contribution to electromyographic evaluation, and Dr. Norio Sakai for performing the genetic diagnosis.

Funding

This report was supported in part by grants from the Research Committee for Charcot–Marie–Tooth Disease, Neuropathy and Applying Health and Technology of Ministry of Health, Welfare and Labour, Japan. This report is also supported by the Research program for conquering intractable disease from Japan Agency for Medical Research and Development, AMED.

Authors' contributions

Conception and design of the report: KY, TM, and MS. Performed the genetic diagnosis: JY and HT Contributed to the writing of the manuscript: KY, JY, TM, HT, and MS. Agreed with manuscript results and conclusions: KY, JY, TM, HT, and MS. All authors read and approved the final manuscript.

Authors' information

K.Y. is an anesthesiologist and a researcher in pain medicine and epidemiology. J.Y. is a neurologist and a researcher in neurogenetics. T.M. is a neurologist and assistant professor in the Department of Neuromodulation, Osaka University Graduate School of Medicine, Japan. H.T. is professor in the Department of Neurology and Geriatrics, Kagoshima University Graduate School of Medical and Dental Sciences, Japan, and a researcher in neurogenetics. M.S. is professor in the Department of Pain Medicine, Osaka University Graduate School of Medicine, Japan.

Competing interests

The authors declare that they have no competing interests.

Author details

[1]Center for Pain Management, Osaka University Hospital, 2-15 Yamadaoka, Suita-shi, Osaka 565-0871, Japan. [2]Public Health, Department of Social Medicine, Osaka University Graduate School of Medicine, 2-2 Yamadaoka, Suita-shi, Osaka 565-0871, Japan. [3]Department of Neurology and Geriatrics, Kagoshima University Graduate School of Medical and Dental Sciences, 8-35-1 Sakuragaoka, Kagoshima 890-8520, Japan. [4]Department of Neuromodulation, Osaka University Graduate School of Medicine, 2-2 Yamadaoka, Suita-shi, Osaka 565-0871, Japan. [5]Department of Pain Medicine, Osaka University Graduate School of Medicine, 2-2 Yamadaoka, Suita-shi, Osaka 565-0871, Japan.

References

1. Rotthier A, Baets J, Timmerman V, Janssens K. Mechanisms of disease in hereditary sensory and autonomic neuropathies. Nat Rev Neurol. 2012;8:73–85.
2. Lafreniere RG, MacDonald MLE, Dube MP, MacFarlane J, O'Driscoll M, Brais B, et al. Identification of a novel gene (HSN2) causing hereditary sensory and autonomic neuropathy type II through the Study of Canadian Genetic Isolates. Am J Hum Genet. 2004;74:1064–73.
3. Roddier K, Thomas T, Marleau G, Gagnon AM, Dicaire MJ, St-Denis A, et al. Two mutations in the HSN2 gene explain the high prevalence of HSAN2 in French Canadians. Neurology. 2005;64:1762–7.
4. Rivière JB, Verlaan DJ, Shekarabi M, Lafrenière RG, Bénard M, Der Kaloustian VM, et al. A mutation in the HSN2 gene causes sensory neuropathy type II in a Lebanese family. Ann Neurol. 2004;56:572–5.
5. Davidson GL, Murphy SM, Polke JM, Laura M, Salih M, Muntoni F, et al. Frequency of mutations in the genes associated with hereditary sensory and autonomic neuropathy in a UK cohort. J Neurol. 2012;259:1673–85.
6. Coen K, Pareyson D, Auer-Grumbach M, Buyse G, Goemans N, Claeys KG, et al. Novel mutations in the HSN2 gene causing hereditary sensory and autonomic neuropathy type II. Neurology. 2006;66:748–51.
7. Potulska-Chromik A, Kabzińska D, Lipowska M, Kostera-Pruszczyk A, Kochański A. A novel homozygous mutation in the WNK1/HSN2 gene causing: hereditary sensory neuropathy type 2. Acta Biochim Pol. 2012;59:413–5.
8. Cho HJ, Kim BJ, Suh YL, An JY, Ki CS. Novel mutation in the HSN2 gene in a Korean patient with hereditary sensory and autonomic neuropathy type 2. J Hum Genet. 2006;51:905–8.
9. Takagi M, Ozawa T, Hara K, Naruse S, Ishihara T, Shimbo J, et al. New HSN2 mutation in Japanese patient with hereditary sensory and autonomic neuropathy type 2. Neurology. 2006;66:1251–2.
10. Wukich DK, Sung W. Charcot arthropathy of the foot and ankle: modern concepts and management review. J Diabetes Complications. 2009;23:409–26.
11. Armstrong DG, Todd WF, Lavery LA, Harkless LB, Bushman TR. The natural history of acute Charcot's arthropathy in a diabetic foot specialty clinic. Diabet Med. 1997;14:357–63.
12. Okuyama T, Wang XS, Akechi T, Mendoza TR, Hosaka T, Cleeland CS, et al. Japanese version of the M.D. Anderson symptom inventory: a validation study. J Pain Symptom Manage. 2003;26:1093–104.
13. Uki J, Mendoza T, Cleeland CS, Nakamura Y, Takeda F. A brief cancer pain assessment tool in Japanese. J Pain Symptom Manage. 1998;16:364–73.
14. Zigmond AS, Snaith RP. The hospital anxiety and depression scale. Acta Psychiatr Scand. 1983;67:361–70.
15. Sullivan MJL, Bishiop SR, Pivik J. The pain catastrophizing scale: development and validation. Psychol Assess. 1995;7:524–32.
16. Yuan J, Matsuura E, Higuchi Y, Hashiguchi A, Nakamura T, Nozuma S, et al. Hereditary sensory and autonomic neuropathy type IID caused by an SCN9A mutation. Neurology. 2013;80:1641–9.
17. Fu Y, Subramanya A, Rozansky D, Cohen DM. WNK kinases influence TRPV4 channel function and localization. Am J Physiol Ren Physiol. 2006;290:F1305–14.
18. Courade JP, Besse D, Delchambre C, Hanoun N, Hamon M, Eschalier A, et al. Acetaminophen distribution in the rat central nervous system. Life Sci. 2001;69:1455–64.
19. Pickering G, Estève V, Loriot M-A, Eschalier A, Dubray C. Acetaminophen reinforces descending inhibitory pain pathways. Clin Pharmacol Ther. 2008;84:47–51.
20. Högestätt ED, Jönsson BAG, Ermund A, Andersson DA, Björk H, Alexander JP, et al. Conversion of acetaminophen to the bioactive N-acylphenolamine AM404 via fatty acid amide hydrolase-dependent arachidonic acid conjugation in the nervous system. J Biol Chem. 2005;280:31405–12.
21. Madenoğlu H, Kaçmaz M, Aksu R, Bicer C, Yaba G, Yildiz K, et al. Effects of naloxone and flumazenil on antinociceptive action of acetaminophen in rats. Curr Ther Res Clin Exp. 2010;71:111–7.
22. Mallet C, Barrière DA, Ermund A, Jönsson BAG, Eschalier A, Zygmunt PM, et al. TRPV1 in brain is involved in acetaminophen-induced antinociception. PLoS One. 2010;5(9):e12748.
23. Singer T, Seymour B, O'Doherty J, Kaube H, Dolan RJ, Frith CD. Empathy for pain involves the affective but not sensory components of pain. Science. 2004;303:1157–62.
24. Danziger N, Willer J-C. Tension-type headache as the unique pain experience of a patient with congenital insensitivity to pain. Pain. 2005;117:478–83.

9

Clinical and electrophysiological features of post-traumatic Guillain-Barré syndrome

Xiaowen Li[1†], Jinting Xiao[1†], Yanan Ding[1], Jing Xu[1], Chuanxia Li[2], Yating He[1], Hui Zhai[1], Bingdi Xie[1] and Junwei Hao[1*]

Abstract

Background: Post-traumatic Guillain-Barré syndrome (GBS) is a rarely described potentially life-threatening cause of weakness. We sought to elucidate the clinical features and electrophysiological patterns of post-traumatic GBS as an aid to diagnosis.

Methods: We retrospectively studied six patients diagnosed with post-traumatic GBS between 2014 and 2016 at Tianjin Medical University General Hospital, China. Clinical features, serum analysis, lumbar puncture results, electrophysiological examinations, and prognosis were assessed.

Results: All six patients had different degrees of muscular atrophy at nadir and in two, respiratory muscles were involved. Five also had damaged cranial nerves and four of these had serum antibodies against gangliosides. The most common electrophysiological findings were relatively normal distal latency, prominent reduction of compound muscle action potential amplitude, and absence of F-waves, which are consistent with an axonal form of GBS.

Conclusions: It is often overlooked that GBS can be triggered by non-infectious factors such as trauma and its short-term prognosis is poor. Therefore, it is important to analyze the clinical and electrophysiological features of GBS after trauma. Here we have shown that electrophysiological evaluations are helpful for diagnosing post-traumatic GBS. Early diagnosis may support appropriate treatment to help prevent morbidity and improve prognosis.

Keywords: Post-traumatic GBS, GBS, Trauma, Electrophysiology, Axonal damage

Background

Guillain-Barré syndrome (GBS) is a multifactorial and lethal inflammatory demyelinating polyradiculopathy and polyneuropathy, characterized by flaccid paralysis and acute demyelinating changes in the peripheral nervous system [1, 2]. Although a range of infectious factors, such as *Campylobacter jejuni* or cytomegalovirus, are associated with this syndrome, GBS has also been reported to be triggered by non-infectious factors such as trauma [3–6].

Trauma is defined as any physical damage to the body caused by violence or accident. The concept of post-traumatic GBS was recently introduced and defined as GBS preceded by no risk factors other than trauma [4]. To date, there appears to have been no systematic analysis of the clinical and electrophysiological features of GBS following trauma. Therefore, here we performed retrospective analyses to investigate those features.

Methods
Subjects
Six patients with GBS that occurred after trauma resulting from surgery or injury were diagnosed in our Department of Neurology between January 2014 and January 2016. All patients in this study met the clinical criteria for GBS (Table 1) [1, 7, 8] and had no risk factors other than trauma. Exclusion criteria for patient selection included a history of prodromal immunization or antecedent infections and prior use of neuromuscular blocking agents or intravenous gangliosides. We performed a retrospective analysis of these six patients' clinical records in our GBS database reviewing their basic characteristics, neurologic status, serum antibodies against gangliosides, reports of cerebrospinal fluid (CSF) analyses, and electrophysiological data. Because of the retrospective nature of the study, there

* Correspondence: hjw@tijmu.edu.cn
†Equal contributors
[1]Department of Neurology and Tianjin Neurological Institute, Tianjin Medical University General Hospital, Tianjin 300052, China
Full list of author information is available at the end of the article

Table 1 Diagnosis of GBS

Features required for diagnosis
Progressive weakness in both arms and legs (might start with weakness only in the legs)
Areflexia (or decreased tendon reflexes)
Features that strongly support diagnosis
Progression of symptoms over days to 4 weeks
Relative symmetry of symptoms
Mild sensory symptoms or signs
Cranial nerve involvement, especially bilateral weakness of facial muscles
Autonomic dysfunction Pain (often present)
High concentration of protein in CSF
Typical electrodiagnostic features
AMAN
None of the features of AIDP except one demyelinating feature allowed in one nerve if dCMAP <10% LLN
Sensory action potential amplitudes normal
AMSAN
None of the features of AIDP except one demyelinating feature allowed in one nerve if dCMAP < 10% LLN
Sensory action potential amplitudes < LLN

dCMAP = compound muscle action potential amplitude after distal stimulation; LLN = lower limit of normal

were no further nerve conduction studies (NCS) or CSF examinations other than those performed at diagnosis.

Evaluation of functional impairment

The clinical severity of the patients' GBS and their neurologic status were evaluated by calculating their Hughes Functional Grading Scale (HFGS) and Medical Research Council (MRC) sum scores [9, 10]. The nadir of disease was defined as the highest HFGS score or the lowest MRC sum score. The therapeutic efficacy was assessed by the improvement in HFGS and MRC sum scores between nadir and 2 weeks after treatment. All cases were followed up.

Electrophysiological study

Electrodiagnoses were made using Viking Quest (EMG & Evoked Potential Response Unit, Nicolet, NE, USA), the standard method at our institute. Electrophysiological examinations included NCS and F-wave assessments, which all patients underwent 10–14 days after the beginning of symptoms [11, 12]. Limb temperature was maintained above 32 °C with a heater, if needed. Using surface electrodes and a stimulator for NCS, we performed motor and orthodromic sensory NCS in eight nerves of the bilateral upper and lower extremities (median, ulnar, tibial, and peroneal nerve). In motor nerves, distal latency (DL), amplitude of compound muscle action potential (CMAP),

and motor nerve conduction velocity (MCV) were measured. Amplitude of sensory nerve action potential (SNAP) and sensory nerve conduction velocity (SCV) were also evaluated. The incidence of F-waves was measured after 20 supramaximal stimulations of motor nerves (median, ulnar, and tibial nerves). Abnormality was defined as values falling outside the mean ± 2.5 standard deviations of our laboratory control. Diagnosis of axonal or demyelinating neuropathy was based on the electrophysiological criteria proposed by Hadden and colleagues [1].

Anti-ganglioside antibody assay

Sera from all patients except patient #5 were examined for anti-ganglioside antibodies by enzyme-linked immunosorbent assay (ELISA) at the acute phase of GBS [11, 13, 14]. The ganglioside antigens used in the ELISA were 200 ng each of GM1, GD1b and GQ1b. Only IgG antibodies were considered pathological in this study.

Results

Characteristics of the patients

The clinical features of the patients are summarized in Table 1. The mean age was 42.5 years (range 29–57 years), and the group included four women and two men. No complications had occurred following the trauma and all patients were alert and oriented, with stable vital signs and without focal neurological deficits, before the first symptoms of GBS occurred. Patient #2 was admitted to another hospital with a closed head injury after falling. The results of cranial CT imaging and magnetic resonance imaging were normal. Patient #4 was admitted with a rib fracture following an accident. The results of chest CT revealed that the lung appeared normal. Patient #6 was admitted with a femoral fracture after a traffic accident.

The average interval between trauma and the onset of GBS symptoms ranged from 8 to 14 days (average of 11.3 days). However, during the following 7–10 days, the symptoms rapidly worsened. Approximately 2 weeks after GBS onset, all patients underwent lumbar puncture with albumino-cytological dissociation. The principal clinical presentation was progressive symmetrical weakness with varying degrees of muscle atrophy, especially in the lower limbs, and hyporeflexia or areflexia. Two of the six patients had numbness of limbs (#3, #6). Five of the six patients exhibited cranial nerve involvement, and most cranial nerves became affected, generally by palsy of the oculomotor and trochlear nerves (#1, #2, #3, #6), followed by abducens (#1, #2, #3) and vagus nerve deficits (#4). Moreover, the incidence of respiratory muscle paralysis was high, as particularly evident in patients #1 and #4, who required mechanical support for breathing (Table 2). HFGS and MRC scores were also used to evaluate clinical severity and were 4.17 ± 0.75 and 24.67 ± 8.27 at nadir, respectively (Fig. 1).

Table 2 Characteristics and clinical presentations of six patients with GBS

Characteristic	Case 1	Case 2	Case 3	Case 4	Case 5	Case 6
Age (y)/Sex	29/F	48/F	29/F	57/M	53/F	39/M
Antecedent events	Abortion	mild Traumatic brain injury	Cesarean section	Chest trauma	Endoscopic endonasal resection of Rathke cyst	Femoral fracture
Time between trauma and symptom onset (days)	14	10	8	10	12	12
Time between treatment initiation and symptom onset (days)	6	5	6	11	9	5
Time to nadir (days)	9	7	10	5	12	7
Time to discharge (days)	33	43	21	56	38	22
Symptoms at nadir						
Motor function	Weakness on both limbs (G2/5)	Weakness on both limbs (G2/5)	Weakness on both limbs (G3/5)	Weakness on both limbs (G1/5)	Weakness on both limbs (G2/5)	Weakness on both limbs (G3/5)
Deep tendon reflexes	Absent (G —)	Absent (G —)	Decreased (G1+)	Absent (G —)	Absent (G —)	Decreased (G1+)
Muscular atrophy at nadir	+	+	+	+	+	+
Cranial nerve function	III, IV, VI, VII	II, III, IV, VI	III, IV, VI	V, IX, X	–	III, IV
Respiratory muscle involvement	–	+	–	+	–	–
Objective sensory function	Normal	Normal	Abnormal	Normal	Normal	Abormal
Serum anti-ganglioside antibody	GQ1b	GM1	GM1,GD1b	–	Missing	GM1,GD1b
Protein (g/L)/AD in CSF	0.98/yes	0.64/yes	1.10/yes	0.92/yes	0.54/yes	0.72/yes
Treatment	IVIG	IVIG; MV	IVIG	IVIG; HC; MV	IVIG	IVIG

GBS Guillain-Barré syndrome, *AD* Albumino-cytological dissociation, *IVIG* Intravenous Immunoglobulin, *MV* Mechanical ventilation, *HC* high-dose corticosteroids

Electrophysiological features

Table 3 shows the patients' electrophysiological features. The mean interval between the time of NCS and the onset of symptoms was 8.5 (range 6–10) days. Abnormalities were clearly more frequent in motor than sensory nerves. In motor nerves, CMAP amplitude reduction was prominent, and unexcitable nerves were more common in lower than upper limbs. DL and NCV were normal or slightly abnormal in motor nerves. The reduction of CMAP amplitudes was more severe than the slowing of motor conduction. In sensory nerves, SNAP amplitude was relatively preserved in both the upper and lower

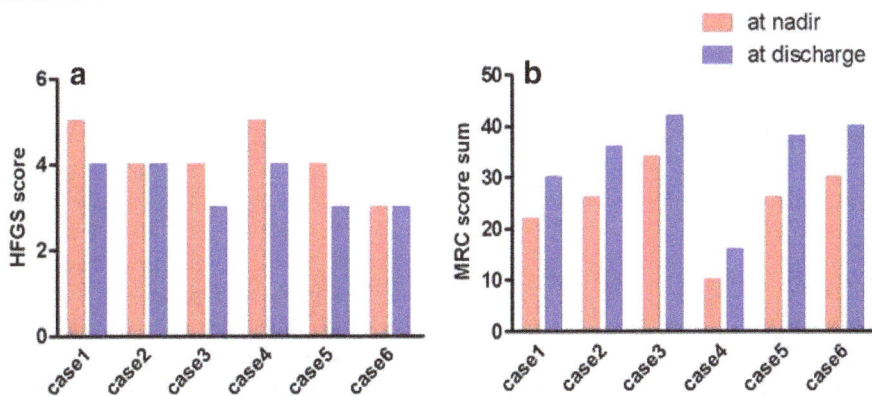

Fig. 1 Neurologic status of patients with post-traumatic GBS. **a** Scores of the Hughes Functional Grading Scale (HFGS) were significantly increased in patients compared to normal values, both at nadir and at discharge. This suggests more severe clinical courses and poorer short-term outcomes. **b** The Medical Research Council sum scores (MRC) were significantly decreased in these patients both at nadir and at discharge

Table 3 Electrophysiological findings of enrolled patients with post-traumatic GBS

		Case 1		Case 2		Case 3		Case 4		Case 5		Case 6	
		L	R	L	R	L	R	L	R	L	R	L	R
CMAP(mV)	Median nerve	2.0	3.5	0.4	2.6	2.2	3.2	2.4	1.2	–	–	2.5	3.4
	Ulnar nerve	1.1	1.8	1.9	3.2	2.0	2.6	1.9	1.2	–	–	1.6	2.8
	Tibial nerve	1.5	2.1	0.8	0.6	1.5	3.2	1.0	1.0	–	–	–	–
	Peroneal nerve	1.2	1.1	1.2	1.0	2.1	2.0	0.6	0.4	–	–	–	–
MCV(m/s)	Median nerve	49	45	65	60	62	58	55	57	–	–	58	50
	Ulnar nerve	50	46	60	56	61	64	52	56	–	–	47	49
	Tibial nerve	44	43	44	43	42	45	50	47	–	–	–	–
	Peroneal nerve	44	44	40	42	41	41	46	45	–	–	–	–
DL(ms)	Median nerve	3.7	3.8	3.8	3.5	3.9	3.3	3.6	3.8	–	–	2.7	3.2
	Ulnar nerve	3.2	3.1	3.8	3.6	2.8	2.9	3.0	2.9	–	–	3.2	2.9
	Tibial nerve	6.2	5.3	5.1	5.1	4.3	4.0	4.3	4.5	–	–	–	–
	Peroneal nerve	4.6	4.4	4.9	5.0	4.1	4.3	4.6	4.3	–	–	–	–
SNAP(uV)	Median nerve	6.3	8.3	15.3	13.5	15.5	13.6	12.6	11.7	11.0	12.5	8.7	10.3
	Ulnar nerve	4.2	6.3	22.6	20.5	14.3	11.5	10.2	11.0	9.2	8.5	7.3	8.2
	Tibial nerve	8.5	8.2	22.1	19.3	12.4	10.6	15.3	11.5	6.3	7.4	8.5	8.7
	Peroneal nerve	12.4	15.3	23.6	20.2	15.8	17.3	21.6	24.3	19.6	15.8	14.7	17.2
SCV(m/s)	Median nerve	59	58	63	60	57	53	51	50	59	56	52	56
	Ulnar nerve	57	55	64	59	62	58	55	51	52	54	55	59
	Tibial nerve	59	59	50	53	56	53	50	49	55	53	50	56
	Peroneal nerve	52	57	53	55	57	52	50	51	54	51	52	57
F-wave(%)	Median nerve	25.0	35.0	0.0	0.0	35.0	30.0	35.0	15.0	–	–	20.0	15.0
	Ulnar nerve	0.0	20.0	0.0	0.0	60.0	45.0	15.0	0.0	–	–	0.0	0.0
	Tibial nerve	0.0	0.0	0.0	0.0	20.0	30.0	30.0	0.0	–	–	–	–

GBS Guillain-Barré syndrome, L left, R right, CMAP compound muscle action potential, MCV motor nerve conduction velocity, DL distal latency, SNAP sensory nerve action potential, SCV sensory nerve conduction velocity, –– disappearance

limbs, and remained normal in some patients (#2, #3, #4). In contrast, all subjects had F-wave abnormalities, the most common of which was reduced F-wave persistence. That is, 62% of examined nerves manifested deleterious F-wave changes, especially in the ulnar nerve.

Anti-ganglioside antibodies

Positivity for anti-ganglioside antibodies was detected in sera from five of the six patients (patient #5 refused the examination). IgG antibodies were also present in four patients: the target antigens were GM1 in patients #2, #3 and #6, GD1b in patients #3 and #6, and GQ1b in patient #1.

Treatment and outcomes

Once GBS was confirmed, treatment with intravenous human immunoglobulin (and a large dose of corticosteroids in patient #4) was performed at a dose of 0.4 g/kg for 5 days. Although this treatment provided clinical improvement, recovery was incomplete, and the outcomes were poor. All patients suffered muscular atrophy, which was apparent to different extents at nadir. High HFGS and low MRC scores were noted both at nadir and at discharge, as shown in Fig. 1.

Discussion

Post-trauma inflammatory neuropathy, including focal neuropathies, multifocal neuropathy, and diffuse polyneuropathy, was recently defined as neurologic deterioration occurring during the early post-traumatic period [15]. GBS is one such neuropathy that is a rare but severe neurologic complication after trauma. Duncan and colleagues described in 1987 the first identified case of post-traumatic GBS [16]. During the past few decades, several reports have described patients presenting with GBS after multiple types of trauma (Table 2) [15, 17–22]. The requirement for establishing a temporal relationship between a traumatic event and subsequent neuropathy is that the neuropathic symptoms must start within 30 days of the trauma. In the six GBS patients described here, no risk factors other than trauma were identified, and the average interval between trauma and the onset of GBS symptoms ranged from 8 to

14 days (average of 11.3 days). Interestingly, most patients in our study exhibited motor dysfunction with muscular atrophy, significant cranial nerve deficits, and worsening paresis resulting in respiratory failure. Additionally, the weakness documented in all four limbs was especially acute and severely disabling. Finally, high HFGS and low MRC scores, both at nadir and at discharge, indicated marked increases in disease severity and poor short-term prognoses.

Electrophysiological investigations can provide an auxiliary diagnosis of GBS and are particularly useful for classifying GBS into the subgroups of acute inflammatory demyelinating polyneuropathy (AIDP), acute motor axonal neuropathy (AMAN), or acute motor sensory axonal neuropathy (AMSAN). In this study, electrophysiological abnormalities mainly affected motor nerve fibers but both terminal and proximal segments of the peripheral nervous system were also involved. Specifically, based on the electrophysiological criteria [8], five of the six patients were diagnosed with AMAN and one with AMSAN. All patients exhibited an axonal rather than demyelinating form of neuropathy, which predicted the severe clinical courses and poor outcomes that followed. Subsequently, we reviewed the electrophysiological features of post-traumatic GBS in the literature and found that after trauma, the axonal subtype of GBS is more common than the demyelinating subtype (Table 4). Yang et al. retrospectively analyzed 36 adult patients with GBS and found that the axonal subtype of GBS in post-trauma patients was proportionally higher than that in non-trauma patients, as seen in the present study [23]. The limited number of case reports of post-traumatic GBS in the literature does not support the conclusion that a causal relationship exists between the clinical phenotype and the history of trauma. It is not easy to affirm whether the co-existence of these two factors is anything more than mere coincidence.

About half of the patients with GBS are positive for serum antibodies to various gangliosides, including GM1, GM1b, GM2, GD1a, GalNAc-GD1a, GD1b, GD2, GD3, GT1a, and GQ1b [24–26]. Previous studies suggest that most of these antibodies are specific for defined subgroups of GBS. For example, GM1, GD1a, GD1b, and GalNAc-GD1a antibodies are associated with axonal variants of GBS, whereas GD3, GT1a, and GQ1b antibodies are related to ophthalmoplegia and Miller-Fisher syndrome [27]. In this study, IgG anti-ganglioside antibodies were detected in four of the five patients tested. Patients #3 and #6, who experienced more serious muscle weakness and hypoesthesia were seropositive for GM1 and GD1b antibodies. This combination of serum-positive anti-ganglioside antibodies and electrophysiological abnormalities further illustrates that GBS with predominant axonal damage is most common after trauma.

The cases reported here highlight the importance of differentiating axonal GBS from critical illness polyneuropathy, which is a common cause of axonal polyneuropathy in trauma patients [19]. However, this can be difficult as axonal GBS can have striking similarities to critical illness polyneuropathy, in terms of clinical

Table 4 Descriptions of post-traumatic GBS in the academic literature

Author/Year	Number of case	Sex/ number	Median age, years(range)	Antecedent events	Time from trauma to symptom onset (days)	EMG	Nerve biopsy
Rattananan et al. (2014) [1]	5	F/3	61 (35–68)	Surgery	within 30 days	Neuropathy with active denervation;	Perivascular inflammatory collections;increased axonal degeneration.
Staff et al. (2010) [2]	21	F/11	65 (24–83)	Surgery	within 30 days	Neuropathy with active denervation;	Increased epineurial perivascular inflammation;17 patients had increased axonal degeneration.
Huang et al. (2015) [3]	4	M/4	57 (50–69)	Spine Surgery:	within 1 week	Neuropathy and 2 cases with active denervation	not done
Scozzafava et al. (2008) [4]	1	M/1	28 (28)	Spinal cord injury	within 1 day	Severe axonal polyneuropathy	not done
Tan et al. (2010) [5]	1	M/1	44 (44)	Head injury	1 week	Neuropathy with active denervation;	Presence of lymphocytes and severe axonal degeneration.
Al-Hashel et al. (2013) [6]	2	F/1	39 (31–47)	Traumatic bone injury	within 1 week	1 with features of mixed axonal and demyelinating neuropathy	not done
Rivas et al. (2008) [7]	1	M/1	55 (55)	Head injury	1 week	An inexcitability of all nerves with active denervation;	A severe loss of myelinated axons without significant demyelination.

GBS Guillain-Barré syndrome, F female, M male, EMG electromyography

presentation and electrodiagnostic data. Cranial nerve involvement, such as that associated with bifacial weakness, and dysautonomia are uncommon in critical illness polyneuropathy. In these patients the degree of sensory symptoms and sensory nerve involvement tends to be mild. Albumino-cytological dissociation in CSF and the presence of certain serum anti-ganglioside antibodies also support a diagnosis of GBS. Finally, critical illness polyneuropathy does not generally respond to IVIG and/ or plasma exchange, whereas GBS does. Despite these features, in the setting of critical illness or trauma, it remains a diagnostic challenge to distinguish axonal GBS from critical illness polyneuropathy.

Given the heterogeneity of the patients with post-traumatic GBS, it is postulated that the underlying mechanisms are based on a trauma-related disruption of the cellular and humoral immune system. Trauma often leads to transient immunosuppression and promotes clinical or subclinical exogenous infection [6, 28]. Immunosuppression could induce an alteration of immune tolerance and exogenous infection could elicit cross-reactive antibodies [3]. Together they could promote an autoimmune attack on peripheral nerves, resulting in the occurrence of axonal-type GBS. Conduction failure in the acute phase of axonal GBS could be attributed to lowered safety factors due to a dysfunction of the ion channels or due to microstructural changes at the nodes of Ranvier or paranodal regions caused by anti-ganglioside antibodies. The specific tissue distribution of these gangliosides in peripheral nerves could result in their characteristic clinical features. Therefore, the proliferation of serum antibodies against gangliosides shown here may represent an indirect trigger of GBS via a response to opportunistic infection rather the hypothesized direct incitement by trauma.

Post-traumatic GBS is a rapidly progressive and severe neurologic complication that occurs after trauma [15, 18, 19]. Thus, when there is unexplainable progressive muscle weakness after trauma, GBS should be taken into consideration and corresponding measures should be taken to relieve the condition. Both general medical care and immunological treatment are essential. All patients with sufficient suspicion of post-traumatic GBS should be monitored for possible respiratory failure and cardiac arrhythmia, and timely transfer to intensive care unit when needed. Reports of GBS in trauma patients is limited to case reports and no systematic research has been found so far discussing its immunological treatment. Therefore, an empiric course of intravenous immunoglobulin or plasma exchange might be valuable as it has been shown to improve prognosis [5, 18, 19]. Moreover, we found that some cases showed some clinical improvement, while others did not, when treated with intravenous methylprednisolone [15, 17]. Therefore, further research regarding the immunological treatment of post-traumatic GBS are required.

The limitations of our study include the relatively small sample size and the failure to identify pathogens. However, this first-ever reported case series of ganglioside-associated post-traumatic GBS may alert us to consider this diagnosis in patients with paralysis after trauma.

Conclusions

The clinical presentations and laboratory findings described here played an important part in the diagnosis of post-traumatic GBS as likely immune-response-related nerve damage. The characteristic outcomes of the six patients studied were extremely severe disease, poor prognosis, and delayed recoveries. Such patients often have axonal damage. Therefore, electrophysiological investigations are important for the diagnosis and identification of different subtypes of GBS. This may facilitate early diagnosis and treatment to help prevent morbidity and improve prognosis.

Abbreviations

AIDP: Acute inflammatory demyelinating polyneuropathy; AMAN: Acute motor axonal neuropathy; AMSAN: Acute motor sensory axonal neuropathy; CMAP: Compound muscle action potential; CSF: Cerebrospinal fluid; DL: Distal latency; ELISA: Enzyme-linked immunosorbent assay; GBS: Guillain-Barré syndrome; HFGS: Hughes Functional Grading Scale; MCV: Motor nerve conduction velocity; MRC: Medical Research Council; NCS: Nerve conduction study; SCV: Sensory nerve conduction velocity; SNAP: Sensory nerve action potential

Acknowledgments

We wish to thank all participants in this study.

Funding

This work was funded by the National Natural Science Foundation of China (81,571,600, 81,322,018, 81,273,287 and 81,100,887 to J.W.H) and the Youth Top-notch Talent Support Program. The funders had no role in study design, data collection and analysis, or preparation of the manuscript.

Authors' contributions

JH and XL conceived and designed the project; XL, JtX, YD, CL, JX, HZ and BX recruited the subjects; JH, XL and JtX analyzed the data; JH, XL and YH wrote the manuscript. All authors reviewed and approved the final manuscript.

Competing interests

None of the authors has potential conflicts of interest to be disclosed.

Author details

[1]Department of Neurology and Tianjin Neurological Institute, Tianjin Medical University General Hospital, Tianjin 300052, China. [2]Department of Neurology, Tianjin Haihe Hospital, Tianjin 300060, China.

References

1. Hadden RD, Cornblath DR, Hughes RA, Zielasek J, Hartung HP, Toyka KV, Swan AV. Electrophysiological classification of Guillain-Barre syndrome: clinical associations and outcome. Plasma Exchange/Sandoglobulin Guillain-Barre Syndrome Trial Group. Ann Neurol. 1998;44(5):780–8.
2. Wakerley BR, Yuki N. Infectious and noninfectious triggers in Guillain-Barre syndrome. Expert Rev Clin Immunol. 2013;9(7):627–39.
3. Gensicke H, Datta AN, Dill P, Schindler C, Fischer D. Increased incidence of Guillain-Barre syndrome after surgery. Eur J Neurol. 2012;19(9):1239–44.
4. Carr KR, Shah M, Garvin R, Shakir A, Jackson C. Post-Traumatic brain injury (TBI) presenting with Guillain-Barre syndrome and elevated anti-ganglioside antibodies: a case report and review of the literature. Int J Neurosci. 2015;125(7):486–92.
5. Landais AF. Rare neurologic complication of bariatric surgery: acute motor axonal neuropathy (AMAN), a severe motor axonal form of the Guillain Barre syndrome. Surg Obes Relat Dis. 2014;10(6):e85–7.
6. Sipila JO, Soilu-Hanninen M. The incidence and triggers of adult-onset Guillain-Barre syndrome in southwestern Finland 2004–2013. Eur J Neurol. 2015;22(2):292–8.
7. Sudulagunta SR, Sodalagunta MB, Sepehrar M, Khorram H, Bangalore Raja SK, Kothandapani S, Noroozpour Z, Aheta Sham M, Prasad N, Sunny SP, et al. Guillain-Barre syndrome: clinical profile and management. Ger Med Sci. 2015;13:Doc16.
8. Hughes RA, Cornblath DR. Guillain-Barre syndrome. Lancet. 2005; 366(9497):1653–66.
9. Hughes RA, Newsom-Davis JM, Perkin GD, Pierce JM. Controlled trial prednisolone in acute polyneuropathy. Lancet. 1978;2(8093):750–3.
10. Kleyweg RP, van der Meche FG, Schmitz PI. Interobserver agreement in the assessment of muscle strength and functional abilities in Guillain-Barre syndrome. Muscle Nerve. 1991;14(11):1103–9.
11. Kawakami S, Sonoo M, Kadoya A, Chiba A, Shimizu T. A-waves in Guillain-Barre syndrome: correlation with electrophysiological subtypes and antiganglioside antibodies. Clin Neurophysiol. 2012;123(6):1234–41.
12. Yadegari S, Nafissi S, Kazemi N. Comparison of electrophysiological findings in axonal and demyelinating Guillain-Barre syndrome. Iran J Neurol. 2014;13(3):138–43.
13. Kaida K, Kusunoki S, Kamakura K, Motoyoshi K, Kanazawa I. Guillain-Barre syndrome with antibody to a ganglioside, N-acetylgalactosaminyl GD1a. Brain. 2000;123(Pt 1):116–24.
14. Uchibori A, Chiba A. Autoantibodies in Guillain-Barre Syndrome. Brain Nerve. 2015;67(11):1347–57.
15. Staff NP, Engelstad J, Klein CJ, Amrami KK, Spinner RJ, Dyck PJ, Warner MA, Warner ME. Post-surgical inflammatory neuropathy. Brain. 2010;133(10):2866–80.
16. Duncan R, Kennedy PG. Guillain-Barre syndrome following acute head trauma. Postgrad Med J. 1987;63(740):479–80.
17. Rattananan W, Thaisetthawatkul P, Dyck PJ. Postsurgical inflammatory neuropathy: a report of five cases. J Neurol Sci. 2014;337(1–2):137–40.
18. Huang SL, Qi HG, Liu JJ, Huang YJ, Xiang L. A Rare Complication of Spine Surgery: Guillain-Barre Syndrome. World Neurosurg. 2015;84(3):697–701.
19. Scozzafava J, Jickling G, Jhamandas JH, Jacka MJ. Guillain-Barre syndrome following thoracic spinal cord trauma. Can J Anaesth. 2008;55(7):441–6.
20. Tan IL, Ng T, Vucic S. Severe Guillain-Barre syndrome following head trauma. J Clin Neurosci. 2010;17(11):1452–4.
21. Al-Hashel JY, John JK, Vembu P. Unusual presentation of Guillain-Barre syndrome following traumatic bone injuries: report of two cases. Med Princ Pract. 2013;22:597–9.
22. Rivas S, Douds GL, Ostdahl RH, Harbaugh KS. Fulminant Guillain-Barre syndrome after closed head injury: a potentially reversible cause of an ominous examination. Case report. J Neurosurg. 2008;108(3):595–600.
23. Yang B, Lian Y, Liu Y, Wu BY, Duan RS. A retrospective analysis of possible triggers of Guillain-Barre syndrome. J Neuroimmunol. 2016;293:17–21.
24. Willison HJ, Jacobs BC, van Doorn PA. Guillain-Barre syndrome. Lancet. 2016; 388(10045):717–27.
25. van Doorn PA, Ruts L, Jacobs BC. Clinical features, pathogenesis, and treatment of Guillain-Barre syndrome. Lancet Neurol. 2008;7(10):939–50.
26. van den Berg B, Walgaard C, Drenthen J, Fokke C, Jacobs BC, van Doorn PA. Guillain-Barre syndrome: pathogenesis, diagnosis, treatment and prognosis. Nat Rev Neurol. 2014;10(8):469–82.
27. Yuki N, Hartung HP. Guillain-Barre syndrome. N Engl J Med. 2012; 366(24):2294–304.
28. Samieirad S, Khajehahmadi S, Tohidi E, Barzegar M. Unusual Presentation of Guillain-Barre Syndrome After Mandibular Fracture Treatment: A Review of the Literature and a New Case. J Oral Maxillofac Surg. 2016;74(1):129e121–6.

10

Mononeuritis multiplex as the first presentation of refractory sarcoidosis responsive to etanercept

Ins Brs Marques *, Gavin Giovannoni and Monica Marta

Abstract

Background: Several disorders may present with mononeuritis multiplex and the etiological diagnosis can be challenging.

Case presentation: We report a 42 year-old female who presented with severe lower limb neuropathic pain, asymmetric weakness and sensory impairment and was diagnosed with mononeuritis multiplex. Biopsy showed a granulomatous vasculitic process with eosinophils, scarce granulomata and axonal neuropathy and granulomatosis with poliangiitis was assumed. Steroids, cyclophosphamide, alemtuzumab, azathioprine, mycophenolate mofetil and rituximab were used, all with transient and insufficient response. Skin biopsy performed in a further exacerbation allowed sarcoidosis diagnosis. Infliximab and, later, adalimumab induced good clinical and laboratorial response, but neutralizing antibodies developed to both drugs, so etanercept was tried with good clinical response.

Conclusions: To the best of our knowledge, this is the first report of sarcoidosis successfully treated with etanercept. This drug may be considered in refractory sarcoidosis after other TNF-α inhibitors failure, having the advantage of not being associated with neutralizing antibodies development.

Background

Mononeuritis multiplex (MM) can be a manifestation of several disorders including infectious, inflammatory, neoplastic, toxic, metabolic and hereditary conditions, and the etiological diagnosis may be challenging. Rarely, it can be a presentation of sarcoidosis, an inflammatory multisystem granulomatous disease that can involve any part of the nervous system.

Peripheral neuropathy is an uncommon manifestation of sarcoidosis patients and presents more frequently with symmetric axonal sensorimotor polyneuropathy, however other manifestations are described, including MM, multifocal motor neuropathy, Guillain-Barr syndrome, polyradiculopathy, lumbosacral plexopathy, small fibre neuropathy and multiple painful sensory mononeuropathies [1-7]. Reports of initial presentation with MM are rare [3,8,9].

Sarcoid neuropathy treatment can also be challenging and, in patients refractory to steroids and imunossupressants, tumor necrosis factor alpha (TNF-α) inhibitors are invaluable [10,11]. According to literature, infliximab and adalimumab, which bind both soluble and membrane bound TNF-α, seem to be more effective in sarcoidosis than etanercept, which binds only to soluble TNF-α with incomplete inhibition of TNF-α bioactivity [12,13].

We report a 42-year old female presenting with MM who was eventually diagnosed with sarcoidosis. Tumor necrosis factor alpha (TNF-α) inhibitors were used after steroid and immunosuppressants failure. As neutralizing antibodies (NAbs) against anti-TNF-α antibodies developed, etanercept was tried with good clinical response.

This case illustrates how sarcoidosis diagnosis and treatment can represent a challenge and is, to the best of our knowledge, the first report of sarcoidosis successfully treated with etanercept.

Case presentation

A 42 year-old Afro-Caribbean female presented with severe pain in the lower limbs associated with distal weakness, with progressive worsening during the previous week.

Her past medical history was remarkable for long-standing pigmented skin nodules in limbs and torso, bilateral breast implants ten years prior and giving birth to her first child at 26 weeks three months before.

Neurological examination revealed tetraparesis (distal upper limbs: grade 4+/5; proximal lower limbs: right =

* Correspondence: i.marques@qmul.ac.uk
Queen Mary University London, Blizard Institute, 4 Newark Street, London E1 1AT, UK

grade 4/5, left = 3/5; distal lower limbs: right = grade 3/5, left = 2/5), absent ankle reflexes, indifferent plantar reflexes, reduced positional sense in left ankle and up to right knee and reduced vibration and superficial pain sense up to both knees. Physical examination identified multiple hyperpigmented small nodules over the limbs and trunk.

Investigations

Blood workup revealed normocytic anemia, thrombocytosis and increased erythrocyte sedimentation rate (ESR) (110 mm/h), C-reactive protein (CRP) (33 mg/L) and angiotensin converting enzyme (ACE) (74 units/L). Biochemistry including ionogram, calcium, renal and liver function was unremarkable. Syphilis, hepatitis A, B and C and Human Immunodeficiency Virus serologies were negative. Autoimmune studies showed positive antinuclear antibodies (titre > 1/640, speckled pattern) and antineutrophil cytoplasmic antibodies (ANCA) with an atypical cytoplasmic-ANCA (c-ANCA) pattern, however without myeloperoxidaseA (MPO) or proteinase 3 (PR3) specificity. Antinuclear antibodies, antibodies against double stranded DNA, antibodies against extractable nuclear antigens, anti-cardiolipin antibodies and lupus anticoagulant test were negative.

Cerebrospinal fluid showed hyperproteinorraquia (500 mg/L), 5 leukocytes, normal glucose, increased ACE (1.47 units/ml). Direct microscopy, acid-fast bacilli smear, cultures, including mycobacterial culture, and Herpesvirus family and Adenovirus DNA were negative.

Brain and spinal cord magnetic resonance imaging revealed slight pachymeningeal thickening and enhancement over the vertex. Chest, abdomen and pelvis computerized tomography recognized left breast implant intracapsular rupture and mildly enlarged bilateral axillary lymph nodes only.

Nerve conduction studies identified patchy asymmetrical involvement of sensory nerves in upper and lower limbs with axonal involvement (both sural and superficial peroneal nerves and left ulnar nerve) and minor denervation in the muscles supplied by the affected nerves, consistent with MM.

Dermatology team diagnosed the skin lesions as nodular prurigo.

Treatment, outcome and follow up

As pain and weakness significantly worsened during the following two weeks and a provisional muscle and nerve biopsy description suggested an inflammatory process, a course of intravenous (iv) cyclophosphamide (15 mg/kg) and oral prednisolone (1 mg/kg/d) were started with marked strength improvement in the following days. Oral cyclophosphamide (150 mg/day) was started two weeks later.

Final biopsy findings described a granulomatous vasculitic process associated with axonal neuropathy. Muscle biopsy showed perivascular inflammation without fibrinoid necrosis and a cluster of cells resembling a loose non-necrotic granuloma. Nerve biopsy revealed florid axonal neuropathy with large and small myelinated fibers active degeneration, dense inflammatory infiltrates including several scattered eosinophils and aggregates of epithelioid macrophages forming loose granulomata in perineurium and endoneurium, without vessel fibrinoid necrosis. Skin biopsy was unremarkable.

Granulomatosis with polyangiitis (GPA) was presumed as histology identified eosinophils and poorly formed granulomata. She was discharged on cyclophosphamide, analgesia and prednisolone taper until 20 mg/day. Clinically she was almost pain free, but suffered severe fatigue.

Within three months, she stopped medication against medical recommendation and worsened in the following eight weeks, with severe neuropathic pain and inability to walk autonomously. Neurological examination revealed grade 3/5 tetraparesis, lower limbs arreflexia and sensory gait ataxia. Inflammatory markers were increased (ESR = 86 mm/h; CRP = 54 mg/L). Cyclophosphamide (150 mg/day) and prednisolone (40 mg/day) were restarted with clinical and laboratorial improvement within one month. Nevertheless, recurrence of severe symptoms occurred two months later and alemtuzumab (20 mg/day, iv, 5 days) was used with only mild improvement within three weeks.

By this time, 150 mg/day azatioprine (AZA) was associated with prednisolone taper, but worsening occurred on every taper attempt. Whole body PET performed during an exacerbation with severe systemic symptoms excluded other areas of inflammatory activity and neoplasms.

After four months of AZA, slow clinical recovery was reported. Stability was achieved for further six months on prednisolone (17,5 mg/20 mg on alternate days) and AZA (175 mg/day). However, severe pain and weakness worsening followed and AZA was switched to mycophenolate mofetil (MMF) (750 mg bd). At that point, breast implants were removed as bilateral breast tumefaction and a large left axillary adenopathy were noticed. Biopsy showed granulomatous lymphadenitis and patchy stromal fibrosis of breast tissue with periaqueductal and perilobular inflammation including occasional poorly formed nonnecrotizing granulomas, without signs of malignancy and with negative acid-fast bacilli and fungi stains.

After four months of stability, neurological symptoms recurrence associated with bilateral uveitis were treated with iv methylprednisolone (1 g, 3 days). Oral prednisolone (40/60 mg on alternate days) and MMF (1 g, bd) were increased. Four rituximab infusions (375 mg/m^2/ week) were performed. Despite improvement of systemic symptoms and inflammatory markers, marked disability persisted due to pain and weakness.

Skin biopsy obtained three months later, during a period of skin lesions exacerbation, showed numerous granulomata in the dermis with perivascular lymphocytic infiltrates, without vasculitic features. This time the clinical and histopathological features suggested sarcoidosis, so our treatment strategy changed.

Infliximab (3 mg/kg, iv, at 0/2/6 weeks and every 6 weeks thereafter) was started in combination with MMF and prednisolone with excellent prompt clinical and laboratorial response. Coinciding with clinical symptoms recurrence, five months later, NAbs againts infliximab were detected. Switch to adalimumab (40 mg, sc, every second week) maintained improvement, however, despite strength improvement, sensory ataxia and neuropathic pain still hindered autonomous walking. Eight months later, another period of treatment efficacy loss followed, associated with NAbs against adalimumab, reducing the choice of TNF-α inhibitors described as beneficial in sarcoidosis. We eventually chose etanercept (50 mg, sc, once a week) still in combination with MMF (1.5 g/day) and prednisolone (40 mg/60 mg on alternate days) which controlled most clinical symptoms with complete motor and cognitive functional recovery. She remains clinically stable after eighteen months on etanercept, presenting full power with fatigability, fluctuant facial asymmetry, marked sensory gait ataxia, areas of sensory deficits with numbness and dysesthesia, absent reflexes in the lower limbs and decreased reflexes in the upper limbs. Despite clinical stability, inflammatory markers remain increased (ESR = 83 mm/h; CRP = 14 mg/L) and skin lesions persist.

Figure 1 represents clinical symptoms and inflammatory markers evolution during the disease course and the treatments performed during this period.

Discussion

Sarcoid neuropathy is a rare manifestation of sarcoidosis, estimated to occur in 15% of cases [14]. Theories to explain sarcoid neuropathy include ischemic axonal degeneration and demyelination resulting from local pressure provoked by epineural and perineural granulomas and granulomatous vasculitis; axonal and myelin damage by proteolytic enzymes secreted by epithelioid cells; and ischemic nerve lesions resultant vessel fibrinoid necrosis [3]. Diagnosis requires histological demonstration of non-caseating granulomas, preferably in biopsy tissue obtained from other organs involved, reserving nerve biopsy for

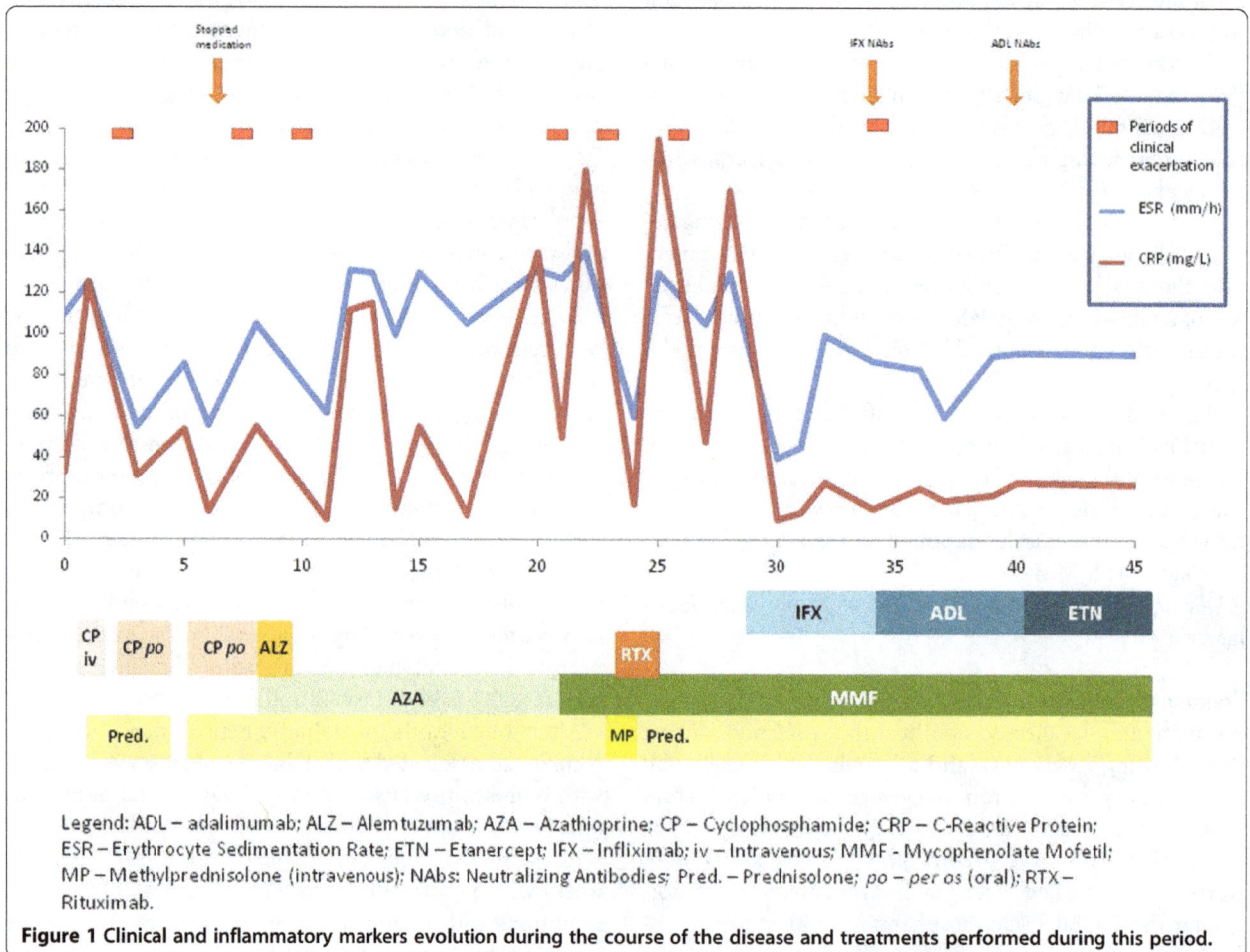

Legend: ADL – adalimumab; ALZ – Alemtuzumab; AZA – Azathioprine; CP – Cyclophosphamide; CRP – C-Reactive Protein; ESR – Erythrocyte Sedimentation Rate; ETN – Etanercept; IFX – Infliximab; iv – Intravenous; MMF - Mycophenolate Mofetil; MP – Methylprednisolone (intravenous); NAbs: Neutralizing Antibodies; Pred. – Prednisolone; po – per os (oral); RTX – Rituximab.

Figure 1 Clinical and inflammatory markers evolution during the course of the disease and treatments performed during this period.

patients without other accessible organs affected. As no histological features differentiate sarcoid granulomas, other granulomatous diseases must be excluded, most importantly acid-fast bacilli and fungi infections. In the case of our patient, MM associated with ANCA antibodies and granulomatous vasculitic process suggested a systemic vasculitis, possibly GPA or Churg-Strauss syndrome (CSS). Despite disparate manifestations, these conditions can present with MM before evident systemic features emerge [15,16]. Histologically, GPA usually shows vasculitis and/or necrotizing granulomas and CSS characteristically reveals eosinophilic infiltrates, vasculitis and granulomas with eosinophilic necrosis [17]. GPA usually associates with c-ANCA PR3 specific and CSS with p-ANCA MPO specific [17]. Atypical ANCA occur in various disorders, including systemic immune-mediated diseases and infections [17]. In our patient, atypical ANCA without PR3/MPO specificity and absence of necrotizing granulomas were uncharacteristic for systemic granulomatous vasculitis.

Infectious granulomatous diseases that may present with MM were also considered in the differential diagnosis. Tuberculoid Leprosy (TL), caused by *Mycobacterium leprae*, usually involves the skin and the peripheral nerves in an asymmetrical pattern and may present as MM [18-20], however the skin lesions are usually anesthetic and present as hypopigmented macules or erythematous plaques with well-defined elevated borders and an atrophic center, and peripheral nerves are usually tender and thickened, making this diagnosis less likely in our patient. TB can also very rarely present with peripheral neuropathy, but usually results from nerve or root compression by regional tubercular lymphadenitis, vertebral collapse or abscess, without direct invasion of the peripheral nerves by the necrotizing granulomas [21-23]. The nerve biopsy of our patient showed dense inflammatory infiltrate in all nerve compartments with granulomata in the perineurium and endoneurium, findings not expected in TB. The negative stains for *acid-fast bacilli* and mycobacterial cultures were also not suggestive of these granulomatous infections.

The recently described Autoimmune/Inflammatory Syndrome Induced by Adjuvants (ASIA) [24], includes immune mediated diseases triggered by an adjuvant stimulus. It results from exposure to external stimuli, including infectious agents, vaccines, silicone, aluminium salts and others, that are thought to stimulate the immune system and trigger an immune response in persons with a favourable genetic background. The most frequently reported symptoms are myalgia, arthralgia, fatigue, sleep disturbances, fever, cognitive impairment and other neurological manifestations, especially associated with demyelination, and this symptoms are thought to improve with removal of the inciting agent [24,25]. As our patient had breast implants, ASIA was considered in the

differential diagnosis, however the clinical manifestations were not the most typical of this syndrome and the disease exacerbations continued after surgical removal of the breast implants.

Sarcoid neuropathy early treatment with oral prednisolone (1 mg/kg/day) or iv methylprednisolone (0.5-1 g/day) is recommended and steroid-sparing medications, such as AZA or MMF, must be considered. In refractory patients, TNF-α inhibitors, mostly infliximab are proposed [26], as TNF-α is thought to be involved in antigen-driven, cell-mediated responses and in granuloma formation. Monoclonal antibodies, infliximab and adalimumab, bind both soluble and membrane bound TNF-α, whereas etanercept binds only soluble TNF-α [13]. Reports of TNF-α inhibitors induced sarcoidosis [27], paradoxically describe etanercept as being more commonly associated with granuloma development [28], possibly because of incomplete TNF-α blockage. NAbs usually reduce anti-TNF-α antibodies efficacy [29], and immunossupressants are suggested to reduce antibody development risk, however our patient developed NAbs despite concomitant MMF. Antibodies to etanercept are usually non-neutralizing and do not affect efficacy or safety [30].

In the case of our patient, steroids, cyclophosphamide, alemtuzumab, azathioprine, mycophenolate mofetil and rituximab were used, all with transient and insufficient response. Alemtuzumab was used for presumed granulomatosis with polyangiitis, before sarcoidosis diagnosis, as it has shown benefit in ANCA-associated refractory vasculitis [31] and clinical trials are ongoing to show evidence. Despite good clinical and laboratorial response was achieved with infliximab and, later, adalimumab, neutralizing antibodies developed to both drugs, so etanercept was tried with good clinical response.

To the best of our knowledge, this is the first report of sarcoidosis responding to etanercept. In our patient, despite significant clinical improvement, inflammatory markers, especially ESR, remain increased. The lack of alternatives with proven efficacy and the reasonable clinical stability achieved support our decision to maintain this treatment.

Conclusions

Mononeuritis multiplex is a rare presentation of sarcoidosis with rare cases described in the literature. The differential diagnosis is extensive and biopsy of the nerve, or other affected organ, is crucial for diagnosis. In refractory patients, TNF-α inhibitors are invaluable, with many successful cases of sarcoidosis treatment with infliximab and adalimumab reported in the literature. This article presents the first report of sarcoidosis treated with etanercept, adding this drug as an option for refractory patients who failed other TNF-α inhibitors, having the advantage of not being associated with development of neutralizing antibodies.

Learning points/take home messages

- Mononeuritis multiplex may be a presentation of sarcoidosis,
- Sarcoidosis diagnosis requires histological demonstration of non-caseating granulomas, preferably in biopsy tissue obtained from organs involved outside of the nervous system,
- TNF-α inhibitors, mostly infliximab and adalimumab, are reported as efficacious in refractory cases,
- Etanercept may be an option in patients who failed other TNF-α inhibitors, having the advantage of not being associated with development of neutralizing antibodies.

Patient consent

Written informed consent was obtained from the patient for publication of this Case report and any accompanying images. A copy of the written consent is available for review by the Editor of this journal.

Competing interests

The authors declare that they have no competing interests.

Authors contributions

IM, GG and MM contributed to data acquisition. IM drafted the manuscript. MM participated in its design and coordination and helped to draft the manuscript. GG and MM revised the draft critically for important intellectual content. All authors approved the version to be published.

References

1. Gainsborough N, Hall SM, Hughes RA, Leibowitz S: Sarcoid neuropathy. J Neurol 1991, 238:177 180.
2. Miller R, Sheron N, Semple S: Sarcoidosis presenting with an acute Guillain-Barr syndrome. Postgrad Med J 1989, 65:765 767.
3. Said G, Lacroix C, Plant-Bordeneuve V, Le Page L, Pico F, Presles O, Senant J, Remy P, Rondepierre P, Mallecourt J: Nerve granulomas and vasculitis in sarcoid peripheral neuropathy: a clinicopathological study of 11 patients. Brain 2002, 125:264 275.
4. Challenor YB, Felton CP, Brust JC: Peripheral nerve involvement in sarcoidosis: an electrodiagnostic study. J Neurol Neurosurg Psychiatry 1984, 47:1219 1222.
5. Koffman B, Junck L, Elias SB, Feit HW, Levine SR: Polyradiculopathy in sarcoidosis. Muscle Nerve 1999, 22:608 613.
6. Hoitsma E, Marziniak M, Faber CG, Reulen JP, Sommer C, De Baets M, Drent M: Small fibre neuropathy in sarcoidosis. Lancet 2002, 359:2085 2086.
7. Dreyer M, Vucic S, Cros DP, Chong PST: Multiple painful sensory mononeuropathies (MPSM), a novel pattern of sarcoid neuropathy. J Neurol Neurosurg Psychiatry 2004, 75:1645 1646.
8. Mattie R, Irwin RW: Neurosarcoidosis presenting as mononeuritis multiplex. Am J Phys Med Rehabil 2014, 93:349 354.
9. Garg S, Wright A, Reichwein R, Boyer P, Towfighi J, Kothari MJ: Mononeuritis multiplex secondary to sarcoidosis. Clin Neurol Neurosurg 2005, 107:140 143.
10. Beegle SH, Barba K, Gobunsuy R, Judson MA: Current and emerging pharmacological treatments for sarcoidosis: a review. Drug Des Devel Ther 2013, 7:325 338.
11. Schutt AC, Bullington WM, Judson MA: Pharmacotherapy for pulmonary sarcoidosis: a Delphi consensus study. Respir Med 2010, 104:717 723.
12. Callejas-Rubio JL, Lpez-Prez L, Ortego-Centeno N: Tumor necrosis factor-alpha inhibitor treatment for sarcoidosis. Ther Clin Risk Manag 2008, 4:1305 1313.
13. Scallon B, Cai A, Solowski N, Rosenberg A, Song XY, Shealy D, Wagner C: Binding and functional comparisons of two types of tumor necrosis factor antagonists. J Pharmacol Exp Ther 2002, 301:418 426.
14. Stern BJ, Krumholz A, Johns C, Scott P, Nissim J: Sarcoidosis and its neurological manifestations. Arch Neurol 1985, 42:909 917.
15. Kararizou E, Davaki P, Spengos K, Karandreas N, Dimitracopoulos A, Vassilopoulos D: Churg-Strauss syndrome complicated by neuropathy: a clinicopathological study of nine cases. Clin Neuropathol 2011, 30:11 17.
16. Wolf J, Bergner R, Mutallib S, Buggle F, Grau AJ: Neurologic complications of Churg-Strauss syndrome a prospective monocentric study. Eur J Neurol 2010, 17:582 588.
17. Seo P, Stone JH: The antineutrophil cytoplasmic antibody-associated vasculitides. Am J Med 2004, 117:39 50.
18. Nascimento OJM: Leprosy neuropathy: clinical presentations. Arq Neuropsiquiatr 2013, 71:661 666.
19. De Freitas MRG, Said G: Leprous neuropathy. Handb Clin Neurol 2013, 115:499 514.
20. Ooi WW, Srinivasan J: Leprosy and the peripheral nervous system: basic and clinical aspects. Muscle Nerve 2004, 30:393 409.
21. Chen H-A, Cheng N-C, Lin K-P, Liao H-T, Chen C-H, Huang D-F: Mononeuropathy multiplex and chylothorax as earlier manifestations of pulmonary tuberculosis. J Intern Med 2005, 257:561 563.
22. Naha K, Dasari MJ, Prabhu M: Tubercular neuritis: a new manifestation of an ancient disease. Australas Med J 2011, 4:674 676.
23. Orrell RW, King RHM, Bowler JV, Ginsberg L: Peripheral nerve granuloma in a patient with tuberculosis. J Neurol Neurosurg Psychiatry 2002, 73:769 771.
24. Shoenfeld Y, Agmon-Levin N: ASIA - autoimmune/inflammatory syndrome induced by adjuvants. J Autoimmun 2011, 36:4 8.
25. Perricone C, Colafrancesco S, Mazor RD, Soriano A, Agmon-Levin N, Shoenfeld Y: Autoimmune/inflammatory syndrome induced by adjuvants (ASIA) 2013: Unveiling the pathogenic, clinical and diagnostic aspects. J Autoimmun 2013, 47:1 16.
26. Santos E, Shaunak S, Renowden S, Scolding NJ: Treatment of refractory neurosarcoidosis with Infliximab. J Neurol Neurosurg Psychiatry 2010, 81:241 246.
27. Tong D, Manolios N, Howe G, Spencer D: New onset sarcoid-like granulomatosis developing during anti-TNF therapy: an under-recognised complication. Intern Med J 2012, 42:89 94.
28. Gonzlez-Lpez MA, Blanco R, Gonzlez-Vela MC, Fernndez-Llaca H, Rodrguez-Valverde V: Development of sarcoidosis during etanercept therapy. Arthritis Rheum 2006, 55:817 820.
29. Van Schouwenburg PA, Rispens T, Wolbink GJ: Immunogenicity of anti-TNF biologic therapies for rheumatoid arthritis. Nat Rev Rheumatol 2013, 9:164 172.
30. Dore RK, Mathews S, Schechtman J, Surbeck W, Mandel D, Patel A, Zhou L, Peloso P: The immunogenicity, safety, and efficacy of etanercept liquid administered once weekly in patients with rheumatoid arthritis. Clin Exp Rheumatol 2007, 25:40 46.
31. Walsh M1, Chaudhry A, Jayne D: Long-term follow-up of relapsing/refractory anti-neutrophil cytoplasm antibody associated vasculitis treated with the lymphocyte depleting antibody alemtuzumab (CAMPATH-1H). Ann Rheum Dis 2008, 67:1322 1327.

11

Guillain-Barré Syndrome - Natural history and prognostic factors: a retrospective review of 106 cases

Inés González-Suárez[*†], Irene Sanz-Gallego[†], Francisco Javier Rodríguez de Rivera[†] and Javier Arpa[†]

Abstract

Background: Guillain-Barre syndrome (GBS) is characterized by acute onset and progressive course, and is usually associated with a good prognosis. However, there are forms of poor prognosis, needing ventilatory support and major deficits at discharge. With this study we try to identify the factors associated with a worse outcome.

Methods: 106 cases of GBS admitted in our hospital between years 2000–2010 were reviewed. Epidemiological, clinical, therapeutical and evolutionary data were collected.

Results: At admission 45% had severe deficits, percentage which improves throughout the evolution of the illness, with full recovery or minor deficits in the 87% of patients at the first year review. Ages greater than 55 years, severity at admission (p < 0.001), injured cranial nerves (p = 0.008) and the needing of ventilator support (p = 0.003) were associated with greater sequels at the discharge and at the posterior reviews in the following months. 17% required mechanical ventilation (MV). Values < 250 L/min in the Peak Flow-test are associated with an increased likelihood of requiring MV (p < 0.001).

Conclusions: Older age, severe deficits at onset, injured cranial nerves, requiring MV, and axonal lesion patterns in the NCS were demonstrated as poor prognostic factors. Peak Flow-test is a useful predictive factor of respiratory failure by its easy management.

Keywords: Guillain-Barre, Natural history, Prognostic factors, Peak flow

Background

The term Guillain-Barré syndrome (GBS) includes a set of clinical syndromes (GBS) with a common pathophysiological basis; an acute inflammatory polyneuropathy with an autoimmune etiology [1-3]. Although usually characterized by a progressive flaccid paralysis with areflexia a wide range of motor, sensory and autonomic symptoms could be seen [1-4]. In general, the diagnosis is based on clinical criteria [4-7]; nevertheless, the presence of suggestive findings in the complementary test as demyelinising changes in the nerve conduction studies (NCS) or albuminocytological dissociation in the cerebrospinal fluid (CSF), help to confirm the diagnosis [1].

The worldwide incidence of GBS is reported to be 0.6-2.4 cases per 100,000 per year [8-15]. The classic form, the acute inflammatory demyelinating polyradiculoneuropathy (AIDP), is the most frequent subtype in Europe, which accounts for 90% of GBS cases [2]. Other subtypes like the axonal forms or the Miller-Fisher syndrome (MFS) [16,17] are less common.

The prognosis is usually good, showing a complete functional recovery or with minimal deficits in the 90% of patients 1 year after the onset of illness [13,18]. Several factors have been identified as predictors of poor outcome [13,14,19-21]. Death rate is described to be between 1-18% [14,15]. This study aimed to describe the epidemiological, clinical, laboratory, and electrodiagnostic features, as well as to identify the predictive factors of worse prognosis in the GBS or its subtypes.

Methods

A retrospective review of the medical records of patients admitted at La Paz University Hospital (Madrid, Spain)

* Correspondence: igonsua@gmail.com
†Equal contributors
Section of Neuromuscular diseases, Department of Neurology, La Paz University Hospital, Paseo de la Castellana, Madrid 261.28046, Spain

with the diagnosis of GBS between 2000–2010 was made. 106 fulfilled levels 1, 2 or 3 of diagnostic certainty for GBS/MFS described by Sejvar et al. [7]. All demographic, clinical, laboratory and electrophysiological data were recorded, as well as outcome and treatment.

Severity at admission was assessed by the Medical Research Council (MRC) sum score, valuing the strength from 0 to 5 in 4 muscles (proximal and distal) in both upper and lower limbs on both sides, so that the score ranged from 40 (normal) to 0 (quadriplegic) and by the GBS disability score advocated by Hughes et al. [22]. Cranial nerve involvement was considered separately by the affectation of oculomotor, facial and bulbar nerves. Respiratory weakness was assessed first by the value obtained at the peak expiratory flow meter (Peak Flow), as well as the need for mechanical ventilation throughout the evolution. Sensory disturbances, autonomic alteration or pain presence were also assessed.

Serological screening for preceding infections was recorded, including Herpes Simplex virus (HSV), Varicella-Zoster (VZV), cytomegalovirus (CMV), Epstein-Barr virus (EBV), *Mycoplasma Pneumoniae*, B and C hepatitis virus, *Haemophilus Influenzae* and, in selected cases, stool and *Campylobacter Jejuni* determination. The CSF was analyzed for cell count, glucose and protein concentration.

Neurophysiological studies were evaluated in accordance with the criteria of Hadden et al. [23,24]. As in a retrospective study, not in all cases were the same nerves measured. Also, electromyography studies (EMG) with concentric needle electrodes were made to evaluate the axonal loss (fibrillation, positive sharp wave...).

The evaluation of the functional impact was graded by the GBS disability score [22] during the discharge from the neurology or the rehabilitation department, and at the third, sixth and twelfth month in the outpatient clinic.

The study was approved by the Research Ethics Committee of La Paz Hospital, Madrid, Spain.

All statistical analyses were performed using the SPSS 12 for Windows program (Chicago, IL, E.U.A.). For univariate analysis, Chi-square test for dichotomic variables was used. For continuous variables, t-Student test in parametric variables or U Mann-Withney with the non-parametric ones were used.

Results

There was no difference between genders (ratio male/female 1.07), with a mean onset age of 43.7 ± 23 years (range 0–85). Demographic and clinical data are summarized in Table 1. There was a seasonal rebound in winter, when 41% of patients were diagnosed. Most patients had an infectious antecedent preceding the onset of the weakness, being the most frequent respiratory tract infection (38%); at least 30% did not present a previous infectious disease [25]. The mean of days since the start of

Table 1 Epidemiological data of GBS patients

	Number of cases	(%)
Gender		
Male	55	51.9
Female	51	48,1
Age (years)		
<15	15	14.2
16-34	24	22.6
35-54	28	26.4
>55	39	36.8
Antecedent events		
Upper respiratory infection	40	37.7
Gastrointestinal infection	29	27.4
Vacunation	2	1.9
Others	3	2.8
None	32	30.2
Season		
Winter	43	40.6
Spring	20	18.9
Summer	21	19.8
Autumn	22	20.8
Motor deficit		
Mild (MRC 31–40)	60	56.6
Moderate (MRC 11–30)	43	40.6
Severe (MRC 0–10)	3	2.8
Cranial nerve involvement	37	35.5
Facial palsy uni/bilateral	27	25.5
MOE	14	13.2
Bulbar nerves	4	3.8
Ataxia	8	7,5
Other symptoms		
Sensory deficit	31	29.2
Pain	33	31.1
SNA	9	8.5
SIADH	7	6.6
Respiratory distress	18	17
GBS disability score		
Minor signs or symptoms	12	11.3
Walk without support	41	38.7
Walk with support	16	15,1
Bedridden or chair bound	19	17.9
Ventilated	18	17
Death attributed to SGB	2	1.9

the infectious sickness until the polyneuropathy debut was 12 ± 8.3 days (range 1–30).

Clinical data

A motor disorder at the admission was referred in 94 patients, with a variable degree. By classifying them according to the GBS disability score, 55% retained the ability to walk (grades 1, 2 and 3), unlike the remaining 45% which showed a severe affectation (grades 4, 5 and 6); Respiratory distress was present in 17% of patients. Pulmonary function was valued by the Peak Flow test in 50 patients, showed that values below 250 L/min were associated with a greater likelihood of requiring MV during the income (p < 0.05), independently of the presence of uni/bilateral facial palsy (p < 0.05). Time between symptom onset and admission was significantly lower in the severe cases (mean 5.17 days) compared with the mild ones (mean 8.87 days), so a faster progression could be postulated in the first ones (p = 0.053). Non-motor symptoms were described; the most frequent, neuropathic pain in 31% of patients, followed by sensory disturbances in 29%. Autonomic dysfunctions were found in 8.5% of cases. In 7% of the patients a syndrome of inappropriate antidiuretic hormone hypersecretion (SIADH) was diagnosed [26].

Laboratory and neurophysiological findings

A lumbar puncture was made in 95 patients (90%) with an average delay of 15 ± 11.71 days (range 1–80) since the beginning of symptoms. Raised concentration of proteins was present in 80 patients (85%) with albuminocytological dissociation in 79 of them (85%).

Serologic studies were made in 101 patients (95%), in 8 (8%) cases CMV was the microorganism responsible for the GBS; in 5 (5%) *Mycoplasma Pneumoniae*, in 1 (1%) EBV and 1 (1%) enterovirus; the remaining 85.1% of serology was negative.

NCS was made in 98 patients (92.5%) with a median period from the onset to the neurophysiological study of 20.73 ± 10.17 days (range 2–62). Resumed data of the neurophysiological test is shown in Table 2. In 57 (58%) a demyelinating pattern was found, 7 (7%) an axonal pattern, 3 (3%) were unexcitable, 2 (2%) were normal, and 29 (30%) didn't fulfil diagnostic criteria for demyelinating lesion, but changes consistent with a peripheral neuropathy were present. Conduction blocks were present in 37 patients (37.8%). F- Responses were altered (absent or delayed) in 29 of 64 median (45%), in 16 of 35 ulnar (46%) in 4 of 8 tibial (50%) and in 34 of 40 (85%) peroneal nerves. H-reflex was affected in 26 of 48 (45%) cases evaluated. In sixth of the Miller Fisher syndromes a NCS was made, 1 of them (17%) was normal, and in the remaining 5 (83%) sensory conduction was affected. In 3 of 5 (60%) H reflex was absent. In the needle EMG examination signs of acute denervation were present in 44 of 86 (51%).

The distribution of the different subtypes of GBS was: AIDP in 83%, acute motor and sensory axonal neuropathy (AMSAN) in 5.7%, acute motor axonal neuropathy (AMAN) in 1.9%, MFS in 8.5% and cranial multineuritis in 0.9%.

Treatment, outcome and prognosis

Some kind of treatment was offered to 89 patients (84%): 88 received IVIg (83%) and 3 plasma exchange (2.8%); in 2 patients both treatments were dispensed sequentially. 16% of cases never started a treatment due to the mild symptoms or the long evolution of the disease.

At discharge, absent or minor deficits were observed in 38 patients (36%), 30 (28%) were able to walk for 10 meters without a help, 28 (26%) needed assistance to walk, 7 (7%) were bedridden and 1 (1%) needed respiratory support. Two patients died of the disease. Patients were followed in the outpatient clinic at 3, 6 and 12 months (Table 3).

Table 2 Neurophysiological data of patients with GBS

	N	CMAP (mV)	MDL (ms)	MCV (m/s)	n	SNAP (µV)	DL(ms)	SCV (m/s)
Median	83	6,8 ± 5,6	6,4 ± 7,8	43,6 ± 17,9	85	7,03 ± 7,8	3,2 ± 3,4	43,6 ± 16,6
Min-Max		0,07-21,30	0,1 ± 61,0	0,10 ± 65,5		0,1-43,2	0,1-27,7	0,1-63,4
Ulnar	32	8,0 ± 7,8	3,4 ± 1,5	46,6 ± 17,4	72	3,9 ± 3,9	2,6 ± 1,9	43,2 ± 16,4
Min-Max		0,1-16,6	0,1-7,5	0,1-8,1		0,1-19,9	0,1-14,2	0,1-59,7
Tibial post	14	4,8 ± 5,9	6,7 ± 2,2	33,5 ± 15,6				
Min-Max		0,2-18,10	4,0-11,0	0,1-50,20				
Peroneal	87	3,6 ± 3,9	6,9 ± 5,1	35,9 ± 14,8				
Min-Max		0,1-15,7	0,1-31,4	0,1-54,1				
Sural					71	6,01 ± 5,4	2,6 ± 1,9	39,2 ± 15,5
Min-Max						0,1-27,4	0,1-18,0	0,1-57,2
Sup Peroneal					39	9,7 ± 8,2	2,2 ± 0,7	39,8 ± 12,7
Min-Max						0,1-37,4	0,1-3,8	0,13-8

Table 3 Proportion of patients, based on the GBS score, during the follow-up

	Discharge		3th month revision		6th month revision		12th month revision	
	N	(%)	N	(%)	N	(%)	N	(%)
Healthy	4	3,8	18	29,5	17	36,2	18	58,1
Minor deficits or symptoms	34	32,1	19	31,1	15	31,9	7	22,6
Walk without support	30	28,3	14	23	8	17	2	6,5
Walk with support	28	26,4	10	16,4	7	14,9	4	12,9
Bedbridden or chairbound	7	6,6	0		0		0	
Ventilated	1	0,9	0		0		0	
Death	2	1,9	0		0		0	

Some factors were analysed as possible predictors of a poor outcome: 1) patients with ages greater than 55 years were most affected at the admission (p = 0.027), with greater deficits at discharge (p = 0.2) and at the third (p = 0.1), sixth (p = 0.001) and twelfth month (p = 0.006); 2) severity at admission, score based on the GBS disability scale (disabling or non-disabling), was also associated with more disability at discharge (p < 0.001), and at the successive medical reviews at the third (p = 0.001) and the sixth month (p < 0.001); 3) cranial nerve involvement was related with greater deficits at discharge (p = 0.008) and 4) mechanical ventilation requirement showed greater sequels at discharge (p = 0.003), in the follow up the results were not statistically significant but a trend to associate with greater deficits was seen. Finally, there seems to be a trend towards a worse prognosis in those patients with axonal lesions in the conduction studies (p = 0.2) which is likely to be maintained throughout the evolution (Table 4).

Discussion

The present work has the limitations of a retrospective study based on hospital case-mix. The incidence is reported to be 0.6-2.4 cases per 100,000 per year [18,19,21]. Changes suffered in the last years in the attendance area of the hospital make incidence calculation complex and inaccurate; however, it appears to be of 1.68-2.46 per 100,000 per year.

There is no difference between gender [1,2]. The bimodal shape wasn't present in our study [8-10], as there is a linear increase in the incidence with age [1,2,9,11,12,24]. GBS is considered a sporadic illness, without a seasonal cluster [1,9]; however, a trend to accrue in winter is shown in our series [11,12]. The infectious event is described to appear in 40-70% of patients [1-3,8-12]. In our series up to 70% of cases have had one, of which respiratory infection was the most frequent.

As in previous series, weakness and hypo/areflexia were the most frequent symptoms, followed by neuropathic pain and numbness. Hyponatremia, as a symptom of SIADH is not a classical manifestation of GBS; however, there are series in which are described to be present in up to 58% of the cases; in our review, it was found in 7% of our patients.

There isn't a consensus about the neurophysiological values defining GBS and its variants [2,4,5,7,23,24,26-29].

Table 4 Possible predictor factors of a poor outcome

	Discharge deficits		3th month revision deficits		6th month revision deficits		12th month revision deficits	
	Disabling	p	Disabling	p	Disabling	p	Disabling	p
Severity at admission		<0.001		0.001		<0.001		0.2
Non disabling	11.3% (6/53)		20.6% (7/34)		7.7% (2/26)		11.8% (2/17)	
Disabling	60.3% (32/53)		63% (17/27)		61.9% (13/21)		28.6% (4/14)	
Age		0.2		0.17		0.01		0.006
<55 years	31.3% (21/67)		34.1% (15/44)		17.6% (6/34)		8% (2/25)	
>55 years	43.6% (17/39)		52.9% (9/17)		69.2% (9/13)		66.7% (4/69)	
MV		0.003		0.13		0.6		1
Yes	66.7% (12/18)		66.7% (6/9)		42.9% (3/7)		25% (1/4)	
No	29.5% (26/88)		34.6% (18/52)		30% (12/40)		18.5% (5/27)	
Axonal lesion at CNS		0.2		0.3		0.06		0.4
Demyelinating	40.7% (22/54)		43.3% (13/30)		30.4% (7/23)		16,7% (3/18)	
Axonal	71.4% (5/7)		66,7% (4/6)		80% (4/5)		33.3% (1/3)	

Statistical analysis of the disabling deficits and the possible poor prognostic factors during the follow-up.

It is accepted as demyelination parameters: motor conduction velocity (MCV) decrease, prolongation of motor distal latency, conduction blocks, temporal dispersion and increased F-wave latency [27]. It is reported that the first electromyographic changes are the alteration of F-wave and H-reflex response [2,22], altered both in our NCS reported as normal, probably due to the earliness of the exploration. In MFS, the CNS are normal in most cases; nonetheless, discrete changes in the sensory conduction or in H-reflex may be present [30-32], some authors postulate a damage in the afferent proprioceptive system as a pathophysiological basis [32].

As classically described, in our study illness prognosis is favourable; 81% of patients presented absent or minimum neurological deficits one year after the onset. Older age, illness severity in the acute phase, prior gastrointestinal infection and axonal injury in the CNS and mechanical ventilation requirement [15,20,33,34] are among the factors that have been advocated for poor prognosis. *Van Koningsveld* et al. defined a clinical prognostic scoring system for GBS outcome at 6 months, the "Erasmus GBS Outcome Score" or EGOS [15], it was based on the punctuation on the GBS disability score at 2 weeks from the admission, the history of diarrhoea and the age. Recently, *Walgaard* et al. have validated a modified EGOS (mEGOS) with the main difference being the use of the MRC sum score at admission and in the 7th day instead the GBS disability score [35], they claimed that the MRC sum score is more accurate, and the possibility of being used at admission could predict the future treatments. However, the mEGOS made on the 7th day after the admission show increased predictive value instead the one made on the first day [35]. However, although useful, the mEGOS passed on the first day of admission showed lower predictive ability than the one performed on the 7th day. In our study we demonstrate that, even in the first day of admission, lower scores on the GBS scale are associated with worse outcome and greater disability at discharge, 3 and 6 months. Respiratory distress is the leading cause of death in the acute phase, 20-30% requiring ventilatory support [20]. Many factors have been proposed as predictors of the future need for respiratory support, like forced vital capacity (FVC) < 60%, bulbar dysfunction, rapid progression of the illness, and difficulty raising the head [19,20]. *Van Doorn* et al. propose a regularly monitoring of the respiratory function initially every 2-4 h, and then every 6-12 h [1]. Although FVC is considered to be the gold standard test for detecting impaired ventilation it has some disadvantages, the requirement of portable spirometers in the acute phase due to the instability of the patient, the need for a minimum of preparation and knowledge of the technique by medical personnel and the higher cost. *Suárez* et al. describe a serie of 79 patients with

neuromuscular diseases in which the Peak Flow test proved to be useful in the monitoring of expiratory muscle weakness [35]. In our hospital, patients were monitored by the Peak Flow test each 6 hours in the acute phase, being observed that values below 250 L/min predict the posterior need of respiratory support ($p < 0.05$), independently of the presence of facial palsy that could hinder the use of the test ($p < 0.05$), making the Peak Flow a safe, inexpensive, and widely-available test in the monitoring of patients with GBS.

Conclusion

Our series is in concordance with those previously published. The seasonal cluster in winter is worth noting on which there is a great controversy. Regarding the outcome, our series reported a worse prognosis in patients with older age, severe deficits at the beginning, injured cranial nerves, requiring MV, and axonal lesion patterns in the NCS. Finally, project the Peak Flow-test as a useful predictive factor of respiratory failure by its availability, and easy management.

Abbreviations
AIDP: Acute inflammatory demyelinating Polyradiculoneuropathy; AMAN: Acute motor axonal neuropathy; AMSAN: Acute motor and sensory axonal neuropathy; CB: Conduction blocks; CMAP: Conduction motor action potential; CMV: Cytomegalovirus; CSF: Cerebrospinal fluid; EBV: Ebstein-Barr virus; EMG: Electromyography studies; GBS: Guillain-Barré syndrome; HSV: Herpes-simplex virus; IVIg: Immunoglobulin; MRC: Medical research council; MFS: Miller-Fisher syndrome; MV: Mechanical ventilation; NCS: Nerve conduction studies; SIADH: Syndrome of inappropriate antidiuretic hormone hypersecretion; VZV: Varicella-Zoster virus.

Competing interests
There are no competing interests in this manuscript.

Authors' contributions
IGS conceived of the study, participated in the design of the study and performed the statistical analysis, and coordination and drafted the manuscript. ISG participated in the design of the study. FJRR participated in the design of the study. JA conceived of the study, participated in the design of the study and coordination and drafted the manuscript. All authors read and approved the final manuscript.

Acknowledgements
Our thanks are due to Mr. Martin J. Smyth, B.A. for correcting the English.

References
1. Van Doorn PA, Ruts L, Jacobs BC: **Clinical features, pathogenesis, and treatment of Guillain-Barré syndrome.** *Lancet Neurol* 2008, **7**:939–950.
2. Vucic S, Kiernan MC, Cornblath DR: **Guillain-Barré syndrome: An update.** *J Cli Neurosci* 2009, **16**:733–741.
3. Tellería-Díaz A, Calzada-Sierra DJ: **Síndrome de Guillain-Barré.** *Rev Neurol* 2002, **34**(10):966–976.
4. Asbury AK, Arnason BGW, Karp HR, McFarlin DF: **Criteria for diagnosis of Guillain-Barré syndrome.** *Ann Neurol* 1978, **3**:565–566.
5. Asbury AK, Cornblath DR: **Assesment of current diagnostic criteria for Guillain-Barré syndrome.** *Ann Neurol* 1990, **27**(Suppl):S21–S24.
6. Hughes RAC, Rees JH: **Clinical and epidemiologic features of Guillain-Barré syndrome.** *J Infect Dis* 1997, **176**(suppl2):S92–S98.
7. Sejvar JJ, Kohl KS, Gidudu J, Amato A, Bakshi N, Baxter R, *et al*: **Guillain-Barré syndrome and Fisher syndrome: case definitions and guidelines for**

collection, analysis, and presentation of immunization safety data. *Vaccine* 2011, **29**:599–612.

8. McGrogan A, Madle G, Seaman HE, De Vries CS: **The epidemiology of Guillain-Barré syndrome worldwide.** *Neuroepidemiology* 2009, **32**:150–163.

9. The Emilia-Romagna Study group on Clinical and Epidemiological Problems in Neurology: **A prospective study on the incidence and prognosis of Guillain-Barré syndrome in Emilia-Romagna region, Italy (1992–1993).** *Neurology* 1997, **48**:214–221.

10. Lyu R-K, Tang L-M, Cheng S-Y, Hsa W-C, Chen S-T: **Guillain-Barré syndrome in Taiwan: a clinical study of 167 patients.** *J Neurol Neurosurgery Psychiatry* 1997, **63**:494–500.

11. Cuadrado JI, de Pedro Cuesta J, Ara JR, Cemillan CA, Díaz M, Duarte J, *et al*: **Guillain-Barré syndrome in Spain, 1985–1997: epidemiological and public health view.** *Eur Neurol* 2001, **46**:83–91.

12. Alandro-Benito Y, Conde-Sendín MA, Muñoz-Fernández C, Pérez-Correa S, Alemany-Rodríguez MJ, Fiuza-Pérez MD, *et al*: **Síndrome de Guillain-Barré en el área norte de Gran Canaria e isla de Lanzarote.** *Rev Neurol (Barc.)* 2002, **35**:705–710.

13. Soysal A, Aysal F, Caliskan B, Dogan Ak P, Mutluay B, Sakalli N, *et al*: **Clinico-electrophysiological findings and prognosis of Guillain-Barré syndrome - 10 years'experience.** *Acta Neurol Scand* 2011, **123**:181–186.

14. The Italian Guillain-Barré Study Group: **The prognosis and main prognostic indicators of GuillainBarré syndrome. A multicentre prospective study of 297 patients.** *Brain* 1996, **119**:2053–2061.

15. Van Koningsveld R, Steyerberg EW, Hughes RAC, Swan AV, Van Doorn PA, Jacobs BC: **A clinical prognostic scoring system of Guillain-Barré syndrome.** *Lancet Neurol* 2007, **6**:589–594.

16. Chodwury D, Arora A: **Axonal Guillain Barré syndrome: a critical review.** *Acta Neurol Scand* 2001, **103**:267–277.

17. Mori M, Kuwaraba S, Fukutake T, Yuki N, Hattori T: **Clinical features and prognosis of Miller Fisher syndrome.** *Neurology* 2001, **56**:1104–1106.

18. Korinthenberg R, Schessl J, Kirschner J: **Clinical presentation and course of childhood Guillain-Barré syndrome: a prospective multicentre study.** *Neuropediatrics* 2007, **38**:10–17.

19. Lawn ND, Fletcher DD, Henderson RD, Wolter TD, Wijdicks EF: **Anticipating mechanical ventilation in Guillain-Barré syndrome.** *Arch Neurol* 2001, **58**:871–872.

20. Durand MC, Porcher R, Orlikowski D, Aboab J, Devaux C, Clair B, *et al*: **Clinical and electrophysiological predictors of respiratory failure in Guillain-Barré syndrome: a prospective study.** *Lancet Neurol* 2006, **5**:1021–1028.

21. Ropper AH, Widjicks EFM, Truax BT (Eds): *Guillain- Barré syndrome.* Philadelphia: F.A. Davis; 1991.

22. Hughes RA, Newsom-Davis JM, Perkin GD, Pierce JM: **Controlled trial prednisolone in acute polineuropathy.** *Lancet* 1978, **2**:750–753.

23. Hadden RDM, Cornblath DR, Hughes RAC, Zielasek J, Hartung HP, Toyka K, *et al*: **Electrophysiological classification of Guillain-Barré Syndrome: clinical associations and outcome.** *Ann Neurol* 1998, **44**:780–788.

24. Hughes RAC, Cornblath DR: **Guillain-Barré syndrome.** *Lancet Neurol* 2005, **366**:1653–1666.

25. Hadden RD, Karch H, Hartung HP, Zielasek J, Weissbrich B, Schubert J: **Preceding infections, immune factors, and outcome in Guillain-Barré syndrome.** *Neurology* 2001, **56**:758–765.

26. Saifudheen K, Jose J, Gafoor VA, Musthafa M: **Guillain-Barré síndrome and SIADH.** *Neurology* 2011, **76**:701–704.

27. Van den Bergh PYK, Piéret F: **Electrodiagnostic criteria for acute and chronic inflammatory demyelinating polyradiculoneuropathy.** *Muscle Nerve* 2004, **29**:565–574.

28. Vucic S, Cairns KD, Black KR, Chong PST, Cros D: **Neurophysiologic findings in early acute inflammatory demyelinating polyradiculoneuropathy.** *Clin Neurophysiology* 2004, **115**:2329–2335.

29. Alam TA, Chaudhry V, Cornblath DR, Electrophysiological studies in the Guillain-Barré syndrome: 30, Alam TA, Chaudhry V, Cornblath DR: **Electrophysiological studies in the Guillain-Barré syndrome: distinguishing subtypes by published criteria.** *Muscle Nerve* 1998, **21**:1275–1279.

30. Jamal GA, Leod Mac WN: **Electrophysiologic studies in Miller Fisher syndrome.** *Neurology* 1984, **34**:685–688.

31. Lo YL: **Clinical and immunological spectrum of the Miller Fisher syndrome.** *Muscle Nerve* 2007, **36**:615–627.

32. Yuki N: **Fisher syndrome and Bickerstaff brainstem encephalitis (Fisher-Bickerstaff syndrome).** *J Neuroimmunol* 2009, **215**:1–9.

33. Rajabally YA, Unicini A: **Outcome and its predictors in Guillain-barré syndrome.** *J Neurol Neurosurg Psychiatry* 2012, **83**:711–718.

34. Walgaard C, Lingsma HF, Ruts L, *et al*: **Early recognition of poor prognosis in Guillain-Barré syndrome.** *Neurology* 2011, **76**:968–975.

35. Suarez AA, Pessolano FA, Monteiro SG, Ferreyra G, Capria ME, Mesa L, *et al*: **Peak flow and peak cough flow in the evaluation of expiratory muscle weakness and bulbar impairment in patients with neuromuscular disease.** *Am J Phys Med Rehabil* 2002, **81**:506–511.

12

Acute autonomic neuropathy with severe gastrointestinal symptoms in children

Ling-Yu Pang[1†], Chang-Hong Ding[2†], Yang-Yang Wang[1], Li-Ying Liu[1], Qiao-Jun Li[3] and Li-Ping Zou[1,4*]

Abstract

Background: Acute autonomic neuropathy (AAN) is rare disorder with anecdotal report, especially for childhood onset patients. Misdiagnosis or delays in treatment can always be found in clinical practice. We conducted this study to give a description of the manifestations and treatment of AAN in children and therefore help clinicians to make the accurate diagnosis early so that the prognosis of the patients can be improved.

Methods: A systematic record from 3 clinical centers was used to identify 11 subject, 3 males and 8 females, with clinical diagnosed AAN.

Result: The age ranged from 2 years and 4 months to 14 years and 6 months (mean, 9 ± 3.6 years old) and the course from onset to diagnosis ranged from 7 days to 8 months. All children shared prominent initial symptoms, 7 with frequent vomiting and 4 with motor dysfunctions. The condition of 9 patients improved after treatment of IVIg and intravenous glucocorticoid.

Conclusion: The clinical manifestations of AAN are diverse, generalized, and non-specific. Gastrointestinal disorders were the most common initial symptoms. Symptoms of gastrointestinal system and abnormal secretion of glands were severe and more common than other symptoms. The mechanism of AAN remains unknown. Although IVIg and intravenous glucocorticoid can be used in clinical practice, there is still no treatment recommendation and further study is needed.

Keywords: Acute autonomic neuropathy, Children, Autonomic nervous system, Gastrointestinal dysfunction, Intravenous immunoglobulin

Background

Acute autonomic neuropathy (AAN), as first described in 1969, mainly involves the peripheral autonomic nervous system without other neurological manifestations [1]. The clinical features of AAN are diverse and generalized including the disturbance of pupillary constriction, gastrointestinal system, urogenital system, cardiovascular system, and gland secretion [2]. Mild sensorimotor symptoms can accompany the autonomic manifestations but not predominant [3]. . The clinical spectrum of ANN ranges from pandysautonomias involving both sympathetic and parasympathetic abnormality to merely cholinergic dysautonomias without noradrenergic dysautonomias, which overshadows the symptoms of somatic motor and sensory abnormalities.

Much as we know about the symptoms, little do we know about the pathogenesis. Some scholars believe that AAN can be considered as an uncommon variant of Guillain–Barré syndrome [3–5] with autonomic manifestations, which can result in mortality and morbidity in some patients and can also be the sole or predominant manifestation.

Most studies on AAN focus on adults instead of children [6–8]. The prominent initial symptoms are often gastrointestinal symptoms (vomiting, abdominal pain, and diarrhea). Thus, patients tend to initially be

* Correspondence: zouliping21@hotmail.com
†Equal contributors
[1]Department of Pediatrics, Chinese PLA General Hospital, Beijing 100853, China
[4]Center of Epilepsy, Beijing Institute for Brain Disorders, Beijing 100069, China
Full list of author information is available at the end of the article

admitted to the gastroenterological department [9], which also adds the difficulty of timely diagnosis.

In this study, we described the symptoms of 11 cases in three pediatric clinical centers in China. We hope to provide more evidence for the clinical diagnosis and treatment of AAN and help improve the prognosis.

Methods

We retrospectively investigated children with acute autonomic neuropathy diagnosed in three pediatric medical centers in China from 2003 to 2014. All clinical data were evaluated by a neurologist.

The following is the diagnostic criteria: (1) acute or sub-acute onset; (2) with clinical and electrophysiological evidence of significant autonomic failure and relative preservation of somatic motor and sensory function; (3) a self-limited course and partial recovery within 1 year to 2 years; (4) without autonomic failure because of central nervous system(CNS)disease; and (5) autonomic neuropathies of known etiology, such as those associated with amyloidosis, diabetes, malignant neoplasm, and neurotoxic drug exposure [3].

We used a series of reproducible, noninvasive, simple, and viable detection methods in the initial diagnosis and the subsequent follow-up.

1. Minor's starch iodine test [10]: The test was administered by applying an alcohol–iodine–oil solution and starch powder. The patient received aspirin and a cup of hot water to promote sweating. The distribution of blue discoloration of the starch iodine mixture was recorded.

2. Skin scratch test [11]: The dermograph reaction indicated normal automatic nerve function if its color changes from white to red in a few minutes. Sympathetic nervous excitement was implicated if the color remained white for more than 5 min. Parasympathetic nervous excitement was implicated if the color remained red.

3. For the Lying-Standing test [12], blood pressure, electrocardiogram (ECG), and heart rate (HR) were measured as the baseline while the patient was in the supine position at resting state. All tests were repeated after standing for 10 min.

4. Oculocardiac reflex [11]: The heart rate was recorded when pressing the eyeball. The HR can decrease 10–12/min under such pressure. A sharp decrease in heart rate (more than 12/min) indicates parasympathetic hyperfunction. The absence of response to the pressure means parasympathetic inadequate function, and an increase in HR means sympathetic hyperfunction.

5. Carotid sinus reflex [11]. The heart rate in response to the pressure on the carotid sinus was recorded. The HR can decrease 6–10/min in such pressure. A sharp decrease (more than 10/min) means parasympathetic hyperfunction. The absence of response to the pressure

means parasympathetic inadequate function, and an increase in HR means sympathetic hyperfunction.

The functional status of the patients was assessed in the initial and subsequent follow-up according to the modified Rankin scale [13].

Results

Demographics

All the 11 patients met our criteria of acute autonomic neuropathy The detailed information can be found in Table 1.

Clinical symptoms

The most frequent symptom is frequent vomiting, followed by motor dysfunctions. In some of them, vomiting was accompanied with lack of appetite, abdominal distention, or diarrhea. An antecedent event was reported in 9 patients before the initial symptoms of neuropathy, including gastrointestinal tract infections ($n = 3$), fever only ($n = 3$), eruption ($n = 2$), and fever with eruption ($n = 1$).

The autonomic manifestations were generalized and severe, affecting multiple systems in the body. Symptoms in the gastrointestinal system and the abnormal secretion of glands were more common than those in the other symptoms. The disturbances of the gastrointestinal system appeared in all patients and the detailed information can be found in Table 2. The weight of 10 patients decreased significantly because of malnutrition. 2 patients were tube feeding dependent.

Symptoms also occur in other systems of the body (Table 3). In the urinary system, uroschesis was observed in 5 patients. Among them, 1 patient needed urethral catheterization because of the severely flaccid bladder. 1 patient showed delayed urination, and 1 patient showed oliguria. Symptoms in the cardiovascular system including orthostatic hypotension occurred in 4 patients. 7 patients exhibited tachycardia. Pupillary reaction to light

Table 1 Demographics and initial symptoms of the 11 patients

Case	Sex	Age	Duration*	Initial symptoms
1	F	3y2 m	38d	limb weakness
2	F	11y5m	7d	vomiting
3	M	14y6 m	3 m	lower limb weakness
4	F	8y10m	39d	limb weakness
5	F	2y4 m	25d	vomiting
6	F	8y7m	2 m	vomiting
7	F	12y	10d	vomiting
8	F	9y7m	2.5 m	vomiting
9	M	11y2 m	6 m	vomiting
10	M	7y4 m	4 m	vomiting
11	F	10y3 m	8 m	limb weakness

*represents the time from the first symptom onset to the definite diagnosis

Table 2 The symptoms of gastrointestinal system and glands secretion

System	N	Symptoms	n[a] (%)
Gastrointestinal system	11 (100%)	Vomiting	8 (72.73%)
		constipation	7 (63.64%)
		Alternate of diarrhea and constipation	2 (18.19%)
		abdominal distension	2 (18.19%)
		diarrhea	1 (9.09%)
Glands secretion	11 (100%)	hyphidrosis,	10 (90.91%)
		oligosialia	7 (63.64%)
		salivate	2 (18.19%)
		hyperidrosis	1 (9.09%)
Malnutrition (marasmus)	10 (90.91%)	Severe	1 (10.00%)
		moderate	7 (70.00%)
		mild	2 (20.00%)

[a]: n/N
Severe malnutrition: weight loss >40%, moderate malnutrition: weight loss 25%–40%; mild malnutrition: weight loss 15%–25%

was absent in 7 patients. Anisocoria was observed in 4 patients. Bilateral mydriasis was present in 3 patients. Abnormal shape of the pupils was observed in 1 patient. All patients showed variable somatic motor or sensory dysfunction. 8 patients experienced variable limb weaknesses. 6 patients were observed with variable loss of limb muscle strength through neurological test. Their myodynamia ranged from III to IV, as indicated by the Medical Research Council grading system (Table 3). The absence/reduction of deep tendon reflexes was observed in 7 patients. Six patients exhibited evidence of distal sensory deficit.

Autonomic function tests
Minor's starch iodine test was performed in 7 patients. 6 of them showed significant areas of anhidrosis, whereas 1 showed hidrosis in the feet and buttocks. The skin scratch test result was abnormal in 8 patients. Oculocardiac and carotid sinus reflexes were performed in 5 patients. However, the HR showed no change in 4 and increment in 1. The result of Lying–Standing test was positive in 4 patients.

Gastrointestinal studies
Gastrointestinal barium meal examination was performed in 2 patients (patients 1 and 2). Patient 1 showed enteroplegia and secondary megacolon. Patient 2 showed incomplete distal esophageal obstruction and cardiospasm. Gastroscopy examination was performed in patient 9 and showed esophageal and gastric ulcers. Chest computerized tomography (CT) scan examination was performed in 2 patients and showed megaesophagus and cardiospasm. 8 patients were found to have low intestinal obstruction by abdominal and pelvic CT scan examination.

Electrophysiological studies
The electrophysiological examination results of 10 patients were summarized in Table 4. The motor nerve conduction was abnormal in 2 patients. The sensory nerve conduction was abnormal in 3 patients. 8 patients showed nerve damages in needle electromyography examination. Fibrillation potentials and positive waves were present in 3 patients in mild muscle contraction. 2 patients showed monophasic pattern in strong muscle contraction.

Table 3 The other symptoms of acute autonomic neuropathy

Case	Pupil	Urinary system	Orthostatic hypotension	Tachycardia	Myodynamia[aa] UL L/R	Myodynamia[aa] LL L/R	Deep tendon reflexes B/P/Ac	Sensory deficits
1	ARL	uroschesis	−	+	IV/IV	III/III	A/A/A	−
2	anisocoria, ARL	uroschesis	Syncope	+	V⁻/V⁻	V⁻/V⁻	N/R/R	tingling
3	ARL	uroschesis	Syncope	+	V/V	IV/IV	N/R/R	−
4	ASP	−	Syncope	+	V/V	IV/IV	R/R/R	−
5	mydriasis, anisocoria, ARL	−	−	+	V/V	V/V	N/N/N	SP tenderness
6	anisocoria, ARL	delayedu- rination	Syncope	+	V⁻/V⁻	V⁻/V⁻	N/N/N	tenderness
7	−	uroschesis	−	+	III/IV	III/IV	R/A/A	−
8	mydriasis, ARL	oliguria	−	−	V/V	V/V	R/R/R	tenderness
9	ARL	uroschesis	−	−	IV/IV	IV/IV	N/N/N	numbness SP
10	mydriasis, anisocoria, ARL	−	−	−	V/V	V/V	A/A/A	tenderness
11	−	−	−	−	III/III	IV/IV	N/N/N	−

+: present; −: absence
Pupil: ARL = absence of reaction to light; ASP = abnormal shape of pupils;
Myodynamia: [aa] = using MRC grading system; LL = lower limb; L = left; R = right; UL = upper limb;
Deep tendon reflexes: A = absent; Ac = Achilles tendon; B = biceps tendon; N = normal; R = reduced; P = patellar tendon
Sensory deficits: SP = spontaneous pain

Table 4 The results of nerve conduction and needle EMG

Table 4 The results of nerve conduction and needle EMG

MCV (n, %)

Nerve	n	CV		AMP	
		N	R	N	R
CPN	10	10 (100%)	0	10 (100%)	0
TN	10	9 (90%)	1 (10%)	10 (100%)	0
MN	10	9 (90%)	1 (10%)	9 (90%)	1 (10%)
UN	10	9 (90%)	1 (10%)	9 (90%)	1 (10%)

SCV (n,%)

Nerve	n	CV		AMP	
		N	R	N	R
SN	10	8 (80%)	2 (20%)	9 (90%)	1 (20%)
MN	10	9 (90%)	1 (10%)	8 (80%)	2 (20%)
UN	10	9 (90%)	1 (10%)	8 (80%)	2 (20%)

Needle EMG (n,%)

Muscle	n	Prolongation of MUAP duration	FP, PSP	Abnormal RP monophase
BB	10	2 (20%)	3 (30%)	2 (20%)
ATM	8	1 (12.5%)	3 (37.5)	2 (25%)
QFM	9	2 (22.22%)	3 (33.33%)	2 (22.22%)
EDCM	9	3 (33.33%)	1 (11.11%)	1 (11.11%)

AMP Amplitude, *ATM* anterior tibial muscle, *BB* biceps brachii, *CPN* common peroneal nerve, *CV* conduction velocity, *EDCM* extensor digitorum communis muscle, *EMG* electromyogram, *FP* fibrillation potential, *MCV* motor conduction velocity, *MN* median nerve, *MUAP* motor unit action potential, *N* normal, *PSP* positive shape potential, *QFM* quadriceps femoris muscle, *R* reduced, *RP* recruitment pattern, *SCV* sensory conduction velocity, *SN* sural nerve, *TN* tibial nerve, *UN* ulnar nerve

The ECG results showed sinus tachycardia in 10 cases, P-R intervals of mild extension in 2 cases, and high-peaked P wave in 2 cases.

Laboratory investigations

The cerebrospinal fluids (CSF) were obtained in 10 of 11 patients. The CSF protein level was elevated in 3 patients (patients 2, 3, and 4). Patient 9 showed dissociation of protein from cell in CSF. 2 patients displayed oligoclonal band in CSF. In one patient, only the value of CSF-IgG elevated, and in another patient, the value of CSF-IgG, IgA, and IgM elevated simultaneously. Infection markers were detected in 2 patients. 1 patient showed C-reactive protein increasing and 1 patient showed elevating erythrocyte sedimentation rate. 1 case was positive for herpes simplex virus IgM antibody. Another was simultaneously positive for Epstein Barr Virus and herpes simplex virus antibody. No other serological or etiological abnormality was noted in laboratory studies.

Treatment and follow-up

The treatments of each patient were listed in Table 5. IVIg combined with intravenous glucocorticoid (methylprednisolone or dexamethasone) was administered to 8 patients. 4 of these patients were additionally administered with gabapentin. Patients 1 and 3 were treated with IVIg alone, whereas patient 6 received other symptomatic treatment. Patients administered with intravenous glucocorticoid were subsequently given glucocorticoid orally. In addition, supportive treatment was administered to all the patients with gastrointestinal symptoms. These treatments included omeprazole to suppress gastric acid secretion, vitamin B6 to ease vomiting, Marzulene-S granules (l-

glutamine and azulene sodium sulfonate) to protect the gastric mucosa, and domperidone or mosapride to promote gastrointestinal motility. Four patients were severely ill, and their functional status was 5 at peak phase. 2 of these patients died within 1 year since the onset of AAN. Cyclophosphamide was administered in patient 11 as symptoms continued to exacerbate during treatment. A slight alleviation of autonomic symptoms was noted in patient 9 after 1 year of follow-up. The functional status of 8 patients was 4 at peak phase. Gradual recovery, especially autonomic symptoms, was observed in these patients after several months of follow-up.

The autonomic abnormalities of different systems recovered differently. Gastrointestinal symptoms were difficult to alleviate, and with high recurrence rate. Abnormal secretion of glands and sensory deficits recovered significantly, although they tended to persist for a long time. Urinary system dysfunction stopped progressing after the initial treatment and recovered completely in the end. 2 patients showed complete recovery from orthostatic hypotension at discharge. The other 2 patients exhibited mild improvement.

Discussion

Gastrointestinal dysfunction was the most common initial symptom. Most patients suffered from gastrointestinal dysfunction especially unexplained vomiting at the onset of this disease. These symptoms showed little improvement even after symptomatic treatment in gastrointestinal department. Some even exacerbated. Most patients presented significant weight loss and suffered from severe malnutrition, even cachexia. Besides, although the initial symptoms of some patients were limb weaknesses, gastrointestinal symptoms appeared and gradually became prominent subsequently. Early diagnosis was difficult through the course of the disease because of the lack of featured symptoms. The duration from onset to diagnosis was more than one month in most patients. The longest duration was eight months. We hope that pediatric gastroenterologist may notice some subtle difference between these symptoms and their classic cases. Therefore, patients can seek for help from specialists earlier.

The main clinical manifestation of AAN is autonomic dysfunction with two main aspects—cholinergic and noradrenergic abnormalities. In our patients, the former is featured with parasympathetic disorder, involving gastrointestinal dysfunction, loss of pupillary constriction, atony of the bladder, impaired salivation, and sweating. The unchanged HR in oculocardiac reflex test and carotid sinus reflex test can also indicate its existence. The latter is featured with orthostatic hypotension and positive Lying–Standing test, and it has been found in 4 patients who also presented cholinergic

Table 5 The treatment and follow-up

Case	Treatment	Modified Rankin Scale		
		peak	discharged	1 year
1	IVIg	4	3	ND
2	IVIg, IVGC	5	5	Dead
3	IVIg	4	4	3
4	IVIg, IVGC	4	3	1
5	IVIg, IVGC	4	3	2
6	ST	4	3	ND
7	IVIg, IVGC	5	4	ND
8	IVIg,IVGC, gabapentn	4	3	1
9	IVIg,IVGC, gabapentn	5	5	4
10	IVIg,IVGC, gabapentn	4	3	1
11	IVIg,IVGC Cyclophosphamide	5	5	Dead

IVIg intravenous immunoglobulin, *IVGC* intravenous glucocorticoid, *ND* not determin

abnormities. The other 7 patients only presented cholinergic abnormalities, which conformed to the typical manifestations of AAN with only cholinergic autonomic dysfunction [14]. Some literatures have pointed that acute cholinergic dysfunction particularly affected younger people [15].

According to the literature, some patients exhibited somatic motor or sensory dysfunction [16]. A few patients complained of limb weakness, distal muscular atrophy, and distal limb sensory disturbance [17]. Distal sensory deficits and variable limb weaknesses were also observed in our study. Nerve conduction was normal in most patients. Needle electromyography showed nerve damages in 8 patents. Some studies revealed that the lesion is peripheral [1]. Thus, we suspected that the reason of motor dysfunction may be dystrophia of muscular tissue caused by denervation. 10 patients showed malnutrition even cachexia and this may be the reason of increasing motor dysfunction.

The treatment of AAN to date is mainly immune regulation involving IVIg and plasma exchange. Meanwhile, supportive treatment remains the cornerstone of management. IVIg treatment was very effective not only for sensory and motor symptoms but also for autonomic symptoms. 10 patients were treated with IVIg in this study. 8 of these patients were given additional intravenous injection of glucocorticoid. The symptoms still progressed in 4 patients even under immunomodulatory treatment. Some patients needed repetitive therapy. 2 of these patients died of severe malnutrition. Progression was ceased in other patients after the treatments. The sensory and motor symptoms recovered significantly, whereas partial autonomic symptoms tended to persist for a long time without interfering daily life.

The limitation of our study was that our sample came from the hospitalized patients, and the characteristics of this sample might be different from the overall characteristics of the affected population. Thus, more systemic studies are needed to help clinicians understand this disease.

Conclusions

The clinical manifestations of AAN are diverse, generalized, and non-specific. Gastrointestinal disorders were the most common initial symptoms. Symptoms of digestive system and abnormal secretion of glands were severe and more common than other symptoms. Most patients suffered from moderate or severe malnutrition. Cholinergic autonomic nervous functions were often disturbed in affected children. Most patients made favorable progress after treatment with IVIg combined with intravenous glucocorticoid. The mechanism of AAN remains unknown. The treatment recommendation is also not available. Further exploration is thus needed.

Abbreviations

AAN: Acute autonomic neuropathy; CNS: Central nervous system; CSF: The cerebrospinal fluids; ECG: Electrocardiogram; HR: Heart rate; IVIG: Intravenous immunoglobulin

Acknowledgments

Thanks to all participating medical centers to help us conduct this study and all the patients and their parents to provide clinical information.

Funding

The acquisition, analysis, and interpretation of the data and the writing of the manuscript were supported by the grants from Major State Basic Research Development Program (973; no. 2012CB517903) and the National Natural Science Foundation of China (nos. 81,471,329, 81,211,140,048, 81,201,013, 81,200,463).

Authors' contributions

LZ participated in the acquisition of data, manuscript drafting, and statistical analysis. CD participated in the design of the study and the acquisition of data. YW participated in the acquisition of data, manuscript revision, and statistical analysis. LL participated in the acquisition of data. QL participated in the acquisition of data. LZ participated in the design of the study, the critical revision of the manuscript for intellectual content. All authors read and approved the final manuscript.

Competing interests

The Authors declare that they have no competing interests.

Author details

[1]Department of Pediatrics, Chinese PLA General Hospital, Beijing 100853, China. [2]Department of Neurology, Beijing Children's Hospital, The Capital Medical University, Beijing, China. [3]Department of Pediatrics, First Affiliated Hospital of the People's Liberation Army General Hospital, Beijing 100048, China. [4]Center of Epilepsy, Beijing Institute for Brain Disorders, Beijing 100069, China.

References

1. Suarez GA, Fealey RD, Camilleri M, Low PA. Idiopathic autonomic neuropathy: clinical, neurophysiologic, and follow-up studies on 27 patients. Neurology. 1994;44(9):1675–82.
2. McDougall AJ, McLeod JG. Autonomic neuropathy, I. Clinical features, investigation, pathophysiology, and treatment. J Neurol Sci. 1996;137(2):79–88.
3. Freeman R. Autonomic peripheral neuropathy. Lancet. 2005;365:1259–70.
4. Feldman EL, Bromberg MB, Blaivas M, Junck L. Acute pandysautonomic neuropathy. Neurology. 1991;41(5):746–8.
5. Ishitobi M, Haginoya K, Kitamura T, Munakata M, Yokoyama H, Iinuma K. Acute dysautonomia: complete recovery after two courses of IVIg. Brain and Development. 2004;26(8):542–4.
6. Besnard M, Faure C, Fromont-Hankard G, et al. Intestinal pseudo-obstruction and acute pandysautonomia associated with Epstein-Barr virus infection. Am J Gastroenterol. 2000;95(1):280–4.
7. Clark MB, Davis T. A pediatric case of severe pandysautonomia responsive to plasmapheresis. J Child Neurol. 2013;28(12):1716–9.
8. Hanai S, Komaki H, Sakuma H, et al. Acute autonomic sensory and motor neuropathy associated with parvovirus B19 infection. Brain and Development. 2011;33(2):161–5.

9. Koike H, Atsuta N, Adachi H, et al. Clinicopathological features of acute autonomic and sensory neuropathy. Brain. 2010;133(10):2881–96.

10. Choi HG, Kwon SY, Won JY, et al. Comparisons of three indicators for Frey's syndrome: subjective symptoms, Minor's starch iodine test, and infrared thermography. Clin Exp Otorhinolaryngol. 2013;6(4):249–53.

11. Jiang Wu JJ. LiYing cui Neurology. 2nd ed. China: People's Medical Publishing House; 2013.

12. Futang Zhu YH, Jiang Z. Textbook of pediatrics. 7th ed. China: People's Medical Publishing House; 2002.

13. van Swieten JC, Koudstaal PJ, Visser MC, Schouten HJ, van Gijn J. Interobserver agreement for the assessment of handicap in stroke patients. Stroke. 1988;19(5):604–7.

14. Takayama H, Kazahaya Y, Kashihara N, et al. A case of postganglionic cholinergic dysautonomia. J Neurol Neurosurg Psychiatry. 1987;50(7):915–8.

15. Hart RG, Kanter MC. Acute autonomic neuropathy. Two cases and a clinical review. Arch Intern Med. 1990;150(11):2373–6.

16. Low PADP, Lambert EH, et al. Acute panautonomic neuropathy. Ann Neurol. 1983;13:412–7.

17. McLeod JG. Invited review: autonomic dysfunction in peripheral nerve disease. Muscle Nerve. 1992;15(1):3–13.

13

Pseudoperipheral palsy: a case of subcortical infarction imitating peripheral neuropathy

Mirza Jusufovic[1*], Astrid Lygren[1,4], Anne Hege Aamodt[1], Bård Nedregaard[2] and Emilia Kerty[1,3]

Abstract

Background: Vascular damage in the central hand knob area can mimic peripheral motor nerve deficits.

Case presentation: We describe the case of a woman presenting with apparent peripheral neuropathy. Brain magnetic resonance imaging and computed tomography angiography revealed an infarct in the precentral hand knob area, with significant stenosis in the right proximal middle cerebral artery trunk. Subsequent 3-Tesla magnetic resonance imaging of the brain suggested cerebral angiitis. The patient experienced improved hand function following combined glucocorticoid and cyclophosphamide treatment.

Conclusion: Vascular damage in the hand knob area should be considered when evaluating peripheral motor nerve deficits in the presence of normal nerve conduction velocities. The diagnosis of cerebral angiitis remains a major challenge for clinicians.

Keywords: Hand knob area, Peripheral motor nerve deficits, Stroke, Cerebral angiitis

Background

Vascular damage involving the central hand control network [1] can produce focal weakness of the fingers, with ulnar presentation [2], and/or a radial/medial distribution [3]. Vascular pathology in the hand knob area should be considered when evaluating peripheral motor nerve deficits in the presence of normal nerve conduction velocities. Here we report a case of subcortical infarct in the hand knob area, suggestive of cerebral angiitis, that presented as apparent peripheral neuropathy.

Case presentation

A 44-year-old, right-handed female presented with sudden hand motor deficits in her left hand. There was no trauma to the arm, she used no medications and she had no vascular risk factors.

Examination revealed severe motor deficits of the left hand with extension of the three ulnar fingers and wrist, muscle atrophy in the first dorsal interosseous muscle, and claw hand deformity without sensory deficits (Fig. 1a, b). According to the Medical Research Council scale examination revealed grade 1 in the left wrist flexor, grade 4 in the left wrist extensor, grade 3 in the left fingers flexor and

grade 4 in the left fingers extensor. Adduction and abduction of the left fingers were also severely impaired (grade 3). Deep tendon reflexes were mildly brisker ipsilateral to the affected hand. No Babinski sign was observed.

Cervical computed tomography (CT) was unremarkable. Peripheral motor nerve conduction velocities were normal. Small, discrete ischemic lesions appeared hyperintense on diffusion-weighted magnetic resonance imaging (MRI) sequence (upper arrows on Fig. 1c). The infarct was located in the right posterior part of the precentral hand knob area (upper arrow on 1d), near the central sulcus (lower arrow on Fig. 1d). CT angiography showed significant stenosis in the right proximal middle cerebral artery (MCA) trunk.

Transesophageal echocardiogram and carotid ultrasound did not suggest an embolic source. Hypercoagulable screening and levels of markers specific to systemic vasculitis were all normal. An embolism arising from the ipsilateral MCA stenosis was subsequently considered as the etiology of the patient's symptoms, and she received acetylsalicylic acid and clopidogrel for secondary stroke prevention.

At the 2-month follow-up, the patient complained of fatigue and progressive headaches. Cerebrospinal fluid analysis was normal. Follow-up 3-Tesla MRI with gadolinium contrast revealed focal wall enhancement in the

* Correspondence: mirza.jusufovic@medisin.uio.no
[1]Dept of Neurology, Oslo University Hospital, Oslo, Norway
Full list of author information is available at the end of the article

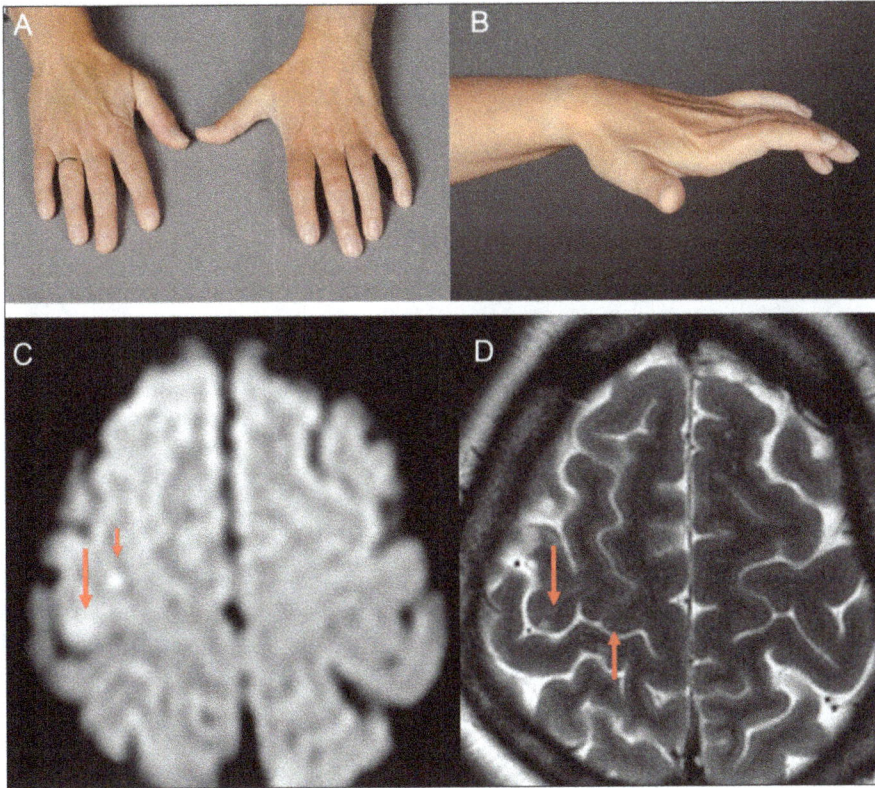

Fig. 1 Clinical photographs of the left hand and MRI of the brain. **a**, **b**. Clinical photographs showing claw hand deformity due to infarct in the hand knob area. **c**. Axial diffusion- and, **d**, T2-weighted MRI showing hyperintense signals (upper arrows on **c**) in the right precentral gyrus near the central sulcus (lower arrow on **d**), indicating an infarct in the hand knob area (upper arrow on **d**)

right proximal MCA (Fig. 2), indicating cerebral angiitis. Multiple stenoses at the same location were seen on digital subtraction angiography (DSA) (Fig. 3). Brain biopsy was not performed.

Cyclophosphamide infusions were administered with glucocorticoids over the subsequent 15 weeks. Left-hand motor function improved, aside from her left fifth finger.

Discussion

It is known that pure motor nerve deficits resulting from acute stroke can occur in the central hand control network [2], but also angular gyrus [4], the ventroposterolateral nuclei of thalamus [5], internal capsule, corona radiate, pontine base and/or ventromedial medulla. It is hypothesised that discrete functional cortical areas for

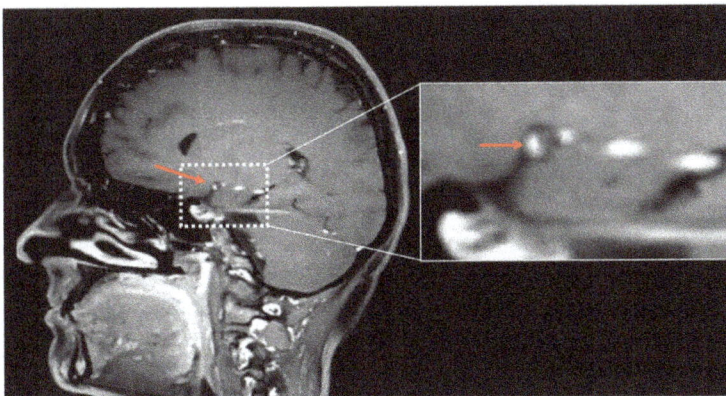

Fig. 2 3-Tesla MRI of the brain. T1-weighted (volumetric T1 turbo spin echo) 3-Tesla MRI of the brain with fat suppression and gadolinium contrast showing focal vessel wall enhancement (arrow) of the right proximal middle cerebral artery

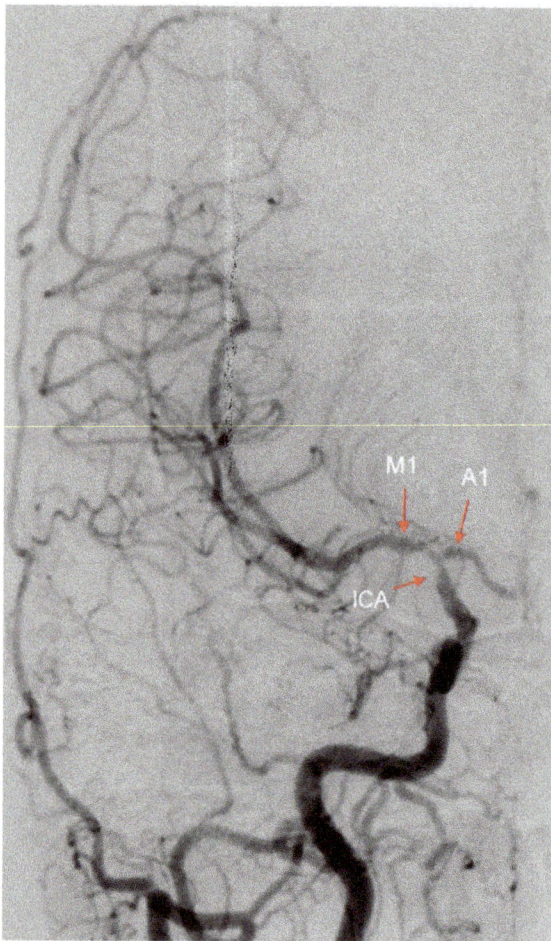

Fig. 3 Digital subtraction angiography of the brain. Multiple stenoses at the internal carotid artery (ICA), middle cerebral artery, M1 segment, and anterior cerebral artery, A1 segment were seen on digital subtraction angiography

neuron lesion and is often accompanied by weakness and fasciculation of the muscles innervated by the affected segments. No radiological evidence for cervical compression was found in our patient.

Functional MRI techniques suggest that the hand knob area, which controls hand motor function [9], is located in the posterior part of the precentral gyrus, near the central sulcus [9–11].

CT of the brain is often insufficient to diagnose the majority of ischemic lesions in the hand knob area, mostly due to the small lesional size and the subcortical location. Diffusion-weighted MRI is more sensitive to confirm the involvement of the precentral knob, and should be included as part of the standard evaluation. The treatment of an infarct in the hand knob area is dependent of the suspected etiology, ranging from arterio-arterial embolism to atherosclerotic infarcts [12]. However, little is known about the underlying pathological mechanisms of this stroke entity [12].

Diagnosis of cerebral angiitis is challenging. Brain biopsy remains the gold standard [13]; however, positive DSA, MRI and cerebrospinal fluid findings are sufficient to diagnose «probable» cerebral angiitis [13, 14]. Recent 3-Tesla MRI studies using increased magnetic field strengths have identified distinct vasculitic patterns, with arterial wall thickening and enhancement in both proximal and distal small intracranial vessels [15–17], that can remain stable for more than 12 months (median follow-up 13.5 months) [16]. 3-Tesla MRI to detect arterial wall inflammation may therefore become the favored criterion for diagnosing cerebral angiitis [17]. Nevertheless, other causes of arterial wall enhancement (e.g., atherosclerosis, radiation vasculopathy, infection, and vasospasm) must be excluded, and studies in a wider range of disorders are required to properly define the role of 3-Tesla MRI in the diagnostic process [17]. It is also possible that our patient had pseudoperipheral palsy due to cerebral angiitis, which was not detected by routine nerve conduction studies.

Although long-term data are scarce, the early-phase prognosis of similar cases is typically good [12], possibly due to the functions carried out by the damaged cortical area being resumed via the recruitment of adjacent areas [18].

Conclusions

The current case underlines that vascular pathology in the hand knob area can cause claw hand deformity, leading the unwary clinician to suspect peripheral nerve problems. However, a subcortical hand knob infarct can imitate peripheral motor nerve deficits, and is easily overlooked. To best of our knowledge, an infaction in the hand knob area associated with cerebral angiitis has not been previously reported.

each finger exist and are sequentially arranged [6], which means that finger movements are controlled by a highly distributed network rather than by functionally and spatially discrete groups of neurons controlling each finger [7]. This is also supported by the findings of one study, in which none of the patients showed hand motor deficits limited strictly to one or a few fingers, but rather both radial and ulnar sided hand motor deficits in varying degrees. The authors suggested this to be a characteristic form of finger motor deficits due to a cortical lesion which is important to differentiate the clinical picture from lesions at other locations [8]. Clinicoradiological signs observed in our patient exhibiting pseudoperipheral neuropathy due to small subcortical infarction well support motor hand area in the motor homunculus in the hand area.

With a muscle hand atrophy, one should also look for compression of the ventral roots or of the anterior horns of grey matter in the cervical regions. The muscle atrophy in such cases is due to a longstanding lower motor

Consent

Written informed consent was obtained from the patient for publication of this Case report and any accompanying images. A copy of the written consent is available for review by the Editor of this journal.

Abbreviations

CT: Computed tomography; DSA: Digital subtraction angiography; ICA: Internal carotid artery; MCA: Middle cerebral artery; MRI: Magnetic resonance imaging.

Competing interests

The authors declare that they have no competing interests.

Authors' contributions

MJ is lead author, analysed and interpreted the case, conducted the literature search and wrote the manuscript. AL performed literature research and drafted the manuscript. AHA was involved in the clinical care of the patient, provided clinical information and commented on the manuscript. BN was involved in the imaging diagnostics of the patient, and commented on the manuscript. EK was involved in the clinical care of the patient, provided clinical information and supervised the writing of the manuscript. All authors read and approved the final manuscript.

Author details

[1]Dept of Neurology, Oslo University Hospital, Oslo, Norway. [2]Dept of Radiology, Oslo University Hospital, Oslo, Norway. [3]Institute of Clinical Medicine, University of Oslo, Oslo, Norway. [4]Dept of Psychiatry, Akershus University Hospital, Lørenskog, Norway.

References

1. Chen PL, Hsu HY, Wang PY. Isolated hand weakness in cortical infarctions. J Formos Med Assoc. 2006;105(10):861–5.
2. Phan TG, Evans BA, Huston J. Pseudoulnar palsy from a small infarct of the precentral knob. Neurology. 2000;54(11):2185.
3. Kim JS. Predominant involvement of a particular group of fingers due to small, cortical infarction. Neurology. 2001;56(12):1677–82.
4. Timsit S, Logak M, Manai R, Rancurel G. Evolving isolated hand palsy: a parietal lobe syndrome associated with carotid artery disease. Brain. 1997;120(Pt 12):2251–7.
5. Lampl Y, Gilad R, Eshel Y, Sarova-Pinhas I. Strokes mimicking peripheral nerve lesions. Clin Neurol Neurosurg. 1995;97(3):203–7.
6. Lee PH, Han SW, Heo JH. Isolated weakness of the fingers in cortical infarction. Neurology. 1998;50(3):823–4.
7. Celebisoy M, Ozdemirkiran T, Tokucoglu F, Kaplangi DN, Arici S. Isolated hand palsy due to cortical infarction: localization of the motor hand area. Neurologist. 2007;13(6):376–9.
8. Takahashi N, Kawamura M, Araki S. Isolated hand palsy due to cortical infarction: localization of the motor hand area. Neurology. 2002;58(9):1412–4.
9. Kim SG, Ashe J, Georgopoulos AP, Merkle H, Ellermann JM, Menon RS, et al. Functional imaging of human motor cortex at high magnetic field. J Neurophysiol. 1993;69(1):297–302.
10. Yousry TA, Schmid UD, Alkadhi H, Schmidt D, Peraud A, Buettner A, et al. Localization of the motor hand area to a knob on the precentral gyrus. A new landmark. Brain. 1997;120(Pt 1):141–57.
11. Yousry TA, Schmid UD, Jassoy AG, Schmidt D, Eisner WE, Reulen HJ, et al. Topography of the cortical motor hand area: prospective study with functional MR imaging and direct motor mapping at surgery. Radiology. 1995;195(1):23–9.
12. Peters N, Muller-Schunk S, Freilinger T, During M, Pfefferkorn T, Dichgans M. Ischemic stroke of the cortical "hand knob" area: stroke mechanisms and prognosis. J Neurol. 2009;256(7):1146–51.
13. Birnbaum J, Hellmann DB. Primary angiitis of the central nervous system. Arch Neurol. 2009;66(6):704–9.
14. Salvarani C, Brown Jr RD, Hunder GG. Adult primary central nervous system vasculitis. Lancet. 2012;380(9843):767–77.
15. Mandell DM, Matouk CC, Farb RI, Krings T, Agid R, terBrugge K, et al. Vessel wall MRI to differentiate between reversible cerebral vasoconstriction syndrome and central nervous system vasculitis: preliminary results. Stroke. 2012;43(3):860–2.
16. Obusez EC, Hui F, Hajj-Ali RA, Cerejo R, Calabrese LH, Hammad T, et al. High-resolution MRI vessel wall imaging: spatial and temporal patterns of reversible cerebral vasoconstriction syndrome and central nervous system vasculitis. AJNR Am J Neuroradiol. 2014;35(8):1527–32.
17. Swartz RH, Bhuta SS, Farb RI, Agid R, Willinsky RA, Terbrugge KG, et al. Intracranial arterial wall imaging using high-resolution 3-tesla contrast-enhanced MRI. Neurology. 2009;72(7):627–34.
18. Butefisch CM, Kleiser R, Korber B, Muller K, Wittsack HJ, Homberg V, et al. Recruitment of contralesional motor cortex in stroke patients with recovery of hand function. Neurology. 2005;64(6):1067–9.

14

Therapeutic options for chronic inflammatory demyelinating polyradiculoneuropathy

Richard J Bright[1,2,3*], Jenny Wilkinson[2] and Brendon J Coventry[3]

Abstract

Background: Chronic inflammatory demyelinating polyradiculoneuropathy is a rare acquired immune-mediated progressive or relapsing disorder causing peripheral neuropathic disease of duration more than two months. Many individuals with chronic inflammatory demyelinating polyradiculoneuropathy fail to make a long-term recovery with current treatment regimes. The aim of this study was to prospectively review the literature to determine the effectiveness of therapies for chronic inflammatory demyelinating polyradiculoneuropathy.

Methods: Articles published from January 1990 to December 2012 were searched for studies to treat adults with chronic inflammatory demyelinating polyradiculoneuropathy. Peer-reviewed full-text articles published in English were included.

Results: Nine placebo-controlled double-blinded randomised trials were reviewed to treat subjects with chronic inflammatory demyelinating polyradiculoneuropathy exhibiting various degrees of effectiveness. The most effect treatments were; three randomised controlled trials using intravenous immunoglobulin, a study comparing pulsed dexamethasone and short term prednisolone and rituximab all showed promising results and were well tolerated.

Conclusion: IVIg and corticosteroids remain first line treatments for CIDP. Therapies using monoclonal antibodies, such as Rituximab and Natalizumab offer the most promise for treatment of Chronic inflammatory demyelinating polyradiculoneuropathy however they also need further research, as does the use of stem cell therapy for treating Chronic inflammatory demyelinating polyradiculoneuropathy. Large randomised controlled trials and better patient selection are required to address responsiveness of CIDP patients to conventional treatments to elucidate mechanisms of action and future directions for therapeutic improvement.

Keywords: Chronic inflammatory demyelinating polyneuropathy, Peripheral neuropathy, Anti-myelin associated glycoprotein, Autoimmune diseases, Treatment, Plasmapheresis, IVIg, Corticosteroids

Background

Chronic inflammatory demyelinating polyradiculoneuropathy (CIDP) is an acquired peripheral neuropathy, with both T and B cell involvement [1]. It is the most common peripheral autoimmune demyelinating neuropathy with a prevalence of 1.2 to 7.7 per 100,000 worldwide, with a slight male predominance [2]. The disease involves progressive loss of immunologic tolerance to peripheral nerve components such as myelin, Schwann cell, the axon, and motor or ganglionic neurons [3,4]. There is increasing evidence that activated macrophages, T cells, and autoantibodies induce an immune attack against peripheral nerve antigens [4]. Complement-fixing immunoglobulin deposits are localised to the myelin sheath surrounding axons and antibodies to various glycolipids and myelin proteins are frequently detected in subjects with CIDP and other autoimmune neuropathies. Activated tissue macrophages comprise the final process in the demyelinating process by invading the lamellae causing focal damage to the myelin sheath [2]. The resulting demyelination affects spinal roots, proximal nerve trunks and major plexi that lead to loss of

* Correspondence: richard.bright@adelaide.edu.au
[1]Faculty of Health Sciences, School of Dentistry, University of Adelaide, Adelaide, Australia
[2]School of Biomedical Sciences, Charles Sturt University, Wagga Wagga, Australia
Full list of author information is available at the end of the article

strength and sensation, which may explain the variability in clinical presentation [4,5]. The common CIDP variants include unifocal or multifocal, pure motor, pure sensory, sensory ataxic and pure distal forms [4]. Relatively little is known about the pathogenesis of CIDP; however there are many theories proposed. The occurrence of CIDP in individuals with melanoma or those who have been administered melanoma vaccine has previously been reported, however this finding is quite rare [6,7]. As numerous carbohydrate epitopes are shared by melanoma cells and myelin molecular mimicry may be a key factor in the initiation of the condition. More commonly, CIDP may develop after bacterial or viral infection particularly viral hepatitis and post vaccination. It has been suggested that viral and bacterial components have antigenic similarities to the body's own proteins leading to an auto-immune reaction, or alterations in T cell function [8,9].

Currently there are no biomarkers or no clear genetic predisposition, although approximately 20% of sufferers have paraproteins in their serum, including anti-myelin associated glycoprotein (MAG) antibodies and elevated cerebrospinal fluid protein levels [3]. Antibodies to GM1 ganglioside have been reported in 23% of patients with CIDP [10], while other researchers have observed increased frequency of other antibodies directed against peripheral nerve antigens and in HLA antigens [11,12]. CIDP can be described as a spectrum of diseases requiring early recognition to enable optimum treatment management. The disease follows a progressive, monophasic or relapsing remitting course with clinical signs of CIDP being proximal and distal weakness (usually symmetrical), sensory involvement (numbness) and areflexia. Nerve conduction in CIDP patients may exhibit prolonged distal motor latency, slowed conduction velocity, partial conduction block and delayed or absent F-wave [13]. Current treatments for CIDP include immunomodulating, anti-inflammatory and immunosuppressive drugs, and these have varying degrees of effectiveness. The most commonly used treatments for CIDP include; corticosteroids, intravenous immunoglobulin (IVIg) and plasma exchange (PE). CIDP may improve spontaneously without any intervention making it difficult to judge drug efficacy in small clinical trials [14,15]. Newer immunotherapies targeting B cells, T cells, transmigration molecules and signal transduction pathways may have potential for treating CIDP. This systematic review evaluates the safety and efficacy of randomised control trials treating chronic inflammatory demyelinating polyradiculoneuropathy.

Methods
Literature search
PubMed, Embase and The Cochrane Neuromuscular Disease Group Trials Specialized Register were searched from January 1990 to December 2012 inclusive for published articles on 'chronic inflammatory demyelinating polyradiculoneuropathy' and 'treatment'. Medical subject heading (MeSH) search terms were used to search PubMed and a keyword search were used if required. Keyword search terms used were; "chronic inflammatory demyelinating polyneuropathy" or "CIDP" or "chronic inflammatory polyneuropathy" or "autoimmune neuropathies" combined with "drug therapy" or "treatment" or "therapy" or "randomised control trial" or "clinical trial". Included in this study were double blind randomised controlled trials for treating CIDP. All current and emerging treatments for CIDP were included in the study and papers were excluded if the diagnosis of CIDP was considered secondary to an underlying disorder.

Study selection and participants
When journal articles did not publish the necessary data for the analyses, attempts were made to contact the authors. This study included adult patients of both sexes diagnosed with CIDP according to the criteria for diagnosis; clinically accepted electrodiagnostic criteria, progression of weakness lasting more than eight weeks and increased cerebrospinal fluid protein [16,17]. However there are numerous sets of accepted criteria for the diagnosis of CIDP, with many variables and there is not one uniform set of criteria. Papers were excluded if subjects had another systemic disease, family history of CIDP or drug or toxin exposure known to cause CIDP. No restrictions were set on suitable settings for involvement in this review.

Assessment of methodological quality
Studies used in the systematic review were assessed for levels of concealment of allocation at randomisation and internal validity to determine if any bias was present. Quality of evidence for each study was graded from very low to high using GRADEprofiler (http://ims.cochrane.org/gradepro). Each paper was assessed for risk of bias, inconsistency, indirectness, imprecision, publication bias, large effect, plausible confounding would change the effect and dose–response gradient. Each item was graded as either; No- negligible, Level 1- Serious or Level 2- Very Serious. GRADEprofiler software utilised these parameters to report a summarised measure of the quality of evidence from; very low, low, moderate to high (Table 1).

Statistical analysis
For the nine randomised controlled trials in this analysis, the proportion of patients with significant improvement in disability or the proportion that exhibited adverse effects for the treatment were used to calculate the odds ratio and 95% confidence intervals for each study. Assumed and corresponding risks (95% confidence interval) were calculated using GRADEprofiler Version 3.6 software. A summary of findings was also created using GRADEprofiler software.

Table 1 Summary of findings and quality assessment for the qualitative analysis using grade profiler software

Outcomes / Intervention and comparison intervention	Randomised clinical studies to treat CIDP- summary of findings			Quality of the evidence (GRADE)	References
	Illustrative comparative risks* (95% CI)		No of participants (studies)		
	Assumed risk With comparator	Corresponding risk With intervention			
Greater than 20% reduction in mean weekly dose of corticosteroids or IVIG					
Methotrexate/placebo (OR OR 1.38, 95% CI 0.5-3.87)	438 per 1000	518 per 1000 (280 to 751)	59 (1 study)	⊕⊕⊕⊝ Moderate	[18]
Disease progression @ 32 weeks					
Interferon/placebo	474 per 1000	343 per 1000 (146 to 620)	54 (1 study)	⊕⊕⊕⊝ Moderate	[20]
Responders					
Immunoadsorption/IVIG	500 per 1000	800 per 1000 (231 to 982)	13 (1 study)	⊕⊝⊝⊝ Very low	[22]
IVIG/placebo	222 per 1000	781 per 1000 (275 to 970)	18 (1 study)	⊕⊕⊕⊝ Moderate	[24]
IVIG/placebo	231 per 1000	266 per 1000 (62 to 671)	28 (1 study)	⊕⊕⊝⊝ Low	[25]
IVIG/placebo	207 per 1000	542 per 1000 (344 to 728)	117 (1 study)	⊕⊕⊕⊕ High	[27]
Rituximab/placebo	77 per 1000	520 per 1000 (49 to 958)	26 (1 study)	⊕⊕⊕⊝ Moderate	[31]
Adverse treatment related effects					
Kiovig (10% liquid immunoglobulin)/Gammagard (5% freeze dried immunoglobulin standard)	692 per 1000	714 per 1000 (321 to 929)	27 (1 study)	⊕⊕⊕⊝ Moderate	[29]
Remission at 12 months					
Pulsed high-dose dexamethasone/standard prednisolone treatment	375 per 1000	417 per 1000 (165 to 723)	40 (1 study)	⊕⊕⊝⊝ Low	[32]

Meta-analysis was performed using OpenMetaAnalyst open-source software (http://www.cebm.brown.edu/open_-meta) on eight of the nine randomised controlled trials. The study by the RMC Trial Group [18] titled *Randomised controlled trial of methotrexate for chronic inflammatory demyelinating polyradiculoneuropathy (RMC trial): a pilot, multicentre study*, did not fit the inclusion criteria for meta-analysis as the outcome measure was a reduction in the weekly dose of IVIg whereas the other studies measured response to the therapies. To assess overall efficacy from all the studies, we calculated odds ratio, and used a binary random-effects model to report an overall effect, heterogeneity and p-value together with 95% CI [19]. Statistical significance was declared if the p value was <0.05. Weighting for each study was also reported (Figure 1).

Data extraction
Titles and abstracts selected were checked by the first author who also determined which studies fit the inclusion criteria. In view of the fact that different studies used different disability scales, the primary outcome measure was defined as the proportion of patients with a clinical response during or after treatment. The strictest criteria to define improvement were used in each study.

Results
The search terms and additional searches resulted in the identification of 540 papers from this 392 were unique (Figure 2). After reviewing the abstracts, a further 351 citations were discarded as they did not meet the inclusion criteria. After examining the full text of the remaining 41 articles a further 32 papers were excluded as they did not use widely accepted case definitions or were review articles. Nine studies met the inclusion criteria for analysis and are summarised in Table 1.

Comparison of methotrexate with placebo
RMC Trial Group [18] compared methotrexate with placebo for the treatment of CIDP. This multicenter, randomised double blinded controlled trial compared oral methotrexate (7.5 mg per week for four weeks, 10 mg for the next four weeks and finally 15 mg for the next 32 weeks) with placebo for CIDP patients who require either IVIg or corticosteroids. Fifty nine patients out of 60 completed the trial with the primary outcome being greater than 20% reduction in weekly dose of IVIg or corticosteroids. Fourteen out of 27 (51.9%) treated with methotrexate and 14 out of 32 (43.8%) treated with the placebo exhibited a greater than 20% reduction in the mean weekly does of corticosteroids

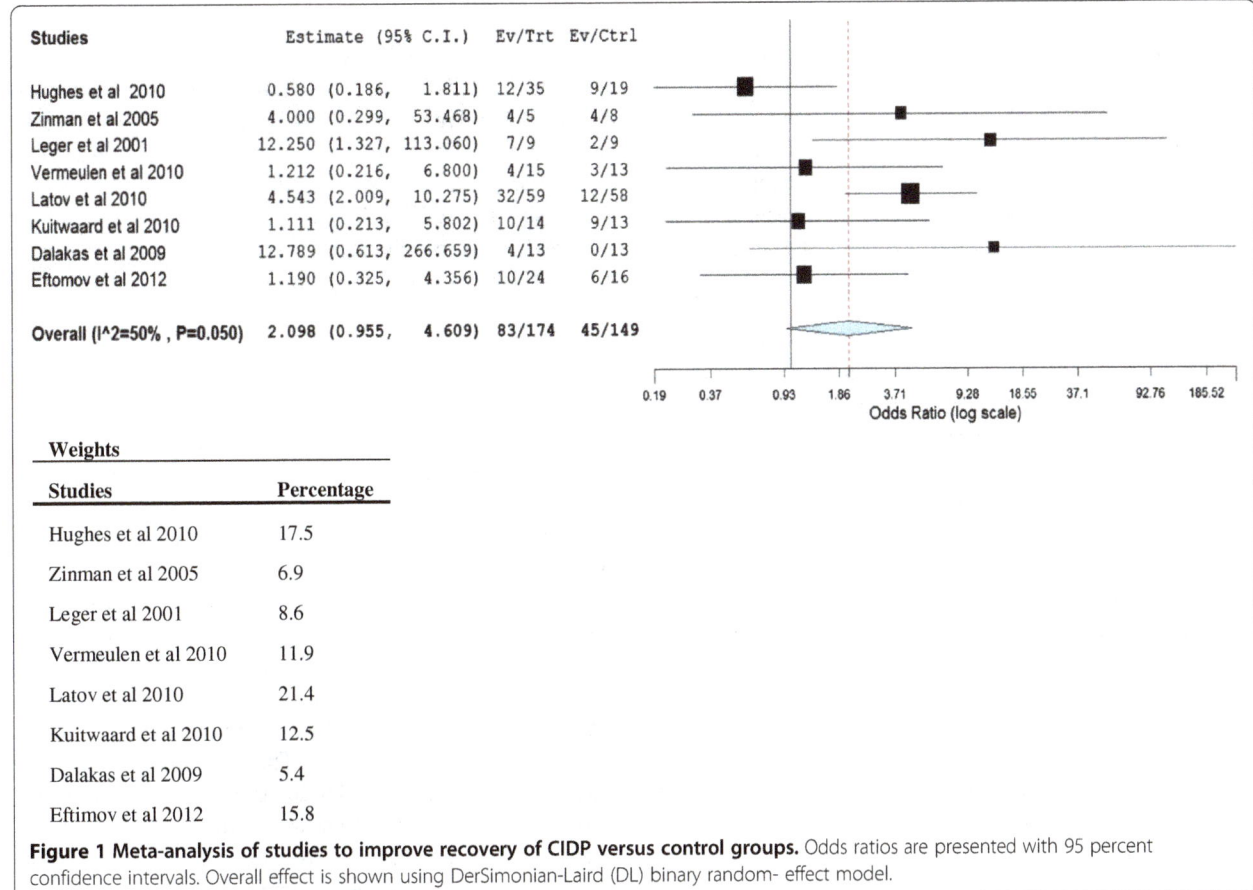

Studies	Estimate (95% C.I.)	Ev/Trt	Ev/Ctrl
Hughes et al 2010	0.580 (0.186, 1.811)	12/35	9/19
Zinman et al 2005	4.000 (0.299, 53.468)	4/5	4/8
Leger et al 2001	12.250 (1.327, 113.060)	7/9	2/9
Vermeulen et al 2010	1.212 (0.216, 6.800)	4/15	3/13
Latov et al 2010	4.543 (2.009, 10.275)	32/59	12/58
Kuitwaard et al 2010	1.111 (0.213, 5.802)	10/14	9/13
Dalakas et al 2009	12.789 (0.613, 266.659)	4/13	0/13
Eftomov et al 2012	1.190 (0.325, 4.356)	10/24	6/16
Overall (I^2=50% , P=0.050)	2.098 (0.955, 4.609)	83/174	45/149

Odds Ratio (log scale): 0.19 0.37 0.93 1.86 3.71 9.28 18.55 37.1 92.76 185.52

Weights

Studies	Percentage
Hughes et al 2010	17.5
Zinman et al 2005	6.9
Leger et al 2001	8.6
Vermeulen et al 2010	11.9
Latov et al 2010	21.4
Kuitwaard et al 2010	12.5
Dalakas et al 2009	5.4
Eftimov et al 2012	15.8

Figure 1 Meta-analysis of studies to improve recovery of CIDP versus control groups. Odds ratios are presented with 95 percent confidence intervals. Overall effect is shown using DerSimonian-Laird (DL) binary random- effect model.

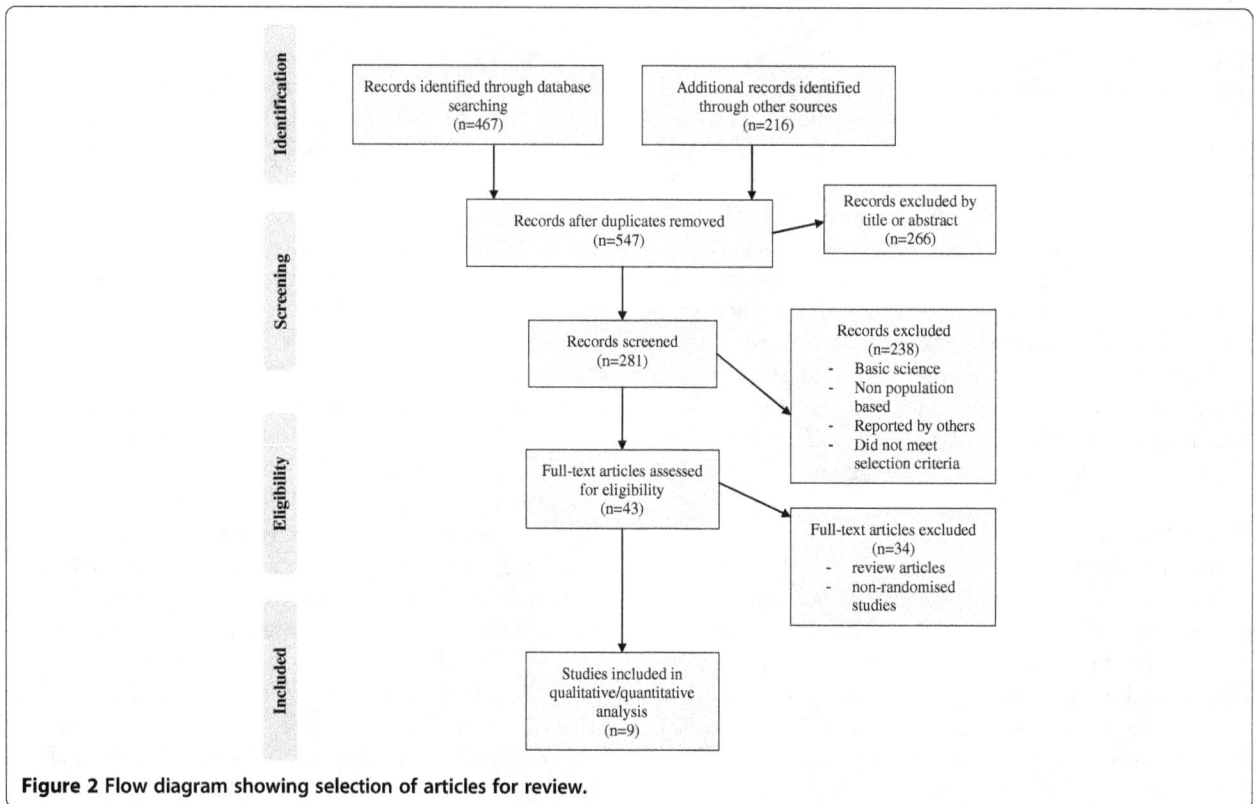

Figure 2 Flow diagram showing selection of articles for review.

or IVIg (OR 1.38, 95% CI 0.5-3.87) (Table 1). There were no serious treatment related effects in either group to methotrexate. Oral methotrexate did not show any significant benefit, however limitations in study design and high response rate in the placebo group may have been due to a higher than necessary dose of IVIg or corticosteroids that had been administered prior to the starting the study.

Interferon versus placebo

A clinical trial comparing interferon (IFNβ 1α) with placebo followed by IVIg was undertaken by Hughes et al. [20]. Forty five patients received either IFNβ 1α (30 μg or 60 μg intramuscular) once or twice a week plus placebo and 22 patients received placebo twice per week. Participants also received their stable IVIg regimen (2 to 5 doses per week, n = 31 received ≤ 0.95 g/kg IVIg and n = 32 received >0.95 g/kg IVIg) from week 1 through to week 16, and subjects who deteriorated post week 16 were re-administered IVIg until stable. The primary outcome was the total IVIg administered from week 16 to week 32, and secondary outcome was time to disease progression. There was no difference in the total IVIg administered after week 16 in both groups (p = 0.75), however the authors suggested IFNβ 1α reduced the total dose of IVIg in patients who required higher dose (>0.95 g/kg/month). The secondary outcome of a ≥ 2 point decrease in medical research council (MRC) sum score [21] and a 1 point

increase in the overall disability status scale (ODSS), was not significant between the treatment and placebo groups (p = 0.67). Twelve out of 35 (34.3%) subjects given IFNβ 1α and 9 out of 19 (47.4%) in the placebo group exhibited disease progression from the time of IVIg withdrawal at week sixteen (OR 0.58, 95% CI 0.19-1.81, p = 0.67) (Figure 1). Adverse effects were observed more commonly in the IFNβ 1α arm, which included flu-like symptoms, headache and fatigue. The dropout rate (>20%) resulted in the study being underpowered for the detection of smaller clinically meaningful differences, and the studies were subsequently classified as a class II. There was no effect on the primary and secondary outcome measures on the four dose regimes of IFNβ 1α therapy combined with IVIg.

Excorim staphylococcal protein immunoadsorption versus IVIg

A pilot study commenced at the Toronto General Hospital from 2003 to 2004 to evaluate the efficacy and safety of immunoglobulin removal by Excorim Immunoadsorption (IA) [22]. Twenty treatment naïve (other than prednisone) subjects with probable CIDP were randomly assigned to IA or IVIg (1 g/kg/day × 2 days). The drop-out rate over the duration of the trial was 35% due to illness and two deaths were reported, however they were unrelated to the treatment. Patients assigned to IA received three treatments over a 7 day period, with a total of 3 plasma volumes processed per treatment. Outcome measures included; nerve conduction parameters, grip strength and the Toronto Clinical Neuropathy Score (TCNS) [23] measured post initiation of treatment at 2 and 6 months. Two months after commencement of the study, 4 out 5 (80%) treated with IA and 4 out of 8 (50%) on the IVIg arm responded well to the treatment (OR 4.0, 95% CI 0.30-53.47) (Table 1 and Figure 1). At 6 months after treatment commencement 100% (4/4) of the IA arm and 50% (3/6) of the IVIg arm continued to exhibit substantial clinical response (p = 0.2). Both treatments were well tolerated, with minimal adverse effects. The study demonstrated the efficacy and safety of IA, however it was not sufficiently powered to detect significant difference between the two treatments. An appropriately powered randomised double-blind controlled clinical trial with stratification for disease duration would be required to determine the usefulness of IA therapy.

Efficacy of IVIg therapy for CIDP

Three randomised controlled clinical trials studying the efficacy and safety of IVIg were identified and included in the review (Table 1). Leger et al. [24] undertook a double-blind, placebo controlled crossover study of nineteen subjects with demyelinating neuropathy and persistent nerve conduction block. Participants were randomly assigned to receive either IVIg (500 mg/kg/day × 5 days) or placebo (1% human albumin) once a month for 3 months. After 3 months participants had a double blind clinical assessment. Responders remained on the same treatment and non-responders switched to the alternative study drug for the remaining three months. The outcome measures were MRC score, nerve conduction and self-evaluation parameters. Follow up evaluation was performed at 4 and 7 months. Eighteen of the 20 subjects were eligible for analysis, 9 in each arm of the study. At four months 77.8% (7/9) of participants who received IVIg first and 22.2% (2/9) who received the placebo responded well to the self-evaluation parameters (OR 12.25, 95% CI 1.33-113.06, p = 0.03). No serious treatment related effects were noted in this study. Although the trial was small and not powered significantly, it did show IVIg was effective treating the symptoms of in CIDP.

Vermeulen and colleagues [25] undertook a double-blind placebo controlled multicentered trial investigating the efficacy of IVIg. Participants were randomised to receive either IVIg (n = 15) or placebo (n = 13) (Table 1). The primary outcome measure was a one point decease on the modified Rankin scale [26]. Weakness of three arm and three leg muscles on both sides of the body were also assessed using the MRC sixty point scales. The assessments were done at day 1, then again between day 16 and 21 and also after the completion of the trial. Four of fifteen (26.7%) and 3 of 13 (23.6%) subjects who received IVIg and placebo respectively improved by one point on the

Rankin scale (OR 1.21, 95% CI 0.21-6.80). No significant difference was observed between the treatment and placebo groups possibly due to patient selection, treatment allocation and type II error may be a consideration due to the small sample size. There may be other factors in the placebo (20% albumin solution) that may have contributed to the clinical response seen in the placebo group, such as immunoglobulins other than IgG and proteins including albumin. It was concluded that better patient selection, selection of an appropriate placebo and larger participant number to statically power the study would be required. Further investigation would also be warranted to identify factors within the albumin fraction that may be beneficial to CIDP patients. The study did not mention adverse treatment related effects. Latov et al. [27] undertook a study investigating the timing, course and clinical characteristics of IVIg treatment for CIDP. One hundred and seventeen subjects with CIDP were randomly assigned to IVIg (Gamunex, n = 59) or placebo (0.1% albumin, n = 58) [27]. Participants receiving the IVIg, were initially administered a loading dose of 2 g/kg IVIg for 2 to 4 days followed by a maintenance dose of 1 g/kg IVIg /3 weeks for a maximum of 24 weeks. The main outcome measure was an improvement of at least one point on the INCAT disability score [28] at week six and maintained through to week twenty four. Fifty four percent (32/59) treated with IVIg were clinical responders versus 20.7% (12/58) of subjects who received the placebo (OR 4.54, 95% CI 2.01-10.28, p < 0.001).

These observations suggest that a loading dose followed by three weekly maintenance doses of IVIg may be required to achieve a maximum therapeutic response. No serious adverse effects were reported. No bias was detected in this study.

Comparison of two different preparations of IVIg

The primary objective of a study reported by Kuitwaard et al. [29] was to compare the efficacy and safety of two different brands of IVIg for the treatment of CIDP. Twenty seven subjects were randomised to receive either the standard 5% IVIg (Gammagard S/D freeze dried IVIg, n = 13) or the new 10% liquid IVIg (Kiovig, n = 14). The primary outcome measure was a change in overall disability sum score (ODSS), and the secondary outcome measure was the MRC sum score. There was no significant difference for all measures of outcome between the two treatments. ODSS difference from analysis of covariance with adjustment for baseline values was 0.004 (Gammagard minus Kiovig) (95% CI –0.4-0.4 p = 0.98) and MRC sum score was –0.58 (95% CI –1.9-0.7 p = 0.37). The number of subjects who reported adverse effects was similar in groups, 71% in the Gammagard group and 69.2% in the Kiovig group (p = 0.86, OR 1.11, 95% CI 0.21-5.80). This study demonstrated similar efficacy and adverse effects between Gammagard and Kiovig.

There was no bias detected in this study however, it was not possible to blind the nursing staff as dosages of the two IVIg preparations (Gammagard 5% IVIg and Kiovig 10% IVIg) had to be the same.

Comparison of Rituximab with placebo

Rituximab is a humanised murine monoclonal antibody directed against CD20, a cell surface protein found on B lymphocytes the precursors of antibody producing plasma cells, thus depleting circulatory B cells. The immunotherapy drug has showed promising results in treating autoimmune diseases and has been approved for the treatment of rheumatoid arthritis [30]. A double-blind placebo controlled trial was conducted to determine the efficacy of rituximab in patients with demyelinating neuropathy [31]. Twenty six subjects with CIDP were randomised to 375 mg/m^2 of rituximab (n = 13) or placebo (n = 13) (Table 1). Rituximab was administered in four, weekly cycles intravenously and the placebo consisted of an isotonic saline solution. The primary outcome measure was an improvement of ≥ 1 INCAT disability score at baseline and 8 months. Intention to treat analysis was not significant (p = 0.96) due to one subject treated with rituximab had a normal (0) INCAT disability score at the beginning of the trial. When participants were removed from the analysis because they did not improve with the study period the remaining data showed a significant improvement over the placebo (p = 0.036). Four out of thirteen (30%) of subjects treated with rituximab improved by ≥ 1 INCAT disability score compared to 0% in the placebo group (OR 12.79, 95% CI 0.61-266.66). No significant changes in the MRC score or nerve conduction studies were reported in the rituximab group. The most common side effects reported in the rituximab treated subjects were mild temperature increases and chills. Although the sample size was small, rituximab improved the clinical response in patients with treatment resistant demyelinating neuropathy.

Pulsed dexamethasone versus short term standard prednisolone

A multicentered retrospective randomised controlled trial compared pulsed dexamethasone prednisolone to treat CIDP [32]. Forty newly diagnosed subjects with CIDP were randomised to receive pulsed courses of oral 40 mg per day dexamethasone for six months (n = 24) or 60 mg prednisolone daily for eight months (n = 16) (Table 1). One participant from the prednisolone arm was lost during follow-up. Based on improvement of the INCAT disability scale and RMI [26,33] the treating neurologists were asked to score treatment effect, remission, stable disease and non-responders. Ten of 24 (41.7%) subjects treated with pulsed dexamethasone and 6 of 16 (37.5%) on daily prednisolone were in remission at follow-up (OR 1.19, 95% CI 0.33-4.36). The median interval from the

beginning of the remission to relapse was 11 months for prednisolone and 17.5 months for pulsed dexamethasone. Adverse treatment related events were low in both groups. There was no difference between treating subjects with either pulsed dexamethasone or standard daily prednisolone, however long-term remission was possible in 25% of sufferers with CIDP after only one or two courses of monthly dexamethasone compared with eight months of daily prednisolone. The authors failed to analyse the treatment related responses for statistical significance due to heterogeneity. At follow-up many of the non-responders were determined to have been misdiagnosed. Randomisation was achieved with a random number generator, however the study failed to conceal allocation and there was an absence of blinding [34].

Discussion

The purpose of this systematic review was to evaluate recent randomised clinical trials to determine the efficacy and safety of current therapies in the recovery of CIDP. Overall all treatment modalities for CIDP favoured a positive response (OR 2.10, 95% CI 0.96-4.61, p = 0.05) (Figure 1). Two important observations arose from this review; firstly, there is a need to use better objective scales to measure disability and assess long-term outcomes and responses to treatments. Secondly there is a need to be able to identify and omit subjects with stable or inactive disease, as they would be naturally less likely to respond to new or novel treatments. Recent research illustrated that up to 40% of subjects with CIDP were in remission or cured, but included in clinical trials, however CIDP patients can exhibit spontaneously improvement. This may explain why there was a high placebo response rate observed in some clinical trials [15,27]. Using a reliable scale such as CIDP Disease Activity Status (CDAS) in patient recruitment for clinical trials would provide more meaningful data with fewer patients. Constructing better powered larger studies would also assist in demonstrating potentially important small differences and in data interpretation. The data from the systematic review identified, that IVIg appeared to provide an effective treatment option for subjects with active CIDP, particularly evident in the studies by Zinman et al. [22], Latov et al. [27] and Leger et al. [24]. Further studies are necessary to investigate plasma factors other than immunoglobulins in IVIg, which may result in an increase in clinical response rates in trials using albumin as placebo. Replacing albumin with isotonic saline would be a better choice for the placebo. As discussed previously, this phenomenon was seen in an IVIg versus placebo trial undertaken by Vermeulen et al. [25], however the high clinical response rate observed in the control arm may also be due to patients being incorrectly diagnosed or possibly spontaneous recovery from the disorder. Rituximab showed promising results [31], however larger randomised clinical trials with long-term follow up would be required. Heterogeneity was moderate between the eight randomised controlled studies included ($Tau^2 = 0.58$, $Q = 14.05$, $I^2 = 50\%$ and $p = 0.05$) and due to the variability of the disease the binary random effect model was used in this study. This was to be expected as the treatments varied considerably and it was not the purpose of this review to combine studies. The systematic review did not include plasma exchange therapy, however two double crossover trials identified did not fit inclusion criteria and had been previously reported [35]. The two clinical trials using plasma exchange for the treatment of CIDP demonstrated a significantly better outcome in the treatment groups [36,37]. Due to the rarity and numerous variants of CIDP, limited large clinical trials have been undertaken. Clinical trials with similar autoimmune inflammatory diseases such as Guillain–Barré syndrome, multiple sclerosis and Crohn's disease may also provide some guidance in treatment options for those suffering from CIDP. Two compounds, Kv1.3 and KCa3.1 (voltage-gated potassium channel and calcium activated potassium channel inhibitors respectively) have shown promising results in animal studies for the treatment of autoimmune diseases such as multiple sclerosis, psoriasis and type-one diabetes may also benefit subjects with CIDP [38,39]. Currently a clinical trial is underway to observe whether alpha lipoic acid, an antioxidant with anti-inflammatory properties may prove effective to treat CIDP symptoms (ClinicalTrials.gov Identifier: NCT00962429). Hematopoietic stem cell transplantation for treating CIDP is also showing some promise [40], with a clinical trial actively recruiting participants (ClinicalTrials.gov Identifier: NCT00278629). With the development of antigen arrays, customised DNA vaccines may have potential to cure CIDP and other autoimmune disorders by tolerizing against an aberrant immune response observed in subjects with CIDP.

Conclusion

This systematic review demonstrated that IVIg and corticosteroids still provide the most effective first line treatment options for patients with active CIDP. The review also revealed there is a pressing need for further basic research into the pathogenesis of CIDP to ultimately develop new therapies for more effective treatment. Larger randomised controlled studies are required to define the validity and efficacy of treatments such as stem cell transplantation and immune-modulating agents. Better definition of CIDP is also required due to wide spectrum and the variability of clinical presentations of CIDP, together with the use of a valid disability scale such as CDAS, to ultimately lead to better subject selection for long-term studies of CIDP therapies.

Abbreviations

IVIg: Intravenous immunoglobulin; CIDP: Chronic inflammatory demyelinating polyradiculoneuropathy; MAG: Anti-myelin associated glycoprotein; PE: Plasma exchange; MRC: Medical research council; ODSS: Overall disability sum score; CDAS: CIDP Disease activity status.

Competing interests

The authors declare that they have no conflicting interests.

Authors' contributions

RB conceived the study and design, all acquisition of data, analysis and interpretation of data and drafting the manuscript. JW & BC critically revised the manuscript. All authors read and approved the final manuscript.

Author details

[1]Faculty of Health Sciences, School of Dentistry, University of Adelaide, Adelaide, Australia. [2]School of Biomedical Sciences, Charles Sturt University, Wagga Wagga, Australia. [3]Faculty of Health Sciences, Immunotherapy Research Laboratory, Royal Adelaide Hospital, Adelaide, Australia.

References

1. Hughes RA, Allen D, Makowska A, Gregson NA: **Pathogenesis of chronic inflammatory demyelinating polyradiculoneuropathy.** *J Peripher Nerv Syst* 2006, **11**(1):30–46.
2. Dalakas MC: **Clinical trials in CIDP and chronic autoimmune demyelinating polyneuropathies.** *J Peripher Nerv Syst* 2012, **17**(Suppl 2):34–39.
3. Dalakas MC: **Advances in the diagnosis, pathogenesis and treatment of CIDP.** *Nat Rev Neurol* 2011, **7**(9):507–517.
4. Koller H, Kieseier BC, Jander S, Hartung HP: **Chronic inflammatory demyelinating polyneuropathy.** *N Engl J Med* 2005, **352**(13):1343–1356.
5. Said G: **Chronic inflammatory demyelinating polyneuropathy.** *Neuromuscul Disord* 2006, **16**(5):293–303.
6. Anthoney DA, Bone I, Evans TR: **Inflammatory demyelinating polyneuropathy: a complication of immunotherapy in malignant melanoma.** *Annals of oncology: official journal of the European Society for Medical Oncology / ESMO* 2000, **11**(9):1197–1200.
7. Bird SJ, Brown MJ, Shy ME, Scherer SS: **Chronic inflammatory demyelinating polyneuropathy associated with malignant melanoma.** *Neurology* 1996, **46**(3):822–824.
8. Briemberg HR, Amato AA: **Inflammatory neuropathies.** *Curr Neurol Neurosci Rep* 2005, **5**(1):66–71.
9. Zeng XL, Nagavalli A, Smith CJ, Howard JF, Su MA: **Divergent effects of T cell costimulation and inflammatory cytokine production on autoimmune peripheral neuropathy provoked by Aire deficiency.** *Journal of immunology* 2013, **190**(8):3895–3904.
10. van Schaik IN, Vermeulen M, van Doorn PA, Brand A: **Anti-GM1 antibodies in patients with chronic inflammatory demyelinating polyneuropathy (CIDP) treated with intravenous immunoglobulin (IVIg).** *J Neuroimmunol* 1994, **54**(1–2):109–115.
11. Feeney DJ, Pollard JD, McLeod JG, Stewart GJ, Doran TJ: **HLA antigens in chronic inflammatory demyelinating polyneuropathy.** *J Neurol Neurosurg Psychiatry* 1990, **53**(2):170–172.
12. van Doorn PA, Schreuder GM, Vermeulen M, D'Amaro J, Brand A: **HLA antigens in patients with chronic inflammatory demyelinating polyneuropathy.** *J Neuroimmunol* 1991, **32**(2):133–139.
13. Czaplinski A, Steck AJ: **Immune mediated neuropathies–an update on therapeutic strategies.** *J Neurol* 2004, **251**(2):127–137.
14. Kuitwaard K, van Doorn PA: **Newer therapeutic options for chronic inflammatory demyelinating polyradiculoneuropathy.** *Drugs* 2009, **69**(8):987–1001.
15. van Schaik IN, Winer JB, de Haan R, Vermeulen M: **Intravenous immunoglobulin for chronic inflammatory demyelinating polyradiculoneuropathy: a systematic review.** *Lancet Neurol* 2002, **1**(8):491–498.
16. Yoon MS, Chan A, Gold R: **Standard and escalating treatment of chronic inflammatory demyelinating polyradiculoneuropathy.** *Ther Adv Neurol Disord* 2011, **4**(3):193–200.

17. Robertson EE, Donofrio PD: **Treatment of chronic inflammatory demyelinating polyneuropathy.** *Curr Treat Options Neurol* 2010, **12**(2):84–94.

18. Group RMCT: **Randomised controlled trial of methotrexate for chronic inflammatory demyelinating polyradiculoneuropathy (RMC trial): a pilot, multicentre study.** *Lancet Neurol* 2009, **8**(2):158–164.

19. DerSimonian R, Laird N: **Meta-analysis in clinical trials.** *Controlled clinical trials* 1986, **7**(3):177–188.

20. Hughes RA, Gorson KC, Cros D, Griffin J, Pollard J, Vallat JM, Maurer SL, Riester K, Davar G, Dawson K, et al: **Intramuscular interferon beta-1a in chronic inflammatory demyelinating polyradiculoneuropathy.** *Neurology* 2010, **74**(8):651–657.

21. Hermans G, Clerckx B, Vanhullebusch T, Segers J, Vanpee G, Robbeets C, Casaer MP, Wouters P, Gosselink R, Van Den Berghe G: **Interobserver agreement of Medical Research Council sum-score and handgrip strength in the intensive care unit.** *Muscle Nerve* 2012, **45**(1):18–25.

22. Zinman LH, Sutton D, Ng E, Nwe P, Ngo M, Bril V: **A pilot study to compare the use of the Excorim staphylococcal protein immunoadsorption system and IVIG in chronic inflammatory demyelinating polyneuropathy.** *Transfus Apher Sci* 2005, **33**(3):317–324.

23. Bril V, Tomioka S, Buchanan RA, Perkins BA: **Reliability and validity of the modified Toronto Clinical Neuropathy Score in diabetic sensorimotor polyneuropathy.** *Diabetic medicine: a journal of the British Diabetic Association* 2009, **26**(3):240–246.

24. Leger JM, Chassande B, Musset L, Meininger V, Bouche P, Baumann N: **Intravenous immunoglobulin therapy in multifocal motor neuropathy: a double-blind, placebo-controlled study.** *Brain* 2001, **124**(Pt 1):145–153.

25. Vermeulen M, van Doorn PA, Brand A, Strengers PF, Jennekens FG, Busch HF: **Intravenous immunoglobulin treatment in patients with chronic inflammatory demyelinating polyneuropathy: a double blind, placebo controlled study.** *J Neurol Neurosurg Psychiatry* 1993, **56**(1):36–39.

26. Bamford JM, Sandercock PA, Warlow CP, Slattery J: **Interobserver agreement for the assessment of handicap in stroke patients.** *Stroke; a journal of cerebral circulation* 1989, **20**(6):828.

27. Latov N, Deng C, Dalakas MC, Bril V, Donofrio P, Hanna K, Hartung HP, Hughes RA, Merkies IS, van Doorn PA: **Timing and course of clinical response to intravenous immunoglobulin in chronic inflammatory demyelinating polyradiculoneuropathy.** *Arch Neurol* 2010, **67**(7):802–807.

28. Merkies IS, Schmitz PI: **Getting closer to patients: the INCAT overall disability sum score relates better to patients' own clinical judgement in immune-mediated polyneuropathies.** *J Neurol Neurosurg Psychiatry* 2006, **77**(8):970–972.

29. Kuitwaard K, van den Berg LH, Vermeulen M, Brusse E, Cats EA, van der Kooi AJ, Notermans NC, van der Pol WL, van Schaik IN, van Nes SI, et al: **Randomised controlled trial comparing two different intravenous immunoglobulins in chronic inflammatory demyelinating polyradiculoneuropathy.** *J Neurol Neurosurg Psychiatry* 2010, **81**(12):1374–1379.

30. Edwards JC, Szczepanski L, Szechinski J, Filipowicz-Sosnowska A, Emery P, Close DR, Stevens RM, Shaw T: **Efficacy of B-cell-targeted therapy with rituximab in patients with rheumatoid arthritis.** *N Engl J Med* 2004, **350**(25):2572–2581.

31. Dalakas MC, Rakocevic G, Salajegheh M, Dambrosia JM, Hahn AF, Raju R, McElroy B: **Placebo-controlled trial of rituximab in IgM anti-myelin-associated glycoprotein antibody demyelinating neuropathy.** *Ann Neurol* 2009, **65**(3):286–293.

32. Eftimov F, Vermeulen M, van Doorn PA, Brusse E, van Schaik IN: **Long-term remission of CIDP after pulsed dexamethasone or short-term prednisolone treatment.** *Neurology* 2012, **78**(14):1079–1084.

33. Collen FM, Wade DT, Robb GF, Bradshaw CM: **The Rivermead mobility index: a further development of the Rivermead motor assessment.** *International disability studies* 1991, **13**(2):50–54.

34. van Schaik IN, Eftimov F, van Doorn PA, Brusse E, van den Berg LH, van der Pol WL, Faber CG, van Oostrom JC, Vogels OJ, Hadden RD, et al: **Pulsed high-dose dexamethasone versus standard prednisolone treatment for chronic inflammatory demyelinating polyradiculoneuropathy (PREDICT study): a double-blind, randomised, controlled trial.** *Lancet Neurol* 2010, **9**(3):245–253.

35. Mehndiratta MM, Hughes RA, Agarwal P: **Plasma exchange for chronic inflammatory demyelinating polyradiculoneuropathy.** *Cochrane Database Syst Rev* 2004, **3**, CD003906.

36. Dyck PJ, Daube J, O'Brien P, Pineda A, Low PA, Windebank AJ, Swanson C: **Plasma exchange in chronic inflammatory demyelinating polyradiculoneuropathy.** *N Engl J Med* 1986, **314**(8):461–465.

37. Hahn AF, Bolton CF, Pillay N, Chalk C, Benstead T, Bril V, Shumak K, Vandervoort MK, Feasby TE: **Plasma-exchange therapy in chronic inflammatory demyelinating polyneuropathy. A double-blind, sham-controlled, cross-over study.** *Brain* 1996, **119**(4):1055–1066.

38. Lam J, Wulff H: **The lymphocyte potassium channels Kv1.3 and KCa3.1 as targets for immunosuppression.** *Drug development research* 2011, **72**(7):573–584.

39. Wulff H, Calabresi PA, Allie R, Yun S, Pennington M, Beeton C, Chandy KG: **The voltage-gated Kv1.3 K + channel in effector memory T cells as new target for MS.** *J Clin Invest* 2003, **111**(11):1703–1713.

40. Remenyi P, Masszi T, Borbenyi Z, Soos J, Siklos L, Engelhardt JI: **CIDP cured by allogeneic hematopoietic stem cell transplantation.** *Eur J Neurol* 2007, **14**(8):e1–e2.

15

Effectiveness of the capsaicin 8% patch in the management of peripheral neuropathic pain in European clinical practice: the ASCEND study

Colette Mankowski[1], Chris D. Poole[1], Etienne Ernault[2*], Roger Thomas[3], Ellen Berni[3], Craig J. Currie[4], Cecil Treadwell[1], José I. Calvo[5], Christina Plastira[6], Eirini Zafeiropoulou[6] and Isaac Odeyemi[1]

Abstract

Background: In randomised studies, the capsaicin 8% patch has demonstrated effective pain relief in patients with peripheral neuropathic pain (PNP) arising from different aetiologies.

Methods: ASCEND was an open-label, non-interventional study of patients with non-diabetes-related PNP who received capsaicin 8% patch treatment, according to usual clinical practice, and were followed for ≤52 weeks. Co-primary endpoints were percentage change in the mean numeric pain rating scale (NPRS) 'average daily pain' score from baseline to the average of Weeks 2 and 8 following first treatment; and median time from first to second treatment. The primary analysis was intended to assess analgesic equivalence between post-herpetic neuralgia (PHN) and other PNP aetiologies. Health-related quality of life (HRQoL, using EQ-5D), Patient Global Impression of Change (PGIC) and tolerability were also assessed.

Results: Following first application, patients experienced a 26.6% (95% CI: 23.6, 29.62; $n = 412$) reduction in mean NPRS score from baseline to Weeks 2 and 8. Equivalence was demonstrated between PHN and the neuropathic back pain, post-operative and post-traumatic neuropathic pain and 'other' PNP aetiology subgroups. The median time from first to second treatment was 191 days (95% CI: 147, 235; $n = 181$). Forty-four percent of all patients were responders (≥30% reduction in NPRS score from baseline to Weeks 2 and 8) following first treatment, and 86.9% ($n = 159/183$) remained so at Week 12. A sustained pain response was observed until Week 52, with a 37.0% (95% CI: 31.3, 42.7; $n = 176$) reduction in mean NPRS score from baseline. Patients with the shortest duration of pain (0–0.72 years) experienced the highest pain response from baseline to Weeks 2 and 8. Mean EQ-5D index score improved by 0.199 utils (responders: 0.292 utils) from baseline to Week 2 and was maintained until Week 52. Most patients reported improvements in PGIC at Week 2 and at all follow-up assessments regardless of number of treatments received. Adverse events were primarily mild or moderate reversible application site reactions.

Conclusion: In European clinical practice, the capsaicin 8% patch provided effective and sustained pain relief, substantially improved HRQoL, improved overall health status and was generally well tolerated in a heterogeneous PNP population.

Keywords: Capsaicin 8% patch, Neuropathy, Pain management, Peripheral neuropathic pain, Topical analgesic, Numeric pain rating scale, Health-related quality of life

* Correspondence: etienne.ernault@astellas.com
[2]Astellas Pharma Europe B.V., Leiden, The Netherlands
Full list of author information is available at the end of the article

Background

Peripheral neuropathic pain (PNP) is caused by a lesion or disease involving the somatosensory system [1]. Common causes of PNP include traumatic nerve injury, surgery, diabetes, herpes zoster infection, cancer, chemotherapy and human immunodeficiency virus (HIV) infection [2]. PNP affects 7–8% of the population in Europe [3, 4] and can negatively impact quality of life, psychological wellbeing, sleep and work productivity [5].

The latest treatment guidance from the Neuropathic Pain Special Interest Group (NeuPSIG) of the International Association for the Study of Pain recommends several options for first line treatment of neuropathic pain (NP), including calcium α_2-δ ligands (e.g. pregabalin, gabapentin), serotonin/norepinephrine reuptake inhibitors and tricyclic antidepressants [6]. Despite proven efficacy, these therapies have limitations including inadequate pain relief, lengthy dose-titration periods, multiple daily dosing, dose-limiting adverse events, suboptimal adherence due to adverse events, and the potential for abuse and addiction [7–9].

NeuPSIG guidance suggests tramadol, the lidocaine 5% patch and the 179 mg (8% w/w) capsaicin patch as second line treatment options for patients with neuropathic pain [6]. Capsaicin is a selective, potent and high-affinity agonist for the transient receptor potential vanilloid type 1 (TRPV1) ion channel complex [10]. Application of high-dose capsaicin at the site of pain can defunctionalise TRPV1 leading to disruption of mitochondrial respiration and retraction of the nerve fibres, thereby reducing the pain response [10]. Localised treatment with the capsaicin 8% patch limits the potential for drug–drug interactions and avoids the need for dose adjustment in the elderly or in patients with renal or hepatic impairment [11].

The capsaicin 8% patch has been shown to reduce pain compared with placebo for patients with post-herpetic neuralgia (PHN), HIV-associated neuropathy (HIV-AN), and painful diabetic peripheral neuropathy [12–17]. In non-diabetic patients with a variety of PNP aetiologies, the capsaicin 8% patch demonstrated non-inferior pain relief versus pregabalin, with a more rapid onset of pain relief and fewer systemic side effects [18]. The capsaicin 8% patch is generally well tolerated with treatment-related side effects mostly limited to application site reactions such as erythema [12, 14].

A 12-week, non-interventional study of a single capsaicin 8% patch treatment demonstrated effectiveness and suggested a benefit of early treatment within six months of diagnosis [19]. The aim of this non-interventional study was long-term monitoring (52 weeks) of non-diabetic patients with PNP undergoing treatment with the capsaicin 8% patch in a real-world setting. This work reports the efficacy, re-treatment pattern, tolerability and health-related quality of life (HRQoL) associated with capsaicin 8% patch treatment in Europe.

Methods

Study design and participants

The ASCEND study (NCT01737294) was a Phase 4, multi-centre, open-label, non-interventional study (NIS) conducted between February 2012 and August 2014 in accordance with the principles of the Declaration of Helsinki, International Conference on Harmonisation Guidelines, and local ethical and legal requirements.

Patients were eligible for inclusion if they were at least 18 years old, recommended capsaicin 8% patch treatment by their treating physician, diagnosed with non-diabetic PNP and had provided written informed consent for participation in the study. Patients were excluded for the following reasons: neuropathic painful areas located only on the face, above the hairline of the scalp and/or in proximity to mucous membranes; history of diabetes mellitus; diagnosis of any major psychiatric disorder, or evidence of cognitive impairment; prior treatment with capsaicin 8% patch; hypersensitivity to capsaicin, capsaicin 8% patch excipients/adhesives, and/or local anaesthetics; participation in any other clinical study and/or receipt of an investigational drug within 30 days prior to screening visit; history of substance abuse (including alcoholism).

A detailed medical history was taken with particular emphasis on the primary PNP diagnosis. Patients were classified into one of six aetiology groups: PHN; HIV-AN; neuropathic back pain (NBP), including cases secondary to radiculopathy, polyneuropathy, plexopathy and ankylosing spondylitis; cancer-related neuropathic pain (CRNP); post-operative and post-traumatic neuropathic pain (PONP); 'other' neuropathies. Prior and concomitant medications were recorded at baseline and patients were categorised by the treating physician as being in the primary (first treatment received for NP), secondary (second treatment received for NP) or tertiary (at least third treatment received for NP) stage of the treatment pathway. The duration of pre-existing PNP was recorded.

Treatment

Study medication was prescribed in routine clinical practice. At each treatment visit, the size and location of the patient's painful area was assessed to determine the required area of treatment. Each capsaicin 8% patch contained 179 mg of capsaicin (640 µg per 1 cm^2) and up to four patches were allowed per treatment. Multiple treatment areas were possible; the recommended treatment time was 30 min for the foot and 60 min for other anatomical sites. Patients were followed up by phone or during clinic visits (Fig. 1). Scheduled follow-up contact

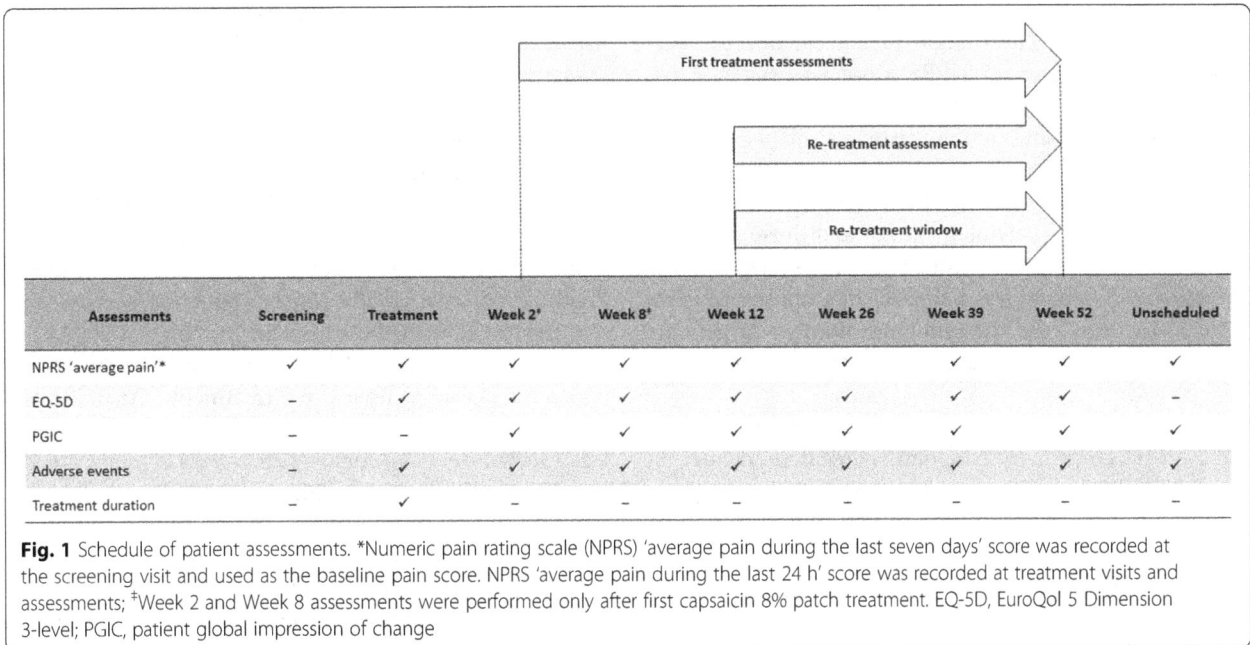

Fig. 1 Schedule of patient assessments. *Numeric pain rating scale (NPRS) 'average pain during the last seven days' score was recorded at the screening visit and used as the baseline pain score. NPRS 'average pain during the last 24 h' score was recorded at treatment visits and assessments; †Week 2 and Week 8 assessments were performed only after first capsaicin 8% patch treatment. EQ-5D, EuroQol 5 Dimension 3-level; PGIC, patient global impression of change

at Week 2 and Week 8 was made after first treatment only. Subsequent follow-up contact was made at Week 12, Week 26, Week 39 and Week 52. Multiple treatments with the capsaicin 8% patch were allowed, although intervals of at least 90 days between each application were recommended, consistent with the summary of product characteristics [20].

Efficacy and tolerability assessments

Patients assessed the intensity of their pain using an 11-point numeric pain rating scale (NPRS) ranging from 0 (no pain) to 10 (worst imaginable pain) [21]. NPRS 'average pain during the last seven days' score was recorded at the screening visit and used as baseline pain in all related analyses. NPRS 'average pain during the last 24 h' score was recorded at each treatment visit/assessment (prior to patch application). Sensitivity analysis was performed to exclude the effect of treatment outside of the recommended application time (<90% and ≥110%) on the pain response. HRQoL was assessed using the EuroQol 5 Dimension 3-level (EQ-5D) questionnaire [22]. The default York MVH A1 value set [23] was used to derive the EQ-5D index for all observations in this study. The change in patients' general state of health was assessed by the patient global impression of change (PGIC) instrument [24] using a 7-point Likert scale, ranging from 1 (very much improved) to 7 (very much worse). Patients were asked to indicate how they felt 'now', compared with how they felt before receiving their most recent capsaicin 8% patch treatment.

The primary endpoints were: (i) the percentage change in mean NPRS 'average pain' score from baseline to the

average of Weeks 2 and 8 following first capsaicin 8% patch treatment; and (ii) the median time between the first and second capsaicin 8% patch treatments. Secondary endpoints were: the percentage change in mean NPRS score from baseline to the average of Weeks 2 and 12 following re-treatment(s); the proportion of patients with a ≥30% or ≥50% reduction in mean NPRS score from baseline to the average of Weeks 2 and 8 for first treatment or the average of Weeks 2 and 12 for re-treatment (defined as ≥30% responders and ≥50% responders, respectively); the percentage change in mean NPRS scores from baseline to each assessment; median time between second and third treatment; number of capsaicin 8% patches used at each treatment; treatment area size at each treatment; the proportion of patients completing ≥90% of the recommended treatment duration at each application (≥27 min for the feet or ≥54 min for all other anatomical sites); change in EQ-5D index from baseline to each assessment; proportion of patients with improved overall health status versus baseline according to the PGIC (i.e. very much improved, much improved or slightly improved) at assessments; proportion of patients reporting adverse events (AEs) and serious AEs (SAEs). All study assessments were performed at scheduled follow-up visits and, with the exception of EQ-5D, at additional, unscheduled visits.

Statistical analyses

All analyses were performed using the full analysis set (FAS), consisting of all patients who received treatment with the capsaicin 8% patch. The planned primary analysis was to test equivalence between the PHN group and each of the other PNP aetiology groups for each co-primary endpoint. The margin of equivalence for percentage change in mean NPRS score was set at ±16% (comparable to a one-point change on the NPRS scale [25]) while for time to re-treatment, it was set at ±1 month according to clinical judgement. The decision to perform inferential equivalence testing between the patients in the PHN aetiology group and those in any of the other PNP aetiology groups for the analysis of the co-primary endpoints was based on the number of PHN patients recruited and the minimum number of patients in any one of the other aetiologies required to achieve 80% power.

Based on the actual number of PHN patients ($n = 89$), for the first co-primary endpoint (percentage change in mean NPRS score from baseline), recruitment in three of the aetiology groups (NBP, PONP and 'other') was sufficient to achieve 80% power. However, recruitment to the CRNP and HIV-AN aetiology groups fell below the minimum threshold; therefore comparison of neither group versus PHN was performed for this co-primary endpoint. An analysis of covariance was used to adjust for gender, country and baseline 'average pain' as fixed-effects covariates. Least squares mean estimates were provided with 95% confidence intervals (CIs). For the second co-primary endpoint (time to re-treatment), recruitment in all PNP aetiology groups fell below the minimum threshold to achieve sufficient power for testing equivalence. Therefore only descriptive time to event statistics derived using the Kaplan-Meier method were provided for each PNP aetiology group. Missing values were presented without imputation for all analyses. A sensitivity analysis was conducted in order to demonstrate consistency with the primary endpoint. Patients treated outside of the recommended application time (<90% [<27 min for the feet; <54 min for all other anatomical sites] and ≥110% [≥33 min for the feet; ≥66 min for all other anatomical sites]) were excluded from this analysis.

Results

Patient characteristics

A total of 429 patents were enrolled in the study and 420 patients received at least one treatment with the capsaicin 8% patch (FAS). Patients were from seven European countries: Austria (7 sites, $n = 65$), Greece (11 sites, $n = 88$), Italy (8 sites, $n = 30$), Portugal (11 sites, $n = 98$), Spain (7 sites, $n = 68$), Switzerland (2 sites, $n = 22$) and United Kingdom (5 sites, $n = 49$). The median age of the study population was 61 (range 21–98) years; 39.8% of patients were male; and the most common diagnoses were PONP (47.1%, $n = 198$) and PHN (21.1%, $n = 89$) (Table 1). The proportion of patients in the primary, secondary or tertiary stage of the treatment pathway

was 19.3%, 42.9% and 37.9%, respectively. Overall, patients had a median follow-up time of 370 days (interquartile range: 360–434).

Treatment exposure

At first treatment, the mean number of patches used was 1.5 (standard deviation [SD] ±0.7) and the mean treatment area was 306.4 (SD ±228.2) cm^2; both values remained consistent through successive applications (Table 2). A total of 239 (56.9%) patients received only one treatment with the capsaicin 8% patch, 181 (43.1%) patients received at least two treatments and 70 (16.7%) patients received at least three treatments. At first treatment, patches were applied to the following body areas: legs (36.2%, $n = 152$); torso (35.0%, $n = 147$); feet (16.2%, $n = 68$); hands (8.6%, $n = 36$); arms (8.3%, $n = 35$); and the head and neck (5.5%, $n = 23$), excluding areas above the hairline of the scalp and/or in proximity to mucous membranes. During first treatment, 388 patients (92.4%) completed ≥90% of the recommended duration of patch application. Similarly, 157 (94.0%) and 63 (98.4%) patients completed ≥90% of the recommended duration of patch application at second and third treatment, respectively.

Pain scores

Following first treatment with the capsaicin 8% patch, there was an overall 26.6% (95% CI: 23.6, 29.6; $n = 412$) reduction in mean NPRS 'average pain' score from baseline to Weeks 2 and 8 (co-primary endpoint) (Table 3; Fig. 2a). The findings of the sensitivity analysis were consistent with this result (-27.7%; $n = 254$). The primary analysis demonstrated equivalence between the PHN group and each of NBP, PONP and 'other' groups as the difference did not exceed the pre-defined margin of equivalence (Fig. 2a). Patients who received second and third treatments had similar reductions in their mean NPRS scores of 28.7% (95% CI: 22.9, 34.5; $n = 161$) and 27.3% (95% CI: 18.1, 36.5; $n = 59$), respectively from baseline to Weeks 2 and 12. Overall, patients had a 24.5% (95% CI: 21.1, 27.9; $n = 401$) reduction in their mean NPRS score from baseline to Week 2 and a 37.0% (95% CI: 31.3, 42.7; $n = 176$) reduction to Week 52 (Fig. 2b).

A total of 44.4% ($n = 183$) and 26.2% ($n = 108$) of patients were classified as ≥30% and ≥50% responders, respectively, after first treatment (Table 4). Of responders at Week 8, 86.9% ($n = 159/183$) retained responder status at Week 12 after first treatment. There was a small increase in the percentage of responders following re-treatment. The percentage of ≥30% responders after second and third treatment was 49.1% ($n = 79$) and 49.2% ($n = 29$), respectively (Table 4). The percentage of ≥50% responders at second and third treatment was

Table 1 Patient demographics and baseline characteristics (FAS)

	PHN (n = 89)	HIV-AN (n = 5)	NBP (n = 50)	CRNP (n = 22)	PONP (n = 198)	Other (n = 56)	Overall (n = 420)
Gender, n (%)							
Male	36 (40.4)	5 (100)	17 (34.0)	5 (22.7)	75 (37.9)	29 (51.8)	167 (39.8)
Female	53 (59.6)	0	33 (66.0)	17 (77.3)	123 (62.1)	27 (48.2)	253 (60.2)
Ethnicity, n (%)							
Caucasian	88 (98.9)	4 (80.0)	49 (98.0)	19 (86.3)	185 (93.4)	55 (98.2)	400 (95.2)
Asian	0	1 (20.0)	0	0	2 (1.0)	0	3 (0.7)
Black/African/Caribbean	1 (1.1)	0	1 (2.0)	1 (4.5)	8 (4.0)	1 (1.8)	12 (2.9)
Mixed/multiple ethnic groups	0	0	0	1 (4.5)	1 (0.5)	0	2 (0.5)
Not recorded	0	0	0	1 (4.5)	2 (1.0)	0	3 (0.7)
Median age, years (min–max)	72 (37–98)	52 (33–59)	63 (27–90)	59 (42–76)	54 (21–83)	60 (24–86)	61 (21–98)
Median duration of pain, years (min–max)	1.0 (0.1–73.2)	0.3 (0.2–13.6)	2.6 (0–40.0)	2.2 (0.2–8.1)	2.6 (0.1–50.1)	2.2 (0.1–29.2)	2.1 (0–73.2)
Treatment pathway, n (%)							
Primary	13 (14.6)	1 (20.0)	20 (40.0)	2 (9.1)	35 (17.7)	10 (17.9)	81 (19.3)
Secondary	48 (53.9)	3 (60.0)	14 (28.0)	13 (59.1)	78 (39.4)	24 (42.9)	180 (42.9)
Tertiary	28 (31.5)	1 (20.0)	16 (32.0)	7 (31.8)	85 (42.9)	22 (39.3)	159 (37.9)
Baseline 'average pain',[a] n (SD)	7.1 (2.0)	6.4 (1.5)	7.3 (2.0)	7.2 (1.5)	6.8 (1.8)	6.9 (1.8)	6.9 (1.8)
Mean number of concomitant medications,[b] n (SD)	1.8 (1.5)	1.4 (1.5)	1.5 (1.6)	2.2 (1.4)	1.9 (1.5)	1.7 (1.4)	1.8 (1.5)

[a]Average pain during the 7 days prior to screening visit; [b]Number of concomitant medications for neuropathic pain at screening visit. *CRNP*, cancer-related neuropathic pain; *FAS*, full analysis set; *HIV-AN*, HIV associated neuropathy; *NBP*, neuropathic back pain; *NPRS*, numeric pain rating scale; *Other*, other non-diabetic PNP; *PHN*, postherpetic neuralgia; *PONP*, post-operative and post-traumatic neuropathic pain; *SD*, standard deviation

30.4% (n = 49) and 30.5% (n = 18), respectively. These findings suggest that the proportion of responders was maintained with each subsequent capsaicin 8% patch treatment.

In a subgroup analysis, patients in the shortest PNP duration quartile of 0–0.72 years had a 36.3% (95% CI: 30.0, 42.6; n = 101) reduction in their mean NPRS score from baseline to Weeks 2 and 8 compared with reductions of 23.6% (95% CI: 17.1, 30.1; n = 104), 25.0% (95% CI: 19.4, 30.6; n = 104), and 21.8% (95% CI: 16.4, 27.2; n = 103), in the 0.72–2.1 years, >2.1–5.4 years and >5.4 years quartiles, respectively. Similarly, 62.4% of patients in the shortest PNP duration quartile (0–0.72 years) were ≥30% responders after first treatment, followed by 39.4% of patients in 0.72–2.1 years, 40.4% in >2.1–5.4 years, and 35.9% in >5.4 years PNP duration quartiles, respectively. In patients classified as being in the primary, secondary and tertiary stages of the treatment pathway, the change in mean NPRS scores from baseline to Weeks 2 and 8 was −30.5% (n = 80), −28.1% (n = 177), and −22.8% (n = 155), respectively.

Time to re-treatment

Patients had a median time from first to second treatment of 191 days (95% CI: 147, 235; n = 181) (co-primary endpoint) and a median time from second to third treatment of 301 days (95% CI: 245, 357; n = 70) (Fig. 3a). The median time to second treatment for the PHN and PONP groups was 180 days (95% CI: 116, 244; n = 40) and 161 days (95% CI: 120, 202; n = 97), respectively (Fig. 3b). Median time to second treatment could not be calculated for NBP and the 'other' aetiology groups within the period of the study and the HIV-AN and CRNP aetiology groups were excluded due to low recruitment.

EQ-5D

The mean EQ-5D health state utility score increased by 0.199 utils at Week 2 (from a baseline score of 0.345 utils), at least two-times greater than the minimally important difference of 0.074 utils [26]. This improvement was maintained to Week 52 following first treatment (Table 5). Responders to capsaicin 8% patch treatment reported the most substantial improvements in HRQoL. At Week 2 after first treatment, ≥30% and ≥50% responders had increases of 0.292 utils and 0.327 utils, respectively in their EQ-5D scores from baseline.

PGIC

Analysis of PGIC demonstrated that the majority of patients experienced an improvement (very much, much or slightly) in health status during the study (Table 6).

Table 2 Treatment exposure (FAS)

	PHN (n = 89)	HIV-AN (n = 5)	NBP (n = 50)	CRNP (n = 22)	PONP (n = 198)	Other (n = 56)	Overall (n = 420)
Patients treated at each application, n (%)							
First treatment	89 (21.2)	5 (1.2)	50 (11.9)	22 (5.2)	198 (47.1)	56 (13.3)	420 (100)
Second treatment	40 (9.5)	2 (0.5)	15 (3.6)	8 (1.9)	97 (23.1)	19 (4.5)	181 (43.1)
Third treatment	16 (3.8)	–	4 (1.0)	4 (1.0)	38 (9.0)	8 (1.9)	70 (16.7)
Mean size of treatment area, cm² (SD)							
First treatment	298.6 (168.1)	380.0 (138.6)	297.7 (196.9)	519.5 (404.9)	271.5 (209.7)	362.0 (263.9)	306.4 (228.2)
Second treatment	286.8 (169.3)	210.0 (99.0)	291.3 (160.6)	566.6 (387.9)	278.6 (206.4)	391.5 (300.5)	306.4 (225.0)
Third treatment	270.0 (190.6)	–	357.5 (230.7)	467.5 (113.5)	229.7 (211.8)	487.4 (412.4)	294.8 (248.8)
Mean number of patches (SD)							
First treatment	1.4 (0.6)	1.4 (0.6)	1.3 (0.6)	2.1 (1.3)	1.4 (0.7)	1.6 (0.8)	1.5 (0.7)
Second treatment	1.4 (0.6)	1.0 (0.0)	1.4 (0.6)	2.3 (1.2)	1.5 (0.7)	1.7 (0.9)	1.5 (0.7)
Third treatment	1.4 (0.7)	–	1.8 (1.0)	2.0 (0.0)	1.4 (0.8)	2.0 (1.3)	1.6 (0.8)
Patients completing ≥90% of recommended treatment duration[a], n (%)							
First treatment	84 (94.4)	5 (100)	47 (94.0)	19 (86.4)	184 (93.9)	49 (87.5)	388 (92.8)
Second treatment	37 (94.9)	2 (100)	12 (85.7)	7 (87.5)	81 (94.2)	18 (100)	157 (94.0)
Third treatment	16 (100)	–	4 (100)	4 (100)	33 (100)	7 (87.5)	63 (98.4)

[a]Recommended treatment duration times were 30 min for foot and 60 min for other anatomical locations. For patients treated on the foot, the treatment time corresponding to the percentage duration was 27–33 min for ≥90% to <110% and >33 min for ≥110%. For patients treated on other locations, the treatment time corresponding to the percentage duration was 54–66 min for ≥90% to <110% and >66 min for ≥110%. CRNP, cancer-related neuropathic pain; FAS, full analysis set; HIV-AN, HIV associated neuropathy; NPRS, numeric pain rating scale; PHN, postherpetic neuralgia; NBP, neuropathic back pain; Other, other non-diabetic PNP; PONP, post-operative and post-traumatic neuropathic pain; SD, standard deviation

Table 3 NPRS 'average pain' scores at baseline and Weeks 2 and 8 (FAS)

NPRS 'average pain' scores	PHN (n = 89)	HIV-AN (n = 5)	NBP (n = 50)	CRNP (n = 22)	PONP (n = 198)	Other (n = 56)	Overall (n = 420)
First treatment							
Baseline, mean (95% CI)	7.1 (6.9, 7.5) n = 88	6.4 (5.1, 7.7) n = 5	7.3 (6.8, 7.9) n = 50	7.2 (6.6, 7.8) n = 22	6.8 (6.6, 7.1) n = 198	6.9 (6.4, 7.4) n = 56	6.9 (6.7, 7.1) n = 419
Weeks 2 and 8, mean (95% CI)	4.9 (4.4, 5.4) n = 89	4.6 (2.0, 7.3) n = 4	4.8 (4.2, 5.5) n = 48	5.8 (4.9, 6.7) n = 21	5.2 (4.9, 5.5) n = 195	4.5 (4.0, 5.1) n = 56	5.0 (4.8, 5.2) n = 412
Percentage reduction, mean (95% CI)	29.7 (23.4, 36.0)	34.5 (7.6, 61.5)	30.9 (21.7, 40.1)	21.0 (11.6, 30.5)	22.3 (17.7, 27.0)	34.3 (27.3, 41.4)	26.6 (23.6, 29.6)
Second treatment							
Baseline, mean (95% CI)	7.1 (6.5, 7.7) n = 39	6.5 (3.6, 9.4) n = 2	7.7 (6.7, 8.7) n = 15	6.9 (5.9, 7.9) n = 8	6.8 (6.4, 7.2) n = 97	6.6 (5.7, 7.5) n = 19	6.9 (6.6, 7.2) n = 180
Weeks 2 and 12, mean (95% CI)	4.7 (4.1, 5.3) n = 39	3 (–) n = 2	4.3 (2.8, 5.8) n = 12	3.4 (1.6, 5.2) n = 6	4.9 (4.4, 5.4) n = 85	5.1 (4.1, 6.1) n = 18	4.8 (4.5, 5.1) n = 162
Percentage reduction, mean (95% CI)	30.5 (19.8, 41.2) n = 38	51.3 (29.2, 73.4) n = 2	44.9 (24.7, 65.1) n = 12	51.0 (24.3, 77.7) n = 6	25.0 (16.5, 33.5) n = 85	21.4 (5.2, 37.6) n = 18	28.7 (22.9, 34.5) n = 161
Third treatment							
Baseline, mean (95% CI)	6.9 (5.9, 7.9) n = 16	–	7.5 (4.6, 10.4) n = 4	7.8 (6.3, 9.3) n = 4	6.3 (5.8, 6.8) n = 38	6.8 (5.6, 8.0) n = 8	6.7 (6.3, 7.1) n = 70
Weeks 2 and 12, mean (95% CI)	3.9 (2.9, 4.9) n = 14	–	5.5 (3.5, 7.5) n = 4	5.0 (2.6, 7.4) n = 4	4.4 (3.7, 5.1) n = 29	5.2 (4.2, 6.2) n = 8	4.5 (4.0, 5.0) n = 59
Percentage reduction, mean (95% CI)	42.3 (26.8, 57.8) n = 14	–	25.4 (15.3, 35.5) n = 4	35.5 (8.8, 62.2) n = 4	23.1 (9.5, 36.7) n = 29	13.6 (−20.8, 48.0) n = 8	27.3 (18.1, 36.5) n = 59

CI, confidence interval; CRNP, cancer-related neuropathic pain; FAS, full analysis set; HIV-AN, HIV associated neuropathy; NBP, neuropathic back pain; NPRS, numeric pain rating scale; Other, other non-diabetic PNP; PHN, postherpetic neuralgia; PONP, post-operative and post-traumatic neuropathic pain

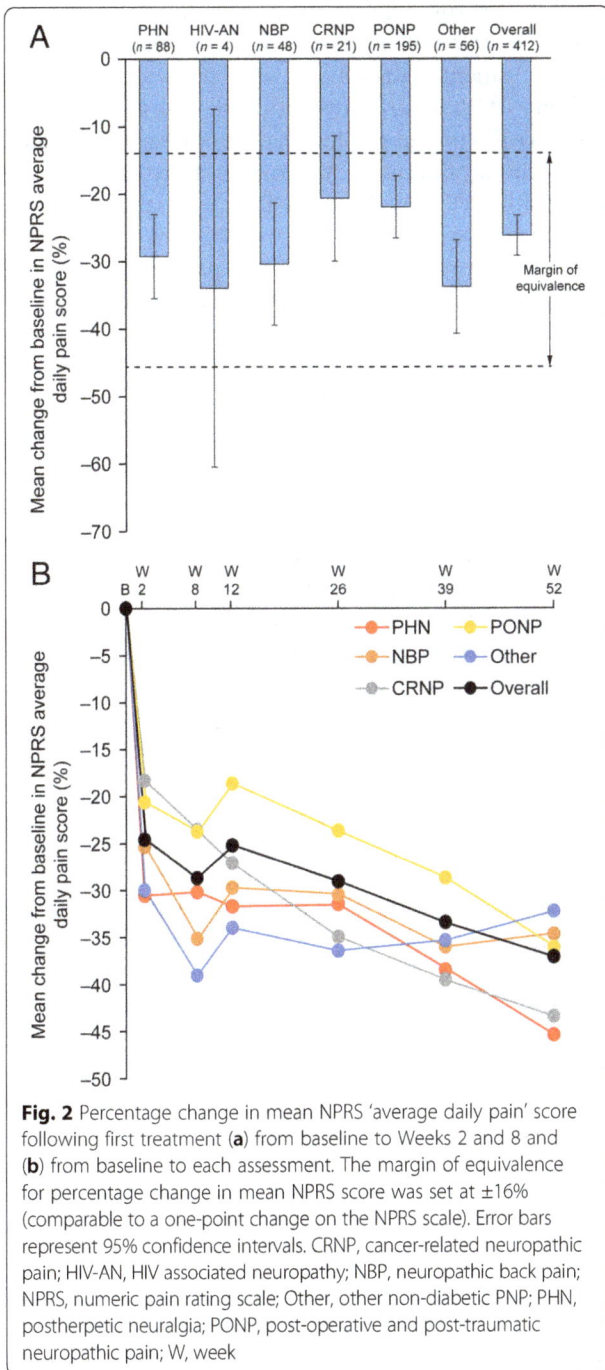

Fig. 2 Percentage change in mean NPRS 'average daily pain' score following first treatment (**a**) from baseline to Weeks 2 and 8 and (**b**) from baseline to each assessment. The margin of equivalence for percentage change in mean NPRS score was set at ±16% (comparable to a one-point change on the NPRS scale). Error bars represent 95% confidence intervals. CRNP, cancer-related neuropathic pain; HIV-AN, HIV associated neuropathy; NBP, neuropathic back pain; NPRS, numeric pain rating scale; Other, other non-diabetic PNP; PHN, postherpetic neuralgia; PONP, post-operative and post-traumatic neuropathic pain; W, week

Table 4 Responders after each capsaicin 8% patch treatment

NPRS 'average pain' score reduction	Responders, n (%)
First treatment (n = 412)	
≥30% reduction from baseline to Weeks 2 and 8	183 (44.4)
≥50% reduction from baseline to Weeks 2 and 8	108 (26.2)
Second treatment (n = 161)	
≥30% reduction from baseline to Weeks 2 and 12	79 (49.1)
≥50% reduction from baseline to Weeks 2 and 12	49 (30.4)
Third treatment (n = 59)	
≥30% reduction from baseline to Weeks 2 and 12	29 (49.2)
≥50% reduction from baseline to Weeks 2 and 12	18 (30.5)

NPRS numeric pain rating scale

Tolerability

Capsaicin 8% patch treatment was generally well tolerated. Over the course of the study, 47 (11.2%) patients reported a total of 91 AEs. The number of patients reporting at least one AE following first, second, third and fourth treatment was 26 (6.2%), 15 (3.6%), 5 (1.2%) and 1 (0.2%), respectively. The most frequently reported AEs were anticipated capsaicin-related application site reactions (8.3%; $n = 35$) including erythema (8.1%; $n = 34$), pain (5.0%; $n = 21$) and pruritus (1.0%; $n = 4$). Twenty-one SAEs were reported in 9 (2.1%) patients; five of these reported for one patient were probably treatment-related (two application site erythema, two application site pruritus and one headache). Four patients died during the study; causes of death were assessed by the treating physicians and were not considered to be treatment-related.

Discussion

ASCEND was the first real-world study to demonstrate that treatment with the capsaicin 8% patch can provide effective, rapid and sustained pain relief in a heterogeneous population with respect to PNP aetiologies, gender, age, and duration of previous neuropathic pain. A pain response was observed as early as Week 2, in common with previous clinical studies [12, 16, 18]. Long-term follow up of patients enabled the observation that the median time to second treatment was more than 26 weeks and increased to over 43 weeks from second to third treatment. There were also clear benefits in HRQoL and in treating patients with a short history of PNP. In line with other analgesics such as pregabalin and gabapentin [27, 28], observations of the capsaicin 8% patch in routine clinical practice were consistent with findings from clinical trials [12–16].

Following first, second and third treatment applications, 61.0% ($n = 224/367$), 74.6% ($n = 112/150$) and 78.7% ($n = 37/47$) of patients, respectively reported improved status at Week 12, while 7.4% ($n = 27/367$), 5.3% ($n = 8/150$) and 4.3% ($n = 2/47$) of patients reported some deterioration. At Week 52, following first, second or third treatment, more than half of all patients had an improvement in PGIC and less than 8% had worsened.

The mean NPRS 'average pain' reduction from baseline to Weeks 2 and 8 (26.6%), and to Weeks 2 and 12 after second and third treatment (28.7% and 27.3%), was consistent with Phase 3 studies of the capsaicin 8% patch

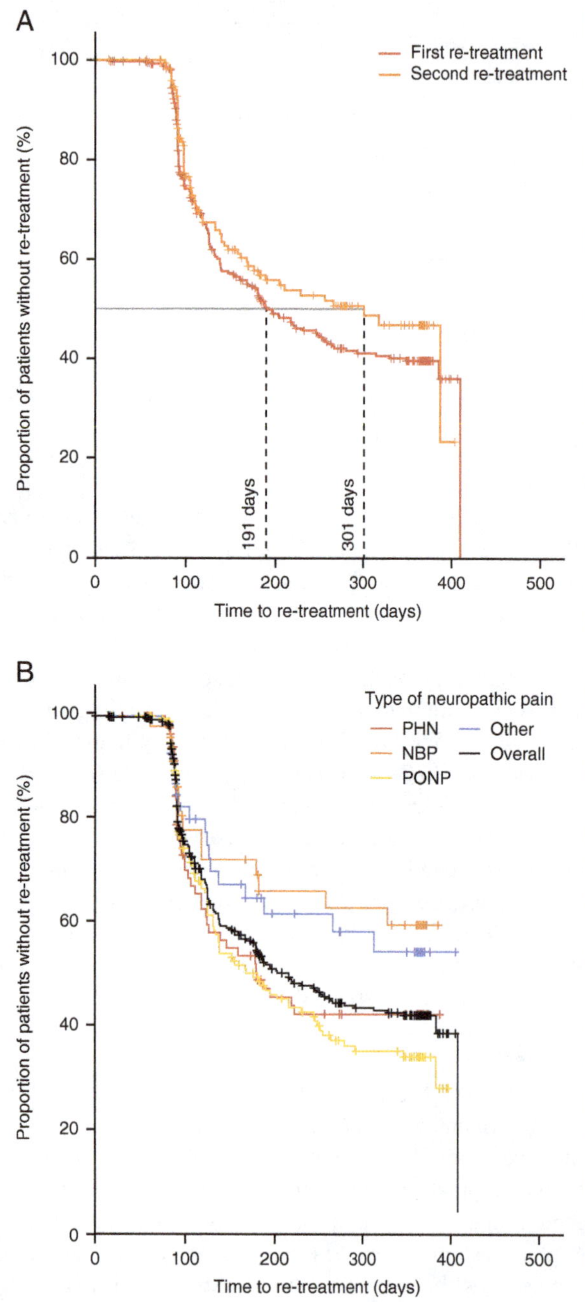

Fig. 3 Capsaicin 8% patch re-treatment intervals between (**a**) first and second treatment and second and third treatment; and (**b**) time between first and second treatment by aetiology group. NBP, neuropathic back pain; Other, other non-diabetic PNP; PHN, postherpetic neuralgia; PONP, post-operative and post-traumatic neuropathic pain

non-inferior pain relief versus pregabalin treatment, with a more rapid onset of action, fewer systemic effects and greater patient satisfaction with treatment [18]. In addition, studies performed in parallel to the ASCEND study have reported positive data for capsaicin 8% patch treatment in patients with painful diabetic peripheral neuropathy [29, 30]. A recent European label extension now allows for the use of the capsaicin 8% patch, either alone or in combination with other pain medications, in adults with diabetic PNP. Together, these data confirm that the capsaicin 8% patch provides consistent pain relief in a broad range of PNP aetiologies.

A potential advantage of the capsaicin 8% patch over other treatments is that a single treatment can provide lasting pain relief. In this study, almost half of all patients achieved a clinically important ≥30% reduction [21] in mean NPRS 'average pain' by Weeks 2 and 8 following first treatment, which was sustained in patients receiving re-treatment. Significantly, 86.9% of ≥30% responders at Weeks 2 and 8 were also classified as responders at Week 12. These results are concordant with a study in patients with HIV-AN [31], where responders (≥30% reduction in 'average pain' from baseline to Weeks 2 and 12) maintained a response for a median time of 17 weeks (95% CI: 13, 27) after a single treatment with the capsaicin 8% patch. Taken together, these data support the conclusion that a clinically important pain response with capsaicin 8% patch treatment is likely to be sustained over time and with successive treatments.

PNP treatment guidelines suggest the use of the capsaicin 8% patch as second-line treatment for localised neuropathic pain [6]. The duration of pre-existing pain and the stage of the treatment pathway, in relation to capsaicin 8% patch treatment, were assessed in this study. Higher levels of pain reduction were observed in patients treated within the primary and secondary stages of the treatment pathway compared with the tertiary stages. Furthermore, the shortest PNP duration quartile (0–0.72 years) had the largest mean percentage reduction in pain intensity from baseline to Weeks 2 and 8, and the highest percentage of responders (≥30% reduction in mean NPRS score). This is consistent with findings from a 12-week non-interventional study (QUEPP), where patients with pre-existing pain of less than 6 months benefited to a greater extent than patients with a longer history of pain [19], indicating that the capsaicin 8% patch may be most effective in earlier stages of PNP treatment or after recent onset of neuropathic pain.

The number of capsaicin 8% patches used per treatment in this study (1.5 patches/treatment) was consistent with the ELEVATE study [18], but considerably lower than that observed in randomised studies (mean

in non-diabetic patients with PHN [12, 14] and HIV-AN [13, 16]. These findings are further supported by a randomised, open-label, non-inferiority study of the capsaicin 8% patch versus pregabalin (ELEVATE study) where non-diabetic patients with PHN, peripheral nerve injury or non-diabetic painful peripheral polyneuropathy had

Table 5 EQ-5D index scores following first 8% capsaicin patch treatment

EQ-5D index score	Responders at Weeks 2 and 8		Non-responders at Weeks 2 and 8		Overall
	≥30%[a]	≥50%[a]	<30%[a]	<50%[a]	
Baseline, mean (SD)	0.392 (0.352) n = 182	0.386 (0.367) n = 108	0.306 (0.349) n = 229	0.329 (0.347) n = 303	0.345 (0.354) n = 419
Change from baseline, mean (SD)					
Week 2	0.292 (0.313) n = 176	0.337 (0.327) n = 104	0.128 (0.297) n = 223	0.152 (0.296) n = 295	0.199 (0.315) n = 400
Week 8	0.323 (0.307) n = 165	0.349 (0.321) n = 99	0.104 (0.323) n = 209	0.147 (0.322) n = 275	0.200 (0.333) n = 375
Week 12	0.289 (0.352) n = 165	0.342 (0.359) n = 97	0.111 (0.320) n = 196	0.138 (0.325) n = 264	0.190 (0.348) n = 363
Week 26	0.288 (0.292) n = 93	0.309 (0.290) n = 62	0.099 (0.339) n = 112	0.131 (0.334) n = 143	0.185 (0.330) n = 206
Week 39	0.306 (0.320) n = 78	0.310 (0.321) n = 52	0.123 (0.335) n = 96	0.161 (0.339) n = 122	0.205 (0.340) n = 174
Week 52	0.307 (0.327) n = 76	0.305 (0.330) n = 52	0.114 (0.376) n = 100	0.153 (0.373) n = 124	0.198 (0.367) n = 176

[a]Percentage reduction in average NPRS score. *EQ-5D*, EuroQol 5 Dimension 3-level; *SD*, standard deviation

Table 6 Patient Global Impression of Change (PGIC) responses

Response	Patients, n (%)		
	First treatment	Second treatment	Third treatment
Week 2	n = 408		
Improved	258 (63.2)		
No change	117 (28.7)		
Worsened	33 (8.1)		
Week 8	n = 368		
Improved	231 (62.8)		
No change	110 (29.9)		
Worsened	27 (7.3)		
Week 12	n = 367	n = 150	n = 47
Improved	224 (61.0)	112 (74.7)	37 (78.7)
No change	116 (31.6)	30 (20.0)	8 (17.0)
Worsened	27 (7.4)	8 (5.3)	2 (4.3)
Week 26	n = 207	n = 101	n = 28
Improved	113 (54.6)	67 (66.3)	23 (82.1)
No change	76 (36.7)	26 (25.7)	3 (10.7)
Worsened	18 (8.7)	8 (7.9)	2 (7.1)
Week 39	n = 177	n = 81	n = 21
Improved	96 (54.2)	50 (61.7)	18 (85.7)
No change	65 (36.7)	24 (29.6)	1 (4.8)
Worsened	16 (9.0)	7 (8.6)	2 (9.5)
Week 52	n = 176	n = 56	n = 7
Improved	93 (52.8)	38 (67.9)	5 (71.4)
No change	71 (40.3)	14 (25.0)	1 (14.3)
Worsened	12 (6.8)	4 (7.1)	1 (14.3)

Improved: slightly, much, very much; Worsened: slightly, much, very much

2.3 patches/treatment) [12, 14], despite comparable treatment area sizes. This may be related to differences in the number of patches per pack between the Phase 3 randomised controlled studies (4 patches/pack) and those used in routine clinical practice (1 patch/pack) or the cost of treatment in routine clinical practice versus a clinical trial. The lower number of patches used in this study did not affect the reported efficacy.

Patients with PNP can experience considerable impairment in HRQoL as highlighted by the EQ-5D index at baseline (0.345 utils), which suggests the typical UK adult would choose to forfeit almost two-thirds of their remaining lifespan in order to avoid this state of health [23]. The capsaicin 8% patch improved HRQoL as demonstrated by an improvement in the EQ-5D index and PGIC. The improvement from baseline in the EQ-5D index at Week 2 (0.199 utils) was maintained up to the final measurement at Week 52. It was also observed that responders had the greatest improvements in EQ-5D. Furthermore, 61.0% of patients reported an improved health status at Week 12 as measured by PGIC, similar to results obtained from previous studies in patients with HIV-AN (67%) and PHN (62%) [13, 14]. This result was sustained over successive treatments and up to Week 52 (52.8%).

The capsaicin 8% patch was shown to be well tolerated across a range of aetiologies with over 92% of patients completing at least 90% of the suggested patch application duration at first or subsequent treatments. Similarly, 98% of patients in a previous study with PHN completed at least 90% of the suggested patch application duration [14]. AEs were reported for 11% of patients and most were anticipated application site reactions. The frequency of adverse events reported in other studies of the capsaicin 8% patch was higher (98–99%), but the majority were also application site reactions [12, 14]. Repeated use of the capsaicin 8% patch did not increase the frequency of AEs, supporting findings from an open-label study in patients with HIV-AN who had up to three applications [31].

The strengths of the ASCEND trial include a large and heterogeneous population, a real-world setting, inclusion of patients with different PNP aetiologies and the monitoring of patients for at least one year after treatment and over multiple treatments. A potential limitation of the trial was low patient numbers in the CRNP and HIV-AN groups, which prevented meaningful subgroup analyses. This could have been improved with stratified sampling to increase recruitment in the subgroups. In addition, controlling for longitudinal change in concomitant medication was not possible in this study and could have affected the outcomes reported with the capsaicin 8% patch.

Conclusions

In conclusion, the use of the capsaicin 8% patch in a real-world, clinical practice setting provided rapid pain relief in patients with various PNP aetiologies. The response to initial treatment and re-treatment was sustained as evidenced by the maintenance of treatment response with re-treatment intervals averaging over 26 weeks. The capsaicin 8% patch was generally well tolerated, usually required less than two patches per treatment, and improved overall HRQoL. Patients in the primary stage of treatment or with short duration of disease had the greatest pain reduction suggesting that patients with PNP may benefit from early treatment with the capsaicin 8% patch. In addition, the capsaicin 8% patch may benefit patients who have inadequate pain relief from systemic therapies or for those suffering intolerable systematic side effects.

Abbreviations

AE: Adverse event; CI: Confidence interval; CRNP: Cancer-related neuropathic pain; EQ-5D: EuroQol 5 Dimension questionnaire (3-level); FAS: Full analysis set; HIV-AN: Human immunodeficiency virus-associated neuropathy; HRQoL: Health-related quality of life; NBP: Neuropathic back pain; NeuPSIG: Neuropathic pain special interest group; NIS: Non-interventional study; NP: Neuropathic pain; NPRS: Numeric pain rating scale; PGIC: Patient global impression of change; PHN: Post-herpetic neuralgia; PNP: Peripheral neuropathic pain; PONP: Post-operative and post-traumatic neuropathic pain; w/w: weight for weight; SAE: Serious adverse event; SD: Standard deviation; TRPV1: Transient receptor potential vanilloid type 1

Acknowledgements

Medical writing support was provided by Kinnari Patel of Bioscript Group, which was funded by Astellas Pharma Europe Ltd.

Funding

This study and medical writing and editing services were funded by Astellas Pharma Europe Ltd.

Authors' contributions

CM, CDP and IO participated in the concept and design of the study. RT, EB, EE and CJC performed the analyses. CT was responsible for medical oversight of the study, and review of clinical data and study reporting. JIC, CP and EZ recruited patients and acquired data. All provided critical revision of the publication for intellectual content. All authors read and approved the final manuscript.

Competing interests

CM and EE are employed by Astellas. IO was employed by Astellas at the time of the study. CDP was employed by Astellas at the time of analysis and is now employed by Digital Health Labs Ltd. CT is employed by Astellas as a contractor. RT and EB are employed by Pharmatelligence. EZ was employed at Evangelismos General Hospital until the completion of the study and is now employed by Novartis (Hellas) S.A.C.I. CJC, JIC and CP have no disclosures.

Author details

[1]Astellas Pharma Europe Ltd, 2000 Hillswood Drive, Chertsey KT16 0PS, UK. [2]Astellas Pharma Europe B.V., Leiden, The Netherlands. [3]Pharmatelligence, Cardiff, UK. [4]Cardiff University, Cardiff, UK. [5]Complejo Hospitalario de Navarra, Pamplona, Spain. [6]Evangelismos General Hospital, Athens, Greece.

References

1. Treede RD, Jensen TS, Campbell JN, Cruccu G, Dostrovsky JO, Griffin JW, et al. Neuropathic pain: redefinition and a grading system for clinical and research purposes. Neurology. 2008;70(18):1630–5.
2. Marchettini P, Lacerenza M, Mauri E, Marangoni C. Painful peripheral neuropathies. Curr Neuropharmacol. 2006;4(3):175–81.
3. Torrance N, Smith BH, Bennett MI, Lee AJ. The epidemiology of chronic pain of predominantly neuropathic origin. Results from a general population survey. J Pain. 2006;7(4):281–9.
4. Bouhassira D, Lanteri-Minet M, Attal N, Laurent B, Touboul C. Prevalence of chronic pain with neuropathic characteristics in the general population. Pain. 2008;136(3):380–7.
5. Doth AH, Hansson PT, Jensen MP, Taylor RS. The burden of neuropathic pain: a systematic review and meta-analysis of health utilities. Pain. 2010; 149(2):338–44.
6. Finnerup NB, Attal N, Haroutounian S, McNicol E, Baron R, Dworkin RH, et al. Pharmacotherapy for neuropathic pain in adults: a systematic review and meta-analysis. Lancet Neurol. 2015;14(2):162–73.
7. Haanpää M, Treede RD. Neuropathic Pain. In Lynch ME, Craig KD & Peng PWH (eds). Clinical pain management: a practical guide. Oxford: Wiley-Blackwell; 2010: 281-9.
8. Wallace JM. Update on pharmacotherapy guidelines for treatment of neuropathic pain. Curr Pain Headache Rep. 2007;11(3):208–14.
9. Gahr M, Freudenmann RW, Hiemke C, Kolle MA, Schonfeldt-Lecuona C. Pregabalin abuse and dependence in Germany: results from a database query. Eur J Clin Pharmacol. 2013;69(6):1335–42.
10. Anand P, Bley K. Topical capsaicin for pain management: therapeutic potential and mechanisms of action of the new high-concentration capsaicin 8% patch. Br J Anaesth. 2011;107(4):490–502.
11. Uceyler N, Sommer C. High-dose capsaicin for the treatment of neuropathic pain: what we know and what we need to know. Pain Ther. 2014;3(2):73–84.
12. Backonja M, Wallace MS, Blonsky ER, Cutler BJ, Malan Jr P, Rauck R, et al. NGX-4010, a high-concentration capsaicin patch, for the treatment of postherpetic neuralgia: a randomised, double-blind study. Lancet Neurol. 2008;7(12):1106–12.
13. Clifford DB, Simpson DM, Brown S, Moyle G, Brew BJ, Conway B, et al. A randomized, double-blind, controlled study of NGX-4010, a capsaicin 8% dermal patch, for the treatment of painful HIV-associated distal sensory polyneuropathy. J Acquir Immune Defic Syndr. 2012;59(2):126–33.
14. Irving GA, Backonja MM, Dunteman E, Blonsky ER, Vanhove GF, Lu SP, et al. A multicenter, randomized, double-blind, controlled study of NGX-4010, a high-concentration capsaicin patch, for the treatment of postherpetic neuralgia. Pain Med. 2011;12(1):99–109.

15. Maihofner C, Heskamp ML. Prospective, non-interventional study on the tolerability and analgesic effectiveness over 12 weeks after a single application of capsaicin 8% cutaneous patch in 1044 patients with peripheral neuropathic pain: first results of the QUEPP study. Curr Med Res Opin. 2013;29(6):673–83.

16. Simpson DM, Brown S, Tobias J, the NGX-4010 C107 Study Group. Controlled trial of high-concentration capsaicin patch for treatment of painful HIV neuropathy. Neurology. 2008;70(24):2305–13.

17. Stoker M, Katz N, Van J, Snijder R, Jacobs H, Long S, et al. Capsaicin 8% patch in painful diabetic peripheral neuropathy: a randomised, double-blind, placebo-controlled study. Diabetologia. 2015;58(Suppl. 1):S32.

18. Haanpää M, Cruccu G, Nurmikko TJ, McBride WT, Docu Axelarad A, Bosilkov A, et al. Capsaicin 8% patch versus oral pregabalin in patients with peripheral neuropathic pain. Eur J Pain. 2016;20(2):316–28.

19. Maihofner CG, Heskamp ML. Treatment of peripheral neuropathic pain by topical capsaicin: Impact of pre-existing pain in the QUEPP-study. Eur J Pain. 2014;18(5):671–9.

20. European Medicines Agency. Qutenza Product Information. Annex 1: Summary of product characteristics. 2015. Available at: http://www.ema.europa.eu/docs/en_GB/document_library/EPAR_-_Product_Information/human/000909/WC500040453.pdf.

21. Farrar JT, Young Jr JP, LaMoreaux L, Werth JL, Poole RM. Clinical importance of changes in chronic pain intensity measured on an 11-point numerical pain rating scale. Pain. 2001;94(2):149–58.

22. Rabin R, de Charro F. EQ-5D: a measure of health status from the EuroQol Group. Ann Med. 2001;33(5):337–43.

23. Dolan P. Modeling valuations for EuroQol health states. Med Care. 1997;35(11):1095–108.

24. Hurst H, Bolton J. Assessing the clinical significance of change scores recorded on subjective outcome measures. J Manipulative Physiol Ther. 2004;27(1):26–35.

25. Grant MD, Samson D. Special report: measuring and reporting pain outcomes in randomized controlled trials. Technol Eval Cent Assess Program Exec Summ. 2006;21(11):1–2.

26. Walters SJ, Brazier JE. Comparison of the minimally important difference for two health state utility measures: EQ-5D and SF-6D. Qual Life Res. 2005;14(6):1523–32.

27. Anastassiou E, Iatrou CA, Vlaikidis N, Vafiadou M, Stamatiou G, Plesia E, et al. Impact of pregabalin treatment on pain, pain-related sleep interference and general well-being in patients with neuropathic pain: a non-interventional, multicentre, post-marketing study. Clin Drug Investig. 2011;31(6):417–26.

28. Markley HG, Dunteman ED, Kareht S, Sweeney M. Real-world experience with once-daily gabapentin for the treatment of postherpetic neuralgia (PHN). Clin J Pain. 2015;31(1):58–65.

29. Simpson DM, Robinson-Papp J, Van J, Stoker M, Jacobs H, Snijder RJ, et al. Capsaicin 8% patch in painful diabetic peripheral neuropathy: a randomized, double-blind, placebo-controlled study. J Pain. 2017;18(1):42–53.

30. Vinik AI, Perrot S, Vinik EJ, Pazdera L, Jacobs H, Stoker M, Long SK, Snijder RJ, van der Stoep M, Ortega E, Katz N. Capsaicin 8% patch repeat treatment plus standard of care (SOC) versus SOC alone in painful diabetic peripheral neuropathy: a randomised, 52-week, open-label, safety study. BMC Neurol. 2016;16:251.

31. Simpson DM, Brown S, Tobias JK, Vanhove GF, the NGX-4010 C107 Study Group. NGX-4010, a capsaicin 8% dermal patch, for the treatment of painful HIV-associated distal sensory polyneuropathy: results of a 52-week open-label study. Clin J Pain. 2014;30(2):134–42.

16

Guillain–Barré syndrome presenting with Raynaud's phenomenon

Sonali Sihindi Chapa Gunatilake[*] and Harith Wimalaratna

Abstract

Background: Guillain–Barré syndrome is an immune mediated acute inflammatory polyradiculo-neuropathy involving the peripheral nervous system. Commonest presentation is acute or subacute flaccid ascending paralysis of limbs. Rarely autonomic dysfunction can be the presenting feature of Guillain–Barré syndrome. Raynaud's phenomenon, although had been described in relation to many disease conditions, has not been described in association with Guillain–Barré syndrome up to date.

Case presentation: We report the first case of Guillain–Barré syndrome presenting with Raynaud's phenomenon in a 21-year-old previously well boy. New onset Raynaud's phenomenon was experienced followed by acute ascending flaccid paralysis of lower limbs and upper limbs together with palpitations and postural giddiness. Nerve conduction studies showed acute inflammatory demyelinating polyneuropathy with cerebrospinal fluid cyto-protein dissociation. He was treated with intravenous immunoglobulin and showed a satisfactory clinical recovery of muscle weakness, Raynaud's phenomenon and autonomic disturbances.

Conclusion: Guillain–Barré syndrome presenting with Raynaud's phenomenon is not being reported in literature previously. Although the underlying mechanism is not fully understood, Raynaud's phenomenon should prompt the physician to consider Guillain–Barré syndrome with a complimentary clinical picture.

Keywords: Guillain–Barré syndrome, Raynaud's phenomenon, Acute inflammatory demyelinating polyneuropathy, Cerebrospinal fluid, Cyto-protein dissociation, Acute ascending flaccid paralysis

Background

Guillain–Barré syndrome is an acute inflammatory polyradiculo-neuropathy, an immune mediated disease affecting the peripheral nervous system. It comprises of a heterogeneous group of clinical entities. Usually it is preceded by an antecedent event in two thirds of the patients, commonly an infection [1,2]. Typical presentation is of acute ascending flaccid paralysis of lower-limbs with absent or diminished reflexes, extending more proximally with time and proximal muscle groups being affected more than the distal. Many patients experience paresthesia with mild degree of sensory involvement. Cranial nerve involvement is also not uncommon. Dysautonomia had been described in 60% of the patients with Guillain–Barré syndrome [3] manifesting with reduced or excess activation of sympathetic or parasympathetic nervous systems. Rarely autonomic involvement can be the presenting symptom in Guillain–Barré syndrome [2,4,5].

Raynaud's phenomenon is an exaggerated vasospastic response to emotion or cold weather giving rise to triphasic color change in the acral regions of the body [5,6]. Classic color changes are white (due to ischaemia from vasospasms), blue (due to deoxygenation of blood) and red (due to reperfusion). Variety of causes and associated diseases have been described to give rise to Raynaud's phenomenon but an extensive literature survey did not reveal Raynaud's phenomenon in association with Guillain–Barré syndrome. Herein, we report the first case of Guillain–Barré syndrome manifesting with Raynaud's phenomenon as the presenting complaint.

Case presentation

A 21-year-old previously healthy male presented to Teaching Hospital, Kandy, Sri Lanka in July 2013 with the complaint of bluish discoloration of hands for 5 days duration and subsequent weakness of limbs.

He had experienced repeated transient episodes of hand discoloration, blanching followed by bluish discoloration.

* Correspondence: sonaligunatilake@gmail.com
Teaching Hospital, Kandy, Sri Lanka

There was similar involvement of the feet. Episodes occurred several times per day with increasing in frequency. It was not associated with pain, numbness or weakness of the limbs, neck pain or radicular pain. Identified precipitant was cold environment, but was not associated with emotional stress. There was no history of trauma. He did not have recent weight loss, anorexia, fever, oral ulcers, hair-loss, skin rashes, joint swelling or joint pain. No similar episodes were observed in the past.

Five days after the onset of hand discoloration, he noticed weakness of both lower limbs with difficulty in walking which progressed to weakness of upper limbs, predominantly the proximal parts. He was able to walk with support without ataxia initially and his hand grip was poor and dropped certain objects. The weakness was progressive. There was no double vision, slurring of speech, dysphagia or dyspnea. There was neither bladder nor bowel involvement. He had tingling sensation of fingers and toes at the onset of the weakness of limbs but remained static. He did not have postural giddiness but experienced intermittent palpitations. He denied excessive sweating or hypersalivation. Raynaud's phenomenon which he experienced earlier was still present during this period of illness. There was no preceding respiratory tract illness or diarrhoeal illness. His past medical history was not significant and there was no exposure to heavy metals. He did not have any foreign travels or exposure to tick bites. The patient denied any long term use of medication and he was a non-smoker and did not consume alcohol. He was unmarried & denied any sexual misbehavior.

On examination, he was otherwise well looking male with a body mass index of 21 kg/m². Generalized weakness of muscle groups were noted involving distal more than the proximal in both upper and lower limbs (upper limb: distal - grade 3/5, proximal – grade 4/5; lower limb: distal – grade 2/5, proximal – 3/5). There was generalized areflexia with hypotonia. Pupils were size 3, equally reacting to light. Sensory system, cerebellar system, cranial nerves and fundi were clinically normal. Raynaud's phenomenon was observed when hands were exposed to cold. There were no digital ulcers or gangrene. Cardiovascular system examination revealed a regular heart rate of 110/min with a postural drop in systolic blood pressure (supine – 130/80; seated – 100/80). All peripheral pulses were present with good volume and there were no subclavian, carotid or femoral bruits. Respiratory, abdominal and locomotor system examinations were normal.

His complete blood count, blood picture, renal and liver profile were normal. Other basic investigations revealed; erythrocyte sedimentation rate – 05 mm in 1st Hour, C-reactive protein – normal, serum electrolytes including Na⁺, K⁺, Ca²⁺ & Mg²⁺ were normal, serum proteins: total– 7.8 g/dl, albumin - 4.6 g/dl, globulin - 3.1 g/dl.

Fasting blood sugar and lipid profile were within normal range. Cerebrospinal fluid (CSF) studies done on day 10 of the illness showed elevated proteins (120 mg/dl; normal < 40 mg/dl) with 01 white cell, 100% being lymphocytes. CSF sugar was within normal limits compared to plasma value. Nerve conduction studies revealed focal segmental demyelinating type of neuropathy with elevated distal motor latency, elongated F-wave, conduction block without axonal abnormalities, concluding as acute inflammatory demyelinating polyneuropathy (AIDP) type Guillain–Barré syndrome.

Further investigations showed negative serology for mycoplasma, campylobacter jejuni, cytomegalovirus, Epstein-Barr virus, hepatitis B & C and human immuno deficiency virus (HIV). Anti-nuclear antibodies, anti-neutrophil antibodies and rheumatoid factor were negative with normal thyroid stimulating hormone levels. Serum protein electrophoresis was normal. X ray cervical spine, thoracic inlet and chest x ray were negative for cervical ribs or any significant pathology. Venous duplex scan of the upper limbs showed good arterial flow without obstruction. Electrocardiogram showed sinus tachycardia and arrhythmias were not noted. He had normal echocardiogram findings with no features suggesting myocarditis.

Based on the clinical and investigation findings, diagnosis of Guillain–Barré syndrome was reached and intravenous immunoglobulin 0.4 g/kg/day was administered for five days. Patient showed good clinical response to treatment and the muscle power improved to 4/5 in all muscle groups during the ward stay, though the patient remained areflexic. His symptoms of Raynaud's phenomenon, palpitations and postural giddiness showed dramatic improvement during the ward stay and on discharge patient was free of symptoms. His pulse rate had reduced to 80 beats per minute and blood pressure was 120/80 mmHg, both supine and erect. He was followed up to six months and had completely recovered with normal muscle power with 1+ reflexes, and had not experienced Raynaud's phenomenon even with exposure to cold weather.

Discussion

Guillain–Barré syndrome is an immune mediated disease, manifesting as an acute polyradiculo- neuropathy involving the peripheral nervous system. Clinical manifestations are preceded by an antecedent event in two thirds of the patients [1,2], commonly an upper respiratory tract infection or a diarrhoeal illness. Pathogenesis involves production of auto antibodies against the infectious agent that cross react against gangliosides and glycolipids (GM1 and GD1b) that are distributed along the myelin sheaths of the peripheral nervous system. This causes defective propagation of electrical impulses thus resulting in marked delay or absence of electrical impulse along the nerve fibers resulting in flaccid paralysis. There are several sub-types of Guillain–Barré syndrome identified depending on clinical presentation, involvement of the particular nerves and pathology; (1) Acute inflammatory demyelinating poluneuropathy, (2) Acute motor axonal neuropathy, (3) Acute motor sensory axonal neuropathy, (4) Miller Fisher syndrome, (5) Acute panautonomic neuropathy and (6) Pure sensory Guillain–Barré syndrome.

Patients with Guillain–Barré syndrome commonly present with acute or sub-acute symmetrical weakness of lower limbs with ascending paralysis extending to upper limbs, neck muscles, bulbar muscles, cranial nerves and respiratory muscles needing ventilatory support [2,7,8]. Muscle involvement is proximal more than the distal muscle groups and commonly with diminished or absent deep tendon reflexes. It is not uncommon to notice mild paresthesia or pain by the patients.

Autonomic dysfunction is also seen in 60% of the patients with Guillain–Barré syndrome [3]. Rarely it can be the presenting manifestation of Guillain–Barré syndrome [2,4,5]. Clinical features of dysautonomia commonly seen in relation to cardiovascular system are sinus tachycardia, sinus bradycardia, other cardiac arrhythmias (both tachy and bradyarrythmias), hypertension, postural hypotension and wide fluctuations of pulse and blood pressure. Tonic pupils, hyper salivation, anhydrosis or excessive sweating, urinary sphincter disturbances, constipation and gastric dysmotility are recognized as a part of autonomic dysfunction [3,9].

Raynaud's phenomenon is the triad of pallor, cyanosis and redness of the acral regions of the body (hands and feet) due to episodic digital vasospasms. Classically it is brought about by cold environment or emotions [10]. Pallor is a result of ischaemia due to vasospasms, cyanosis due to deoxygenation of blood and redness being the result of reperfusion following reversal of the spasms. Two subtypes are described, primary Raynaud's which is not associated with any other illness and secondary Raynaud's phenomenon, where vasospasms are associated with another disease, commonly autoimmune diseases, mixed connective tissue disease and scleroderma. Pathogenesis of primary Raynaud's phenomenon is not fully understood but vascular, intravascular and neural mechanisms are proposed [6,11]. Of the neural mechanisms, central impairment of the autonomic function resulting in Raynaud's phenomenon is suggested by the research done by Koszewicz et al. [12]. Mallipeddi et al. concluded that primary Raynaud's phenomenon is associated with sympathetic denervation in chronic autonomic failure [10]. Sympathetic over-activity provoking vasospasm by exaggerated vascular response is also suggested as one of the mechanisms causing Raynaud's phenomenon [11,13]. Hyperactivity of the α2c adrenoreceptors is also postulated as one of the mechanisms [6]. But experiments done by Fagius et al. showed neither hypersensitivity of the vessels

to sympathetic bursts nor abnormal increase in sympathetic outflow was present in patients with Raynaud's phenomenon [14]. Further studies are required for a better knowledge regarding the contribution of sympathetic nervous system or dysautonomia in Raynaud's phenomenon.

Although several etiologies are described in-relation to Raynaud's phenomenon as primary Raynaud's's disease, occupational, haematological, autoimmune, connective tissue diseases, vasculitis, thrombo-embolic disease, carpal tunnel syndrome, thoracic outlet syndrome, reflex sympathetic dystrophy, pheochromocytoma, acromegaly, lung adenocarcinoma and Fabry s disease, extensive literature survey did not reveal Raynaud's phenomenon in association with Guillain–Barré syndrome. Common pathological features in both conditions are dysautonomia with altered sympathetic activation.

The patient in this case report presented with Raynaud's phenomenon and subsequently developed features of Guillain–Barré syndrome with further supportive evidence from CSF and nerve conduction studies. He also had other features of autonomic dysfunction as postural hypotension. Weakness and neurological symptoms resolved following treatment for Guillain–Barré syndrome and Raynaud's phenomenon also resolved permanently.

Conclusion

We report the first case of Guillain–Barré syndrome presenting with Raynaud's phenomenon, which highlights the importance of considering the possibility of Guillain–Barré syndrome in a patient presenting with de novo Raynaud's phenomenon. More classic features of Guillain-Barre syndrome may follow soon after. This is important for close observation and prompt treatment. The exact pathophysiological mechanisms linking above two entities can be postulated as dysautonomia but need further evaluation with experimental studies.

Consent

Written informed consent was obtained from the patient for publication of this case report. A copy of the written consent is available for review by the Editor-in-chief of this journal.

Abbreviations

AIDP: Acute inflammatory demyelinating polyneuropathy; ANCA: Anti-neutrophil cytoplasmic antibodies; CSF: Cerebrospinal fluid; HIV: Human immunodeficiency virus.

Competing interests

The authors declare that they have no competing interests.

Authors' contributions

HW made the clinical diagnosis and supervised the manuscript drafting. SSCG drafted the first manuscript, reviewed the literature and involved in direct management of the patient. Both authors read and approved the final manuscript.

Authors' information

HW (MBBS, MD, FRCP (Edin), FRCP (Lond), FCCP) is a Consultant Physician working at Teaching Hospital, Kandy, Sri Lanka. SSCG (MBBS) is a Registrar in Medicine attached to the Teaching Hospital, Kandy, Sri Lanka.

References

1. Winer JB, Hughes RA, Anderson MJ, Jones DM, Kangro H, Watkins RP: **A prospective study of acute idiopathic neuropathy. II Antecedent events.** *J Neurol Neurosurg Psychiatry* 1988, **51**:613–618.
2. Seneviratne U: **Guillain-Barré syndrome.** *Postgrad Med J* 2000, **76**:774–782.
3. Patel MB, Goyal SK, Punnam SR, Pandya K, Khetarpal V, Thakur RK: **Guillain-Barré syndrome with asystole requiring permanent pacemaker: a case report.** *J Med Case Rep* 2009, **3**:5.
4. Ferraro-Herrera AS, Kern HB, Nagler W: **Autonomic dysfunction as the presenting feature of Guillain-Barré syndrome.** *Arch Phys Med Rehabil* 1997, **78**(7):777–779.
5. Cortelli P, Contin M, Lugaresi A, Baruzzi A, Montagna P: **Severe dysautonomic onset of Guillain-Barré syndrome with good recovery. A clinical and autonomic follow-up study [abstract].** *Ital J Neurol Sci* 1990, **11**(2):159–162.
6. Herrick AL: **Pathogenesis of Raynaud's phenomenon.** *Rheumatology* 2005, **44**(5):587–596.
7. Flachenecker P: **Autonomic dysfunction in Guillain-Barré syndrome and multiple sclerosis.** *J Neurol* 2007, **254**(2):96–101.
8. Pikula JR: **Guillain-Barre syndrome: a case report.** *J Can Chiropr Assoc* 1995, **39**(2):80–83.
9. Zochodne DW: **Autonomic involvement in Guillain-Barré syndrome: a review.** *Muscle Nerve* 1994, **17**(10):1145–1155.
10. Mallipeddi R, Mathias CJ: **Raynaud's phenomenon after sympathetic denervation in patients with primary autonomic failure: questionnaire survey.** *BMJ* 1998, **316**:438.
11. Coffman JD: **Pathogenesis and treatment of Raynaud's phenomenon.** *Cardiovasc Drugs Ther* 1990, **4**(1):45–51.
12. Koszewicz M, Gosk-Bierska I, Bilińska M, Podemski R, Budrewicz S, Adamiec R, Slotwinski K: **Autonomic dysfunction in primary Raynaud's phenomenon.** *Int Angiol* 2009, **28**(2):127–131.
13. Urbano FL: **Raynaud's phenomenon.** *Hosp Physician* 2001, 27–30. http://www.turner-white.com/pdf/hp_sep01_raynaud.pdf.
14. Fagius J, Blumberg H: **Sympathetic outflow to the hand in patients with Raynaud's phenomenon.** *Cardiovasc Res* 1985, **19**(5):249–253.

17

Trial design and rationale for APOLLO, a Phase 3, placebo-controlled study of patisiran in patients with hereditary ATTR amyloidosis with polyneuropathy

David Adams[1*], Ole B. Suhr[2], Peter J. Dyck[3], William J. Litchy[3], Raina G. Leahy[4], Jihong Chen[4], Jared Gollob[4] and Teresa Coelho[5]

Abstract

Background: Patisiran is an investigational RNA interference (RNAi) therapeutic in development for the treatment of hereditary ATTR (hATTR) amyloidosis, a progressive disease associated with significant disability, morbidity, and mortality.

Methods: Here we describe the rationale and design of the Phase 3 APOLLO study, a randomized, double-blind, placebo-controlled, global study to evaluate the efficacy and safety of patisiran in patients with hATTR amyloidosis with polyneuropathy. Eligible patients are 18–85 years old with hATTR amyloidosis, investigator-estimated survival of ≥2 years, Neuropathy Impairment Score (NIS) of 5–130, and polyneuropathy disability score ≤IIIb. Patients are randomized 2:1 to receive either intravenous patisiran 0.3 mg/kg or placebo once every 3 weeks. The primary objective is to determine the efficacy of patisiran at 18 months based on the difference in the change in modified NIS+7 (a composite measure of motor strength, sensation, reflexes, nerve conduction, and autonomic function) between the patisiran and placebo groups. Secondary objectives are to evaluate the effect of patisiran on Norfolk-Diabetic Neuropathy quality of life questionnaire score, nutritional status (as evaluated by modified body mass index), motor function (as measured by NIS-weakness and timed 10-m walk test), and autonomic symptoms (as measured by the Composite Autonomic Symptom Score-31 questionnaire). Exploratory objectives include assessment of cardiac function and pathologic evaluation to assess nerve fiber innervation and amyloid burden. Safety of patisiran will be assessed throughout the study.

Discussion: APOLLO represents the largest randomized, Phase 3 study to date in patients with hATTR amyloidosis, with endpoints that capture the multisystemic nature of this disease.

Keywords: Patisiran, APOLLO, RNA interference, hATTR amyloidosis, mNIS+7, Methods, Polyneuropathy

Background

Hereditary ATTR (hATTR) amyloidosis, formerly known as familial amyloid polyneuropathy (FAP), is a progressive, life-threatening disease caused by misfolded transthyretin (TTR) protein that accumulates as amyloid fibrils in multiple organs, including the nerves, heart, and gastrointestinal tract [1, 2]. hATTR amyloidosis is a multisystemic disease with a heterogeneous clinical presentation, including sensory, motor, autonomic, and cardiac symptoms that are often concurrent [3–6]. The unrelenting disease course begins with unimpaired ambulation (FAP stage 1 [7]), then requirement for assistance with ambulation (FAP stage 2), which proceeds to wheelchair confinement (FAP stage 3), with patients experiencing a range of life-impacting symptoms that include burning neuropathic pain, loss of sensation in hands and feet, diarrhea/constipation, sexual impotence, and dizziness/fainting [8–10]. The median survival for

* Correspondence: david.adams@aphp.fr; adams.david@neuf.fr
[1]CHU Hôpital Bicêtre, Le Kremlin-Bicêtre CEDEX, Paris, France
Full list of author information is available at the end of the article

patients with hATTR amyloidosis with polyneuropathy is reported as 5–15 years from diagnosis [9, 11–13].

To date >120 *TTR* mutations have been reported [14]; some mutations are more strongly associated with polyneuropathy (e.g. V30M [8]), and others with cardiomyopathy (e.g. V122I [15]). However, this genotype–phenotype association likely represents an over-simplification, with wide variation in presentation reported between genotypes and a mixed phenotype commonly observed [3, 16].

Effectively quantifying the disease burden in hATTR amyloidosis remains challenging, as there is no single test that captures the constellation of symptoms and the multisystemic nature of the condition. Indeed, even assessment of all signs and symptoms of polyneuropathy requires numerous measures, which recent data suggest are not adequately captured in current tests [17]. For example, the Neuropathy Impairment Score (NIS)-Lower Limb (NIS-LL) is based on examination of lower limbs only, so dysfunction occurring in other areas as the disease progresses cannot be captured. The widely used NIS overcomes this limitation through clinical examination of lower limbs, upper limbs, and cranial nerves, although this tool does not include nerve conduction scores, which are critical to assess the axonal neuropathy which progresses during the disease course [6, 8, 12]. In addition, the NIS does not adequately address sensory loss over the body, which is a hallmark of the disease [18]. Ultimately, scoring the full range of neuropathic impairment likely requires a combined measure of the type, severity, and distribution of neurologic signs and symptoms [17]. There is also a limited set of tools that have demonstrated utility in assessment of quality of life (QoL) and physical functioning in hATTR amyloidosis, primarily the Norfolk Quality of Life-Diabetic Neuropathy (QOL-DN), EuroQoL 5-Dimensions (EQ-5D™), and Short-Form 36 (SF-36) Health Survey questionnaires [19–24]. Consequently, the need remains for clinical trials that include a comprehensive set of measures to investigate disease progression and the effects of treatment on patient well-being and function.

As TTR is produced predominantly in the liver [25, 26] orthotopic liver transplantation (OLT) is a well-recognized and effective treatment strategy for replacing mutant TTR protein [27, 28]. However, OLT is only recommended for patients with early-stage hATTR amyloidosis, and survival varies according to modified body mass index (mBMI), disease duration/severity, and *TTR* mutation [8, 28, 29]. The procedure itself is also limited by issues such as cost, donor availability, cardiac involvement, and toxicities associated with immunosuppression [2, 30]. Furthermore, disease progression can continue after OLT as a result of amyloid fibril deposition from wild-type TTR [31, 32]. More recently, the pharmacotherapies tafamidis and diflunisal, which stabilize the TTR complex and prevent protein misfolding (TTR tetramer stabilizers), have been utilized. Tafamidis was approved in Europe for patients with hATTR amyloidosis with early-stage neurologic disease (FAP stage 1), despite limited data, with authorization under "exceptional circumstances" due to the clinical unmet need [33]. Subsequent approvals for treatment of symptomatic polyneuropathy have followed in regions of Latin America and Asia. Diflunisal, a non-steroidal anti-inflammatory drug, has been used off label for management of hATTR amyloidosis [34]. In clinical studies, both compounds have slowed progression of neurologic impairment and were generally well tolerated [19, 24, 35]. However, progression of neuropathy symptoms or disability is still observed in some patients [24, 35–37], and tafamidis may have reduced efficacy in patients with more severe disease [38]. Thus, there remains a need for novel treatment options for hATTR amyloidosis.

Patisiran is an investigational RNA interference (RNAi) therapeutic in clinical development for hATTR amyloidosis. Patisiran is a small interfering RNA (siRNA) that targets a sequence of mRNA conserved across wild-type and all TTR variants and can thereby reduce serum levels of both wild-type and pathogenic (mutated) protein [39]. It is formulated as lipid nanoparticles which direct it to the liver, the primary source of circulating TTR [39]. The benefits of lowering mutant TTR levels in patients with hATTR amyloidosis have been demonstrated by OLT [40, 41], and data from other amyloidoses show that clinical outcomes can be improved by reducing amyloidogenic protein [42–44]. In a Phase 2 study (NCT01617967) of 29 patients with hATTR amyloidosis, two doses of patisiran 0.3 mg/kg every 3 weeks reduced mean serum TTR levels by approximately 80% [45]. This potent TTR knockdown was observed for both wild-type and mutant (V30M) forms of TTR, and in patients who were concurrently receiving TTR tetramer stabilizers [45]. An ongoing open-label extension study (NCT01961921) has provided encouraging data, with stable measures of neuropathy impairment and patisiran being generally well tolerated through 24 months of treatment [46].

Collectively, these data support the hypothesis that TTR reduction has the potential to stabilize the progression of – or even reverse – neuropathy in patients with hATTR amyloidosis. To date, APOLLO is the largest Phase 3 clinical study in patients with hATTR amyloidosis, designed to assess the safety and efficacy of patisiran on neurologic function and QoL.

Methods

Study oversight

This study is conducted according to the guidelines of the International Conference on Harmonisation, the

World Health Organization's Declaration of Helsinki, and the Health Insurance Portability and Accountability Act of 1996. Written informed consent is obtained from all patients who participate in the study, prior to assessment of eligibility. The study protocol was approved by the local Institutional Review Boards and Ethics Committees, and all subsequent protocol amendments underwent the same approval procedure. A clinical monitor, as a representative of Alnylam, will follow the study through periodic site visits and frequent telephone/written contact. A Data Monitoring Committee will be implemented for the study and provide independent evaluation to ensure patient safety. This trial is registered at www.clinicaltrials.gov (NCT01960348).

Study overview and setting

APOLLO is a randomized, multicenter, international, double-blind, placebo-controlled, Phase 3 study designed to evaluate the efficacy of patisiran and establish the safety of chronic dosing in adult patients with symptomatic hATTR amyloidosis with polyneuropathy. A study schematic is shown in Fig. 1. Patients are recruited from 46 sites across 19 countries (United States, France, Taiwan, Spain, Japan, Germany, Mexico, Portugal, South Korea, Sweden, Bulgaria, Italy, Canada, Turkey, Cyprus, Brazil, Netherlands, United Kingdom, and Argentina). All but two of the sites are academic hospitals.

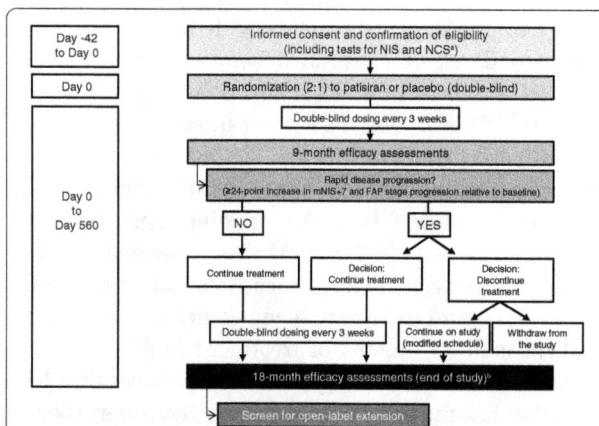

Fig. 1 APOLLO study schematic. [a]Karnofsky performance status, New York Heart Association class, safety, and TTR genotyping also assessed as part of eligibility criteria. [b]18-month efficacy assessments: mNIS+7, NIS+7, FAP score, polyneuropathy disability stage, nerve fiber density, dermal amyloid burden, modified body mass index, timed 10-m walk test, grip strength test, Composite Autonomic Symptom Score-31 questionnaire, Norfolk Quality of Life-Diabetic Neuropathy questionnaire, EuroQol 5-Dimensions questionnaire, Rasch-built Overall Disability Scale, echocardiogram, and cardiac biomarkers. *FAP* familial amyloidotic polyneuropathy; *IV* intravenous; *mNIS+7* modified NIS+7; *NCS* nerve conduction study; *NIS* Neuropathy Impairment Score

Eligibility

At screening, patients are 18–85 years old, with a diagnosis of hATTR amyloidosis, a documented *TTR* mutation, and investigator-estimated survival of ≥2 years. Eligible patients have an NIS of 5–130, polyneuropathy disability (PND) score ≤IIIb, and adequate biochemical liver function. The NIS range of 5–130 was selected to include patients with disease sufficiently advanced to show progression in the placebo group, but not so advanced as to preclude detection of a change in disease status. Patients with previous OLT or sensorimotor/ autonomic neuropathy due to other known causes are not included in the study. The key inclusion and exclusion criteria are summarized in Table 1.

Study design

Patients are randomized to receive either patisiran 0.3 mg/kg or placebo (normal saline 0.9%) once every 3 weeks for 18 months. Study drug is administered as an intravenous infusion over 70 min (1 mL/min for the first 15 min, then 3 mL/min thereafter).

Patients have the option of discontinuing study drug if they experience a protocol-defined rapid disease progression at 9 months, defined as ≥24-point increase in mNIS+7 from baseline (estimated 24-point increase in mNIS+7 score in the placebo group expected by 18 months based on natural history study [47]), and FAP stage [7] progression relative to baseline, confirmed by an external adjudication committee. Such patients may receive alternative therapy (local standard of care) and will be monitored based on a modified visit schedule if they decide to stay on study. All patients who complete the final 18-month assessment are eligible to screen for an open-label extension study of long-term patisiran treatment (NCT02510261).

Premedication

To reduce the likelihood of infusion-related reactions, patients are to receive the following premedications or equivalent at least 60 min before each study drug infusion: dexamethasone; oral acetaminophen/paracetamol; an H_2 blocker (e.g., ranitidine or famotidine); and an H_1 blocker (e.g., diphenhydramine).

Concomitant medications

The use of tafamidis, diflunisal, doxycycline, tauroursodeoxycholic acid, or any investigational agent other than patisiran is prohibited during study participation. These agents may have been used before screening, but a wash-out period is mandated (14 days for tafamidis, doxycycline, or tauroursodeoxycholic acid; 3 days for diflunisal). Palliative and supportive-care medications are permitted during the study.

Table 1 Key inclusion and exclusion criteria for the APOLLO study

Inclusion criteria	Exclusion criteria
• Diagnosis of hATTR amyloidosis with documented mutation • Anticipated survival ≥2 years • Aged 18–85 years (inclusive) • NIS of 5–130 • PND score ≤IIIb • NCS sum of the sural SNAP, tibial CMAP, ulnar SNAP, ulnar CMAP, and peroneal CMAP of ≥2 points • Karnofsky performance status ≥60% • Absolute neutrophil count ≥1500 cells/mm³ • Platelet count ≥50,000 cells/mm³ • Adequate biochemical liver function[a] • Serum creatinine ≤2 × ULN	• Previous liver transplantation, or liver transplantation planned during study period • Sensorimotor or autonomic neuropathy not related to hATTR amyloidosis • Primary or leptomeningeal amyloidosis • Type 1 diabetes • Type 2 diabetes for ≥5 years • Active hepatitis B or C, or HIV infection • NYHA heart failure classification >2 • Acute coronary syndrome within past 3 months • Uncontrolled cardiac arrhythmia or unstable angina • Severe reaction to a liposomal product or hypersensitivity to oligonucleotides • Unable to take premedications • Received an investigational agent within 30 days/5 half-lives (whichever is longer) of study drug administration • Currently taking tafamidis, diflunisal, doxycycline, or tauroursodeoxycholic acid

CMAP compound muscle action potential; *hATTR amyloidosis* hereditary transthyretin-mediated amyloidosis; *NCS* nerve conduction study; *NIS* Neuropathy Impairment Score; *NYHA* New York Heart Association; *PND* polyneuropathy disability; *SNAP* sensory nerve action potential; *ULN* upper limit of normal
[a]Aspartate transaminase and alanine transaminase levels ≤2.5 × ULN; total bilirubin levels within normal limits; international normalized ratio ≤2.0

Stratification, randomization, and blinding

Patients are randomized in a 2:1 (patisiran:placebo) ratio using an interactive response system. Treatment arms are balanced at study entry for: NIS (5–49 vs 50–130), early-onset V30M disease (age < 50 years at onset) vs all other mutations (including late-onset V30M), and previous use of tafamidis or diflunisal. Patients and study personnel who monitor patients during infusions and perform clinical assessments are blinded to the study treatment. Unblinded personnel and pharmacists prepare the drug for administration, but are not involved in patient management or safety or efficacy assessments. Details of patients who discontinue study drug at 9 months due to rapid disease progression remain blinded throughout the study.

Efficacy assessments

Primary outcome measure: mNIS+7

The primary objective is to determine the difference between the patisiran and placebo groups in change from baseline in mNIS+7 at 18 months (Table 2). The mNIS+7 used in APOLLO has been modified from the original NIS+7 to better characterize and quantify sensation all over the body, autonomic function, and nerve conduction changes associated with hATTR amyloidosis progression [17]. A summary of the scoring components of the NIS+7 and mNIS+7 is provided in Table 3.

The mNIS+7 assessment tool [17] used in this study is a 304-point composite measure of neurologic impairment that includes: neurologic examination of lower limbs, upper limbs, and cranial nerves (NIS-weakness and reflexes); electrophysiologic measures of small and large nerve fiber function (including nerve conduction studies [NCS] Σ5 of ulnar, peroneal, and tibial compound muscle action potential [CMAP] amplitudes and sural and ulnar sensory nerve action potential [SNAP] amplitudes; and smart somatotopic quantitative sensory testing [S ST QSTing; including touch pressure and heat pain]) at defined body surface locations (Fig. 2); and autonomic function (postural hypotension). Scoring for NCS and postural hypotension is based on grading of function: normal (<95th percentile) = 0 points; mildly reduced (≥95th to <99th percentile) = 1 point; and very reduced (≥99th percentile) = 2 points. The mNIS+7 is measured in replicates during the pre-randomization phase (at screening/baseline [21 days before the first dose of study drug] and at baseline [≥24 h after screening/baseline measure]), and at 9 and 18 months. Two independent assessments are taken at each time point, performed at least 24 h apart, but no greater than 7 days apart. An increase in mNIS+7 score, or in any of its components, indicates worsening impairment.

To standardize the efficacy assessment and minimize variability across the multiple centers, neuromuscular physicians were trained to perform the mNIS+7 evaluation at a central center (Dyck Peripheral Nerve Research Laboratory, Mayo Clinic, Rochester, MN, USA).

Secondary and exploratory clinical outcome measures

The secondary and exploratory objectives are to determine the effect of patisiran on a variety of clinical parameters, based on their change from baseline to 18 months (Table 2). Unless stated, parameters are assessed at screening/baseline, baseline, 9, and 18 months.

Neurologic and cardiac function

Neurologic function is measured using the NIS+7 tool [48] based on two independent readings as described for mNIS+7. For both mNIS+7 and NIS+7, the individual components of the scores will be reported. Specific motor function assessments include the timed 10-m walk test and hand grip strength test (dynamometer), with measurements performed on separate days. Cardiac function is assessed through echocardiograms and cardiac biomarkers (troponin I and N-terminal pro-brain-type natriuretic peptide).

Table 2 Study objectives

Objective	
Primary	• Determine the efficacy of patisiran by evaluating the difference between the patisiran and placebo groups in the change from baseline of mNIS+7 at 18 months
Secondary (hierarchical ordering)	• Norfolk Quality of Life-Diabetic Neuropathy questionnaire • NIS-weakness score • Level of disability (Rasch-built Overall Disability Scale) • Timed 10-m walk test • mBMI[a] • Composite Autonomic Symptom Score questionnaire
Exploratory	• NIS + 7 score • Grip strength • EuroQol 5-Dimensions questionnaire (EQ-5D-5L index, EQ VAS) • Large versus small nerve fiber function[b] • Sensory and autonomic innervation and analysis of nerve fiber density and sweat gland nerve fiber density • Dermal amyloid content on skin biopsy • FAP stage and PND score • Cardiac measures (echocardiogram, troponin I, and NT-proBNP levels) • Pharmacodynamic biomarkers (TTR, RBP, and vitamin A) • Proportion of patients with rapid disease progression at 9 months • Lower limb nerve injury via voluntary magnetic resonance neurography • Columbia-Suicide Severity Rating Scale (C-SSRS)

FAP familial amyloidotic polyneuropathy; mBMI modified body mass index; mNIS modified Neuropathy Impairment Score; NIS Neuropathy Impairment Score; NT-proBNP N-terminal pro-brain-type natriuretic peptide; PND polyneuropathy disability; RBP retinol-binding protein; TTR transthyretin
[a]mBMI calculated as kg/m^2 × albumin (g/L)
[b]Nerve fiber function assessed through nerve conduction studies of 5 attributes (Σ5): quantitative sensory testing by body surface area including touch pressure and heat pain, vibration detection threshold, heart rate response to deep breathing, and postural blood pressure

Quality of life/symptoms and health status

QoL assessments include the Norfolk QOL-DN questionnaire [49], a 35-item measure sensitive to small fiber, large fiber, and autonomic nerve function, which has been shown to be a reliable indicator of disease severity in patients with hATTR amyloidosis [20] (increase in score = worsening QoL), and the EQ-5D™ questionnaire [50] (decrease in score = worsening QoL). Autonomic symptoms are evaluated using the 31-question Composite Autonomic Symptom Score (COMPASS)-31 questionnaire, which covers six autonomic domains (orthostatic intolerance, vasomotor, secretomotor, gastrointestinal, bladder, and pupillomotor) [51] (increase in score = worsening symptoms). Activity and social function are assessed through the Rasch-built Overall Disability Scale (R-ODS), a 24-item scale to capture limitations on everyday activities [52] (decrease in score = worsening disability). Nutritional status is gauged using mBMI (kg/m^2 × albumin [g/L]), taken at baseline, and days 84, 189, 357, 462, and 546.

(18-month assessment). Changes in ambulation are assessed according to FAP stage [7] and PND score [53] (increase in stage/score = worsening impairment), and the timed 10-m walk test (increase in duration = worsening impairment). Lower limb nerve injury is serially evaluated via voluntary magnetic resonance neurography approximately every 6 months in patients providing voluntary consent.

Pathologic nerve fiber and amyloid evaluation

Nerve fibers and amyloid deposits in the skin are quantified through measurement of intraepidermal nerve fiber density, sweat gland nerve fiber density, and dermal amyloid burden using tandem 3 mm skin punch biopsies in patients providing voluntary consent. At each time point, one set of biopsies is taken from the lower leg and another from the distal thigh.

Pharmacodynamic assessments

Levels of serum TTR protein, vitamin A, and retinol-binding protein (RBP) are measured at baseline, pre-dose on day 0, and on days 21, 126, 252, 253–272 (9 months), 273, 399, 546, and 553–560 (18 months). Serum TTR is measured using an enzyme-linked immunosorbent assay and a turbidimetric assay. Serum RBP is quantified using nephelometry. Serum samples are evaluated by a high-performance liquid chromatography assay to determine vitamin A levels. Pharmacodynamic samples are not taken at 18 months for patients who discontinue treatment at 9 months (modified schedule).

Pharmacokinetic assessments

Plasma samples for pharmacokinetic analysis are taken pre-dose and post-dose on days 0, 21, 126, 252, 399, and 546. Pharmacokinetic parameters for plasma siRNA are evaluated using a validated ATTO™-probe high-performance liquid chromatography assay.

Safety assessments

Adverse events (AEs) are assessed throughout the study, and reported according to the Medical Dictionary of Regulatory Activities (version 18.0 or later). AEs are graded based on their severity (mild, moderate, or severe) and the causal relationship to study drug or premedication recorded. Clinical laboratory and chemistry tests, thyroid function parameters, urinalysis, anti-drug antibodies, electrocardiograms, physical and vital signs, and ophthalmology examinations (including electroretinography) are also monitored. The Columbia-Suicide Severity Rating Scale (C-SSRS) is used to assess mental status as it relates to suicidal ideation and behavior.

Table 3 Comparison of the neurologic impairment scores used in the evaluation of hATTR amyloidosis

	NIS-LL	NIS	NIS+7	mNIS+7	mNIS+7$_{Ionis}$
Total score	88	244	270	**304**	346.3
Assessment (score)					
Motor strength/ weakness	Neurologic exam [lower limbs only] (64)	Neurologic exam (192)	Neurologic exam (192)	**Neurologic exam (192)**	Neurologic exam (192)
Reflexes	Neurologic exam [lower limbs only] (8)	Neurologic exam (20)	Neurologic exam (20)	**Neurologic exam (20)**	Neurologic exam (20)
Sensation	–	–	–	**QST – heat pain and touch pressure at multiple sites (80)**	QST – heat pain and touch pressure at multiple sites (80)
	Neurologic exam [lower limbs only] (16)	Neurologic exam (32)	Neurologic exam (32)	–	Neurologic exam (32)
	–	–	Vibration detection threshold (3.7)	–	–
Composite nerve conduction score	–	–	Σ5 – sural SNAP/ fibular nerve CMAP, tibial motor nerve distal latency, motor nerve conduction velocity, motor nerve distal latency (18.6)[a]	**Σ5 – ulnar CMAP and SNAP, peroneal[c] CMAP, tibial CMAP, sural SNAP (10)[b]**	Σ5 – ulnar CMAP and SNAP, peroneal[c] CMAP, tibial CMAP, sural SNAP (18.6)[a]
Autonomic function	–	–	Heart rate response to deep breathing (3.7)[a]	**Postural blood pressure (2)[b]**	Heart rate response to deep breathing (3.7)[a]

CMAP compound muscle action potential; *exam* examination; *mNIS+7* modified NIS+7; *NIS* Neuropathy Impairment Score; *NIS-LL* NIS based on examination of lower limbs only; *QST* quantitative sensory testing; *SNAP* sensory nerve action potential

[a]Score expressed as normal deviates (0–3.72) based on healthy-subject parameters
[b]Score graded according to defined categories: normal (95th percentile) = 0 points; mildly reduced (≥95th to <99th percentile) = 1 point; and very reduced (≥99th percentile) = 2 points
[c]May also be referred to as fibular [62]

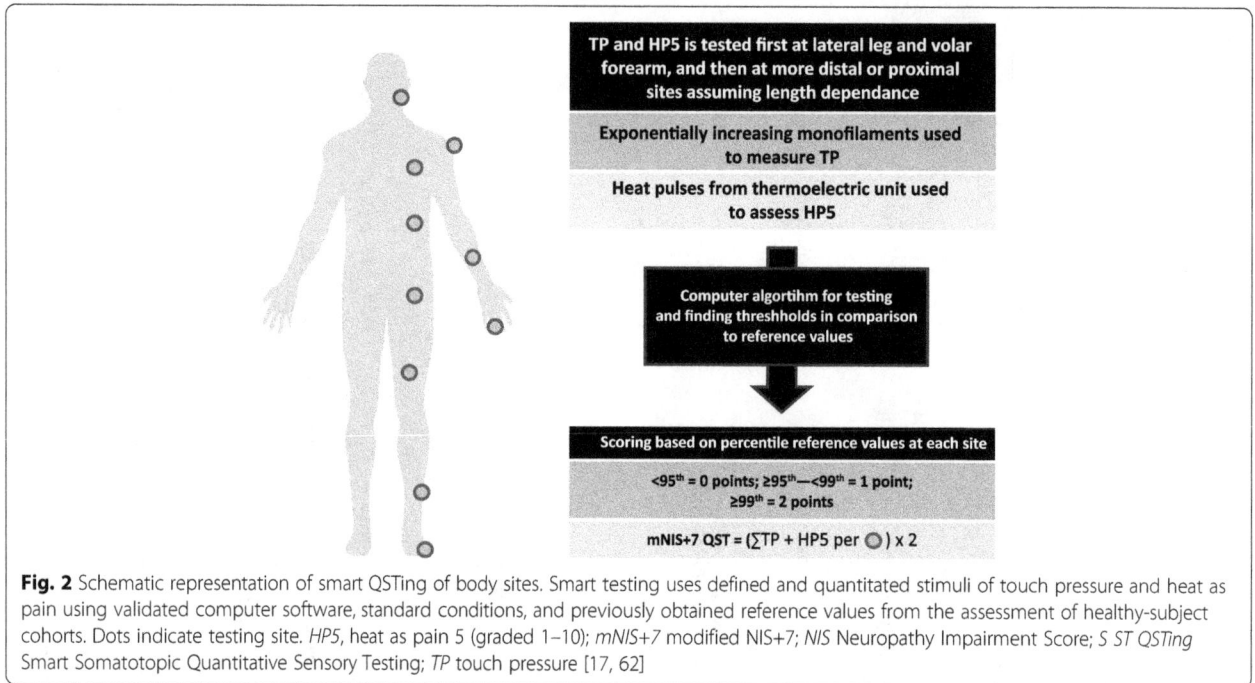

Fig. 2 Schematic representation of smart QSTing of body sites. Smart testing uses defined and quantitated stimuli of touch pressure and heat as pain using validated computer software, standard conditions, and previously obtained reference values from the assessment of healthy-subject cohorts. Dots indicate testing site. *HP5*, heat as pain 5 (graded 1–10); *mNIS+7* modified NIS+7; *NIS* Neuropathy Impairment Score; *S ST QSTing* Smart Somatotopic Quantitative Sensory Testing; *TP* touch pressure [17, 62]

Statistical analyses

A sample size of approximately 200 patients will provide 90% power to test a treatment difference of 8.95 points (37.5%) in mNIS+7 change from baseline (primary endpoint) with a two-sided $\alpha = 0.05$. The sample size of approximately 200 is based on an assumed premature discontinuation rate of 25%.

The populations analyzed in the study are: the modified intent-to-treat (mITT) population (all patients who were randomized and received at least one dose of study drug); the per-protocol population (all patients who completed all efficacy assessments and did not have any major protocol violations); and the safety population (all patients who received at least one dose of study drug).

The analysis of efficacy endpoints will be conducted for the mITT population. Formal statistical hypothesis testing will be performed on the primary and secondary efficacy endpoints with all tests conducted at the nominal two-sided, 0.05 level of significance.

Discussion

The APOLLO study examines the efficacy and safety of the investigational RNAi therapeutic patisiran in a broad hATTR amyloidosis population, including patients with any amyloidogenic *TTR* mutation and with a wide range of neuropathy severity and age at baseline. The composite primary endpoint of APOLLO (mNIS+7) is well suited for use in hATTR amyloidosis because it encompasses multiple aspects of the polyneuropathy and can capture changes during disease progression. In addition,

QoL, motor function, health status, autonomic symptoms, cardiac assessments, and everyday functioning are included as secondary or exploratory endpoints to assess the impact of patisiran on a range of disease involvement.

The mNIS+7 used to assess neurologic impairment in this study is more robust and comprehensive than the tools used in the trials of tafamidis (NIS-LL) [19] or diflunisal (NIS+7) [24], with the modifications outlined in Table 3. One of the key attributes of the mNIS+7 versus NIS+7 is the measurement of sensation, with S ST QSTing used in preference to NIS-sensation evaluation and vibration detection threshold. Indeed, the NIS-sensation score is not included in mNIS+7 in APOLLO, as the study of Suanprasert et al. in 97 patients with hATTR amyloidosis suggested that this score did not adequately capture sensation loss [17]. Compared with NIS-sensation, S ST QSTing provides an improved balance between large and small sensory nerve fibers and measures sensation loss over the whole body rather than at distal sites such as big toes and fingers. Whilst S ST QSTing is time-consuming and requires specialist training and standardized protocols to avoid procedural variability [54, 55], these demands are necessary to assess sensation loss somatopically and accurately [56]. Aside from sensation, the other major alteration from the NIS+7 is in the measurement of nerve conduction. Here, the combined NCSΣ5 in the mNIS+7 includes only action potential amplitudes, which are more suited to capture changes in disease course for hATTR amyloidosis as this disease has a primarily axonal pathophysiology. A further change from the NIS+7 is the new autonomic measure: postural hypotension was included because heart rate decrease with deep breathing was considered an inconsistent assessment of autonomic function as it is unevaluable in patients with cardiac pacemakers and frequently unevaluable in patients with arrhythmias [17, 56]. It is recognized however, that pharmacologic interventions (e.g., fludrocortisone and midodrine) can be used to treat postural hypotension [57], and the use of any such strategies should be considered when gauging the effect of patisiran on this measure. With the modifications to the NIS+7, the total score was increased to 304 points for the mNIS+7 used in this study. Measurement of muscle weakness and stretch reflexes were considered adequate with the original NIS+7, so these elements have not been modified [17].

However, it should be noted that the mNIS+7 described by Suanprasert et al., which is used in APOLLO, is different from that currently being used in the study investigating the anti-TTR antisense oligonucleotide IONIS-TTR$_{Rx}$ (mNIS+7$_{Ionis}$). The critical difference between these two versions of the mNIS+7 is in the measurement of sensation: mNIS+7$_{Ionis}$ includes the NIS-sensation testing score from the original NIS+7, in addition to S ST QSTing [56] (Table 3). As discussed, NIS-sensation may not provide a true reflection of sensation impairment, with inclusion of the original NIS+7-sensation testing potentially being redundant. Indeed, this may lead to double counting for assessments of sensation. The other notable difference is that the mNIS+7$_{Ionis}$ does not include postural hypotension, and instead retains the heart rate decrease with deep breathing measure of the NIS+7 for assessment of autonomic function, which has the limitations discussed above for patients with pacemakers or cardiac arrhythmias. Both mNIS+7 and mNIS+7$_{Ionis}$ include only CMAPs and SNAPs as nerve conduction measures (Table 3). Regarding assessment of NCS, it is worth noting that these are expressed as normal deviates in the mNIS+7$_{Ionis}$, whereas they are graded by defined categories in mNIS+7 (Table 3).

The features of the mNIS+7 described above have been introduced to create a tool suitable for use in hATTR amyloidosis clinical studies. As assessment of neuropathic measures is subject to variability between investigators, extensive training is provided to support the use of a standardized and validated methodology and ensure that scoring is consistent and accurate. Specifically, specialized training is provided for neuromuscular physicians, with certification upon completion. For clinical assessment of neuropathy signs and symptoms, neuromuscular experts are trained to use only unequivocal abnormalities (accounting for age, sex, physical fitness, and anthropomorphic variables) rather than more

traditional clinical criteria, and not to grade for concomitant neuromuscular disease. Previous analyses have shown that this strategy, when used by trained specialists, leads to increased reproducibility and a notable improvement in proficiency when scoring clinical measures, such as weakness and reflexes, as used in APOLLO [58, 59]. Variability between centers has also been noted for NCS, which is countered in this study through specialist training on techniques and reference values, and evaluation of tracings at a central reading center; these methodologies have been shown to reduce inter-investigator variability [60, 61]. Of the other mNIS+7 measures, the S ST QSTings used in APOLLO are also standardized and referenced, to ensure generation of accurate and comparable data across the study [62].

The clinical relevance of NIS has been previously demonstrated, with total NIS correlated with FAP stage, PND score, and QoL (Norfolk QOL-DN and SF-36) in patients with hATTR amyloidosis [47, 56]. In addition, rapid worsening of NIS was observed in untreated patients in a natural history study of patients with hATTR amyloidosis [47], fitting with the relentless progression expected for this disease [8]. The estimated rate of NIS progression for a patient with a baseline NIS of 32 was 14.3 points per year [47], and a separate analysis has indicated a worsening in NIS-LL of up to 7.4 points over 12 months in patients with a baseline NIS-LL of 20–30 [63]. The rapid neurologic deterioration observed in patients with hATTR amyloidosis contrasts with lower rates of NIS progression seen in other neuropathies [64, 65]. For example, in patients with mild-to-moderate diabetic distal symmetric sensorimotor polyneuropathy, NIS and NIS-LL increased by only 0.61 and 0.43 points, respectively, over 4 years of placebo treatment [64]. Furthermore, a study of disease progression in Charcot–Marie–Tooth disease type 1A reported an annual NIS increase of 1.37 points [65].

Based on the described modifications to the NIS, it is anticipated that the mNIS+7 will more accurately capture the degree of polyneuropathy and neurologic impairment in patients with hATTR amyloidosis. Indeed, rapid disease progression in untreated patients has also been demonstrated using the mNIS+7, with an increase of approximately 24 points anticipated after 18 months [47]. The clinical value of the mNIS+7 was further demonstrated in recent analyses of the baseline data from APOLLO, which showed an association between mNIS+7 and FAP stage and PND score (Fig. 3). In addition, investigation of the mNIS+7$_{Ionis}$ showed that clinical polyneuropathy signs and symptoms correlated strongly with assessments of action potential amplitudes and somatotopic touch pressure [56], which are also included in the mNIS+7. Of the other measures taken in

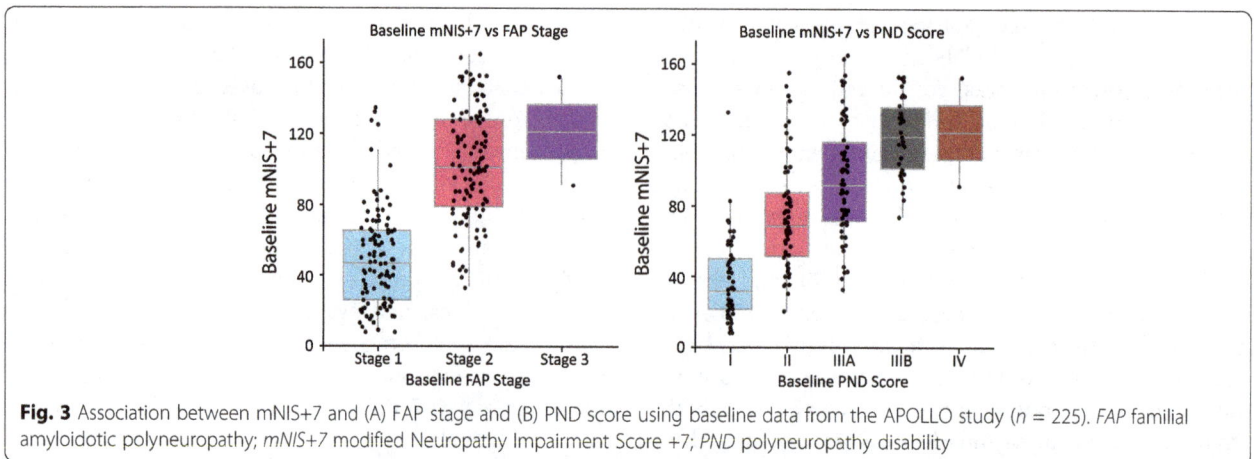

Fig. 3 Association between mNIS+7 and (A) FAP stage and (B) PND score using baseline data from the APOLLO study (*n* = 225). *FAP* familial amyloidotic polyneuropathy; *mNIS+7* modified Neuropathy Impairment Score +7; *PND* polyneuropathy disability

APOLLO, a correlation between mNIS+7 and TTR knockdown was demonstrated in the Phase 2 open-label extension study of patisiran [66], supporting the hypothesis that reducing levels of amyloidogenic protein leads to clinical benefit in hATTR amyloidosis (e.g., via OLT [28]).

hATTR amyloidosis is associated with symptoms across multiple systems [2, 67]. In addition to the neurologic symptoms, patients often present with a mixed phenotype including concurrent cardiac symptoms. Cardiomyopathy associated with hATTR amyloidosis can lead to heart failure and death, highlighting the need for vigilance around cardiac amyloid fibril accumulation. The APOLLO study therefore includes echocardiographic and biochemical cardiac parameters to assess the impact of patisiran on cardiac progression.

The impact of the diverse disease symptoms may not be fully captured by clinical and laboratory examinations, so QoL measures were included as key endpoints in the studies of tafamidis and diflunisal [19, 24]. APOLLO uses the Norfolk QOL-DN and EQ-5D questionnaires to assess QoL. The Norfolk QOL-DN questionnaire evaluates small and large nerve fiber function in addition to autonomic impairment and activities of daily living. It has demonstrated utility in patients with hATTR amyloidosis with polyneuropathy both as a measure of disease severity and as a clinical endpoint to assess response to treatment [20, 21]. The EQ-5D questionnaire has been used as part of the international Transthyretin Amyloidosis Outcomes Survey (THAOS), which demonstrated worsening QoL with disease progression [22]. Autonomic symptoms, particularly gastrointestinal events, are common in patients with hATTR amyloidosis [23] underpinning the comprehensive assessment of autonomic function using the COMPASS-31 questionnaire [51]. Other measures in APOLLO include the R-ODS survey [52] for assessment of the effects of patisiran on activities of daily living. The R-ODS

has already been used to demonstrate that hATTR amyloidosis can affect activities such as washing dishes or fastening buttons [68], and has been validated in patients with V30M hATTR amyloidosis [69].

The pharmacotherapies currently approved or available for hATTR amyloidosis can slow or sometimes stabilize disease, but there is little evidence that complete stabilization or reversal of nerve damage can be achieved. Sensory and autonomic innervation in skin punch biopsies are being evaluated in APOLLO to determine whether patisiran can increase nerve fiber density. Increases in sweat gland fiber density were observed in the Phase 2 open-label extension study of patisiran [46], and APOLLO will provide an opportunity for these findings to be validated in a placebo-controlled setting. Of interest, sweat gland nerve fiber density has previously been associated with ambulation in patients with hATTR amyloidosis [70]. In addition to nerve fiber density, these skin biopsies are also being evaluated in both the Phase 2 open-label extension study and APOLLO for changes in dermal amyloid burden.

Aside from clinical endpoints related to efficacy, safety and pharmacodynamics will also be assessed throughout the APOLLO study and subsequent open-label extension. Longer-term data from the Phase 2 open-label extension study suggest patisiran is well tolerated, but APOLLO will allow comparison against a placebo-controlled arm. In particular, the safety of prolonged lowering of vitamin A levels, associated with TTR reduction, will be assessed. TTR reduction itself provides a convenient biomarker to assess patisiran activity, and reduction in the pathogenic protein may also relate to clinical parameters.

Recruitment for APOLLO started in December 2013 and was completed in January 2016, with 225 patients enrolled. This trial represents the largest Phase 3 study of an RNAi strategy for the treatment of hATTR amyloidosis, with clinical endpoints that strive to assess the multiple ways in which this disease affects patient well-being and function. The Patisiran Global open-label extension study was initiated in July 2015, and will provide further data on long-term safety and efficacy of patisiran in patients with hATTR amyloidosis.

Abbreviations
AE: Adverse event; CMAP: Compound muscle action potential; COMPASS-31: 31-question Composite Autonomic Symptom Score; EQ-5D: EuroQol 5-Dimensions; FAP: Familial amyloid polyneuropathy; hATTR amyloidosis: Hereditary ATTR amyloidosis; mBMI: Modified body mass index; mITT: Modified intent-to-treat; mNIS+7: Modified Neuropathy Impairment Score; mNIS+7$_{\text{Ionis}}$: mNIS+7 being used in the study investigating the anti-TTR antisense oligonucleotide IONIS-TTR$_{\text{Rx}}$; NCS: Nerve conduction study; NIS: Neuropathy Impairment Score; NIS-LL: NIS-Lower Limb; OLT: Orthotopic liver transplantation; PND: Polyneuropathy disability score; QoL: Quality of life; QOL-DN: Norfolk Quality of Life-Diabetic Neuropathy; RBP: Retinol-binding protein; RNAi: RNA interference; R-ODS: Rasch-built Overall Disability Scale; SF-36: Short-Form 36; siRNA: Small interfering RNA; SNAP: Sensory nerve action potential; S ST QSTing: Smart somatotopic quantitative sensory testing; TTR: Transthyretin

Acknowledgements
Editorial support was provided by Adelphi Communications Ltd., UK, funded by Alnylam.

Funding
This study is funded by Alnylam Pharmaceuticals.

Authors' contributions
Authorship was decided based on ICJME criteria. DA, OS, PD, WL, RL, JC, JG, and TC were involved in the conception and design of the study. DA, OS, PD, WL, RL, JC, JG, and TC critically reviewed the manuscript and approved the final version. RL, JC, and JG are employed by the study funder. All authors have read and approved the final manuscript, and agreed to its publication.

Competing interests
Adams: Research funding and consultancy fees from Alnylam Pharmaceuticals, and personal symposium fees from Pfizer Inc. Suhr: Personal fees and non-financial support from Alnylam Pharmaceuticals, and personal fees from Prothena Pharmaceuticals and Pfizer Inc. Dyck: Compensation for training and quality assurance associated with clinical trials from Alnylam Pharmaceuticals and IONIS Pharmaceuticals; honoraria from Diabetes journal as Associate Editor. Litchy: Compensation for travel and training of investigators from Alnylam Pharmaceuticals and IONIS Pharmaceuticals. Leahy: Employment by Alnylam Pharmaceuticals. Chen: Employment by Alnylam Pharmaceuticals. Gollob: Employment by Alnylam Pharmaceuticals. Coelho: Compensation for training from Pfizer Inc. and Alnylam Pharmaceuticals, and compensation for travel from Pfizer Inc., Alnylam Pharmaceuticals, and IONIS Pharmaceuticals.

Author details
[1]CHU Hôpital Bicêtre, Le Kremlin-Bicêtre CEDEX, Paris, France. [2]Department of Public Health and Clinical Medicine, Umeå University Hospital, Umeå, Sweden. [3]Department of Neurology, Mayo Clinic, Rochester, MN, USA. [4]Alnylam Pharmaceuticals, Cambridge, MA, USA. [5]Hospital Santo António, Centro Hospitalar do Porto, Porto, Portugal.

References
1. Hanna M. Novel drugs targeting transthyretin amyloidosis. Curr Heart Fail Rep. 2014;11(1):50–7.
2. Hawkins PN, Ando Y, Dispenzeri A, Gonzalez-Duarte A, Adams D, Suhr OB. Evolving landscape in the management of transthyretin amyloidosis. Ann Med. 2015;47(8):625–38.
3. Coelho T, Maurer MS, Suhr OB. THAOS - The Transthyretin Amyloidosis Outcomes Survey: initial report on clinical manifestations in patients with hereditary and wild-type transthyretin amyloidosis. Curr Med Res Opin. 2013;29(1):63–76.
4. Mohty D, Damy T, Cosnay P, Echahidi N, Casset-Senon D, Virot P, Jaccard A. Cardiac amyloidosis: updates in diagnosis and management. Arch Cardiovasc Dis. 2013;106(10):528–40.
5. Conceicao I, Gonzalez-Duarte A, Obici L, Schmidt HH, Simoneau D, Ong ML, Amass L. "Red-flag" symptom clusters in transthyretin familial amyloid polyneuropathy. J Peripher Nerv Syst. 2016;21(1):5–9.
6. Shin SC, Robinson-Papp J. Amyloid neuropathies. Mt Sinai J Med. 2012;79(6):733–48.
7. Coutinho P, DeSilva A, Lima J, Barbosa A. Forty years of experience with type I amyloid neuropathy: review of 483 cases. In: Glenner G, Costa P, de Freitas A, editors. Amyloid and Amyloidosis. Amsterdam: Excerpta Medica; 1980. pp. 88–98.
8. Ando Y, Coelho T, Berk JL, Cruz MW, Ericzon BG, Ikeda S, Lewis WD, Obici L, Plante-Bordeneuve V, Rapezzi C, et al. Guideline of transthyretin-related hereditary amyloidosis for clinicians. Orphanet J Rare Dis. 2013;8:31.
9. Koike H, Tanaka F, Hashimoto R, Tomita M, Kawagashira Y, Iijima M, Fujitake J, Kawanami T, Kato T, Yamamoto M, et al. Natural history of transthyretin Val30Met familial amyloid polyneuropathy: analysis of late-onset cases from non-endemic areas. J Neurol Neurosurg Psychiatry. 2012;83(2):152–8.
10. Planté-Bordeneuve V, Said G. Familial amyloid polyneuropathy. Lancet Neurol. 2011;10(12):1086–97.
11. Benson MD, Teague SD, Kovacs R, Feigenbaum H, Jung J, Kincaid JC. Rate of progression of transthyretin amyloidosis. Am J Cardiol. 2011;108(2):285–9.
12. Mariani LL, Lozeron P, Theaudin M, Mincheva Z, Signate A, Ducot B, Algalarrondo V, Denier C, Adam C, Nicolas G, et al. Genotype-phenotype correlation and course of transthyretin familial amyloid polyneuropathies in France. Ann Neurol. 2015;78(6):901–16.
13. Sattianayagam PT, Hahn AF, Whelan CJ, Gibbs SD, Pinney JH, Stangou AJ, Rowczenio D, Pflugfelder PW, Fox Z, Lachmann HJ, et al. Cardiac phenotype and clinical outcome of familial amyloid polyneuropathy associated with transthyretin alanine 60 variant. Eur Heart J. 2012;33(9):1120–7.
14. Rowczenio DM, Noor I, Gillmore JD, Lachmann HJ, Whelan C, Hawkins PN, Obici L, Westermark P, Grateau G, Wechalekar AD. Online registry for mutations in hereditary amyloidosis including nomenclature recommendations. Hum Mutat. 2014;35(9):E2403–12.
15. Ruberg FL, Berk JL. Transthyretin (TTR) cardiac amyloidosis. Circulation. 2012;126(10):1286–300.
16. Maurer MS, Hanna M, Grogan M, Dispenzieri A, Witteles R, Drachman B, Judge DP, Lenihan DJ, Gottlieb SS, Shah SJ, et al. Genotype and phenotype of transthyretin cardiac amyloidosis: THAOS (Transthyretin Amyloid Outcome Survey). J Am Coll Cardiol. 2016;68(2):161–72.
17. Suanprasert N, Berk JL, Benson MD, Dyck PJ, Klein CJ, Gollob JA, Bettencourt BR, Karsten V, Dyck PJ. Retrospective study of a TTR FAP cohort to modify NIS+7 for therapeutic trials. J Neurol Sci. 2014;344(1–2):121–8.
18. Andrade C. A peculiar form of peripheral neuropathy; familiar atypical generalized amyloidosis with special involvement of the peripheral nerves. Brain. 1952;75(3):408–27.
19. Coelho T, Maia LF, Martins da Silva A, Waddington Cruz M, Plante-Bordeneuve V, Lozeron P, Suhr OB, Campistol JM, Conceicao IM, Schmidt HH, et al. Tafamidis for transthyretin familial amyloid polyneuropathy: a randomized, controlled trial. Neurology. 2012;79(8):785–92.
20. Vinik EJ, Vinik AI, Paulson JF, Merkies IS, Packman J, Grogan DR, Coelho T. Norfolk QOL-DN: validation of a patient reported outcome measure in transthyretin familial amyloid polyneuropathy. J Peripher Nerv Syst. 2014;19(2):104–14.
21. Coelho T, Vinik A, Vinik EJ, Tripp T, Packman J, Grogan DR. Clinical measures in transthyretin familial amyloid polyneuropathy. Muscle Nerve. 2017;55(3):323–32.
22. Inês M, Coelho T, Conceição I, Ferreira L, de Carvalho M, Costa J. Transthyretin familial amyloid polyneuropathy impact on health-related quality of life. Orphanet J Rare Dis. 2015;10(Supp. 1):O28.

23. Wixner J, Mundayat R, Karayal ON, Anan I, Karling P, Suhr OB, THAOS investigators. THAOS: gastrointestinal manifestations of transthyretin amyloidosis - common complications of a rare disease. Orphanet J Rare Dis. 2014;9:61.

24. Berk JL, Suhr OB, Obici L, Sekijima Y, Zeldenrust SR, Yamashita T, Heneghan MA, Gorevic PD, Litchy WJ, Wiesman JF, et al. Repurposing diflunisal for familial amyloid polyneuropathy: a randomized clinical trial. JAMA. 2013;310(24):2658–67.

25. Mita S, Maeda S, Shimada K, Araki S. Analyses of prealbumin mRNAs in individuals with familial amyloidotic polyneuropathy. J Biochem. 1986;100(5):1215–22.

26. Holmgren G, Steen L, Ekstedt J, Groth CG, Ericzon BG, Eriksson S, Andersen O, Karlberg I, Norden G, Nakazato M, et al. Biochemical effect of liver transplantation in two Swedish patients with familial amyloidotic polyneuropathy (FAP-met30). Clin Genet. 1991;40(3):242–6.

27. Adams D, Samuel D, Goulon-Goeau C, Nakazato M, Costa PM, Feray C, Plante V, Ducot B, Ichai P, Lacroix C, et al. The course and prognostic factors of familial amyloid polyneuropathy after liver transplantation. Brain. 2000;123(Pt 7):1495–504.

28. Ericzon BG, Wilczek HE, Larsson M, Wijayatunga P, Stangou A, Pena JR, Furtado E, Barroso E, Daniel J, Samuel D, et al. Liver transplantation for hereditary transthyretin amyloidosis: after 20 years still the best therapeutic alternative? Transplantation. 2015;99(9):1847–54.

29. Suhr OB, Larsson M, Ericzon BG, Wilczek HE, on behalf of the FAPWTR's investigators. Survival after transplantation in patients with mutations other than Val30Met: extracts from the FAP World Transplant Registry. Transplantation. 2016;100(2):373–81.

30. Carvalho A, Rocha A, Lobato L. Liver transplantation in transthyretin amyloidosis: issues and challenges. Liver Transpl. 2015;21(3):282–92.

31. Adams D, Buades J, Suhr O, Obici L, Coelho T. Preliminary assessment of neuropathy progression in patients with hereditary ATTR amyloidosis after orthotopic liver transplantation. Orphanet J Rare Dis. 2015; 10(Suppl. 1):P19.

32. Liepnieks JJ, Zhang LQ, Benson MD. Progression of transthyretin amyloid neuropathy after liver transplantation. Neurology. 2010;75(4):324–7.

33. EMA. Vyndaqel [http://www.ema.europa.eu/ema/index.jsp?curl=pages/medicines/human/medicines/002294/human_med_001498.jsp&mid=WC0b01ac058001d124].

34. Amyloidosis Patient Information Site. National Amyloidosis Centre. ATTR Anyloidosis. [http://www.amyloidosis.org.uk/introduction-to-attr-amyloidosis/2015].

35. Coelho T, Maia LF, da Silva AM, Cruz MW, Plante-Bordeneuve V, Suhr OB, Conceicao I, Schmidt HH, Trigo P, Kelly JW, et al. Long-term effects of tafamidis for the treatment of transthyretin familial amyloid polyneuropathy. J Neurol. 2013;260(11):2802–14.

36. Plante-Bordeneuve V, Gorram F, Salhi H, Nordine T, Ayache SS, Le Corvoisier P, Azoulay D, Feray C, Damy T, Lefaucheur JP. Long-term treatment of transthyretin familial amyloid polyneuropathy with tafamidis: a clinical and neurophysiological study. J Neurol. 2017;264(2):268–76.

37. Cortese A, Vita G, Luigetti M, Russo M, Bisogni G, Sabatelli M, Manganelli F, Santoro L, Cavallaro T, Fabrizi GM, et al. Monitoring effectiveness and safety of Tafamidis in transthyretin amyloidosis in Italy: a longitudinal multicenter study in a non-endemic area. J Neurol. 2016;263(5):916–24.

38. Lozeron P, Theaudin M, Mincheva Z, Ducot B, Lacroix C, Adams D, French Network for FAP (CORNAMYL). Effect on disability and safety of Tafamidis in late onset of Met30 transthyretin familial amyloid polyneuropathy. Eur J Neurol. 2013;20(12):1539–45.

39. Coelho T, Adams D, Silva A, Lozeron P, Hawkins PN, Mant T, Perez J, Chiesa J, Warrington S, Tranter E, et al. Safety and efficacy of RNAi therapy for transthyretin amyloidosis. N Engl J Med. 2013;369(9):819–29.

40. Okamoto S, Wixner J, Obayashi K, Ando Y, Ericzon BG, Friman S, Uchino M, Suhr OB. Liver transplantation for familial amyloidotic polyneuropathy: impact on Swedish patients' survival. Liver Transpl. 2009;15(10):1229–35.

41. Tashima K, Ando Y, Terazaki H, Yoshimatsu S, Suhr OB, Obayashi K, Yamashita T, Ando E, Uchino M, Ando M. Outcome of liver transplantation for transthyretin amyloidosis: follow-up of Japanese familial amyloidotic polyneuropathy patients. J Neurol Sci. 1999;171(1):19–23.

42. Gillmore JD, Lovat LB, Persey MR, Pepys MB, Hawkins PN. Amyloid load and clinical outcome in AA amyloidosis in relation to circulating concentration of serum amyloid a protein. Lancet. 2001;358(9275):24–9.

43. Lachmann HJ, Gallimore R, Gillmore JD, Carr-Smith HD, Bradwell AR, Pepys MB, Hawkins PN. Outcome in systemic AL amyloidosis in relation to changes in concentration of circulating free immunoglobulin light chains following chemotherapy. Br J Haematol. 2003;122(1):78–84.

44. Gillmore JD, Stangou AJ, Tennent GA, Booth DR, O'Grady J, Rela M, Heaton ND, Wall CA, Keogh JA, Hawkins PN. Clinical and biochemical outcome of hepatorenal transplantation for hereditary systemic amyloidosis associated with apolipoprotein AI Gly26Arg. Transplantation. 2001;71(7):986–92.

45. Suhr OB, Coelho T, Buades J, Pouget J, Conceicao I, Berk J, Schmidt H, Waddington-Cruz M, Campistol JM, Bettencourt BR, et al. Efficacy and safety of patisiran for familial amyloidotic polyneuropathy: a phase II multi-dose study. Orphanet J Rare Dis. 2015;10:109.

46. Suhr O, Adams D, Coelho T, Waddington Cruz M, Schmidt H, Buades J, Campistol J, Pouget J, Berk J, Polydefkis M, et al. Phase 2 open-label extension study of patisiran, an investigational RNAi therapeutic for the tereatment of hereditary ATTR amyloidosis with polyneuropathy. In: The XVth International Symposium on Amyloidosis (International Society of Amyloidosis) Uppsala: Abstract PA80; 2016.

47. Adams D, Coelho T, Obici L, Merlini G, Mincheva Z, Suanprasert N, Bettencourt BR, Gollob JA, Gandhi PJ, Litchy WJ, et al. Rapid progression of familial amyloidotic polyneuropathy: a multinational natural history study. Neurology. 2015;85(8):675–82.

48. Dyck PJ, Herrmann DN, Staff NP, Dyck PJ. Assessing decreased sensation and increased sensory phenomena in diabetic polyneuropathies. Diabetes. 2013;62(11):3677–86.

49. Vinik EJ, Hayes RP, Oglesby A, Bastyr E, Barlow P, Ford-Molvik SL, Vinik AI. The development and validation of the Norfolk QOL-DN, a new measure of patients' perception of the effects of diabetes and diabetic neuropathy. Diabetes Technol Ther. 2005;7(3):497–508.

50. EuroQol Group. EuroQol–a new facility for the measurement of health-related quality of life. Health Policy. 1990;16:199–208.

51. Sletten DM, Suarez GA, Low PA, Mandrekar J, Singer W. COMPASS 31: a refined and abbreviated composite autonomic symptom score. Mayo Clin Proc. 2012;87(12):1196–201.

52. van Nes SI, Vanhoutte EK, van Doorn PA, Hermans M, Bakkers M, Kuitwaard K, Faber CG, Merkies IS. Rasch-built overall disability scale (R-ODS) for immune-mediated peripheral neuropathies. Neurology. 2011;76(4):337–45.

53. Suhr O, Danielsson A, Holmgren G, Steen L. Malnutrition and gastrointestinal dysfunction as prognostic factors for survival in familial amyloidotic polyneuropathy. J Intern Med. 1994;235(5):479–85.

54. Backonja MM, Attal N, Baron R, Bouhassira D, Drangholt M, Dyck PJ, Edwards RR, Freeman R, Gracely R, Haanpaa MH, et al. Value of quantitative sensory testing in neurological and pain disorders: NeuPSIG consensus. Pain. 2013;154(9):1807–19.

55. Cruz-Almeida Y, Fillingim RB. Can quantitative sensory testing move us closer to mechanism-based pain management? Pain Med. 2014;15(1):61–72.

56. Dyck PJ, Kincaid JC, Dyck PJB, Chaudhry V, Goyal NA, Alves C, Salhi H, Wiesman JF, Labeyrie C, Robinson-Papp J, et al. Assessing mNIS+7_{Ionis} and international neurologists' proficiency in a familial amyloidotic polyneuropathy trial. Muscle Nerve. 2017. doi:10.1002/mus.25563. [Epub ahead of print].

57. Lanier JB, Mote MB, Clay EC. Evaluation and management of orthostatic hypotension. Am Fam Physician. 2011;84(5):527–36.

58. Dyck PJ, Overland CJ, Low PA, Litchy WJ, Davies JL, Dyck PJ, O'Brien PC, CI vs. NPhys Trial Investigators, Albers JW, Andersen H, et al. Signs and symptoms versus nerve conduction studies to diagnose diabetic sensorimotor polyneuropathy: CI vs. NPhys trial. Muscle Nerve. 2010;42(2):157–64.

59. Dyck PJ, Overland CJ, Low PA, Litchy WJ, Davies JL, Dyck PJ, Carter RE, Melton LJ, Andersen H, Albers JW, et al. "Unequivocally abnormal" vs "usual" signs and symptoms for proficient diagnosis of diabetic polyneuropathy: CI vs N Phys trial. Arch Neurol. 2012;69(12):1609–14.

60. Dyck PJ, Albers JW, Wolfe J, Bolton CF, Walsh N, Klein CJ, Zafft AJ, Russell JW, Thomas K, Davies JL, et al. A trial of proficiency of nerve conduction: greater standardization still needed. Muscle Nerve. 2013;48(3):369–74.

61. Litchy WJ, Albers JW, Wolfe J, Bolton CF, Walsh N, Klein CJ, Zafft AJ, Russell JW, Zwirlein M, Overland CJ, et al. Proficiency of nerve conduction using standard methods and reference values (cl. NPhys trial 4). Muscle Nerve. 2014;50(6):900–8.

62. Dyck PJ, Argyros B, Russell JW, Gahnstrom LE, Nalepa S, Albers JW, Lodermeier KA, Zafft AJ, Dyck PJ, Klein CJ, et al. Multicenter trial of the proficiency of smart quantitative sensation tests. Muscle Nerve. 2014;49(5):645–53.

63. Li H, Schwartz J, Keohane D. Impact of baseline neurologic score on disease progression in transthyretin familial amyloid polyneuropathy. In: International Society of Amyloidosis (ISA). Uppsala: Poster PB2; 2016.

64. Ziegler D, Low PA, Litchy WJ, Boulton AJ, Vinik AI, Freeman R, Samigullin R, Tritschler H, Munzel U, Maus J, et al. Efficacy and safety of antioxidant treatment with alpha-lipoic acid over 4 years in diabetic polyneuropathy: the NATHAN 1 trial. Diabetes Care. 2011;34(9):2054–60.

65. Shy ME, Chen L, Swan ER, Taube R, Krajewski KM, Herrmann D, Lewis RA, McDermott MP. Neuropathy progression in Charcot-Marie-tooth disease type 1A. Neurology. 2008;70(5):378–83.

66. Coelho T, Suhr O, Conceicao I, Waddington Cruz M, Schmidt H, Buades J, Campistol J, Pouget J, Berk J, Ziyadeh N, et al. Relationship between TTR knockdown and change in mNIS+7: preliminary correlation findings from the Phase 2 open-label extension study of patisiran, an investigational RNAi therapeutic for hereditary ATTR amyloidosis with polyneuropathy. In: The XVth International Symposium on Amyloidosis (Internation Society of Amyloidosis). Uppsala: Poster PA83; 2016.

67. Ueda M, Ando Y. Recent advances in transthyretin amyloidosis therapy. Transl Neurodegener. 2014;3:19.

68. Amyloidosis Foundation: Understanding the patient voice in hereditary transthyretin-mediated amyloidosis. Chicago: Amyloidosis Foundation & Amyloidosis Support Groups Annual Meeting; 2015.

69. Pruppers MH, Merkies IS, Faber CG, Da Silva AM, Costa V, Coelho T. The Val30Met familial amyloid polyneuropathy specific Rasch-built overall disability scale (FAP-RODS(c)). J Peripher Nerv Syst. 2015;20(3):319–27.

70. Chao CC, Huang CM, Chiang HH, Luo KR, Kan HW, Yang NC, Chiang H, Lin WM, Lai SM, Lee MJ, et al. Sudomotor innervation in transthyretin amyloid neuropathy: pathology and functional correlates. Ann Neurol. 2015;78(2):272–83.

18

Acute-onset multiple acyl-CoA dehydrogenase deficiency mimicking Guillain-Barré syndrome

Daojun Hong[1], Yanyan Yu[2], Yuyao Wang[2], Yan Xu[1] and Jun Zhang[1]* (iD)

Abstract

Background: Multiple acyl-CoA dehydrogenase deficiency (MADD) showed great clinical heterogeneity and poses a challenge to diagnosis. Guillain-Barré syndrome (GBS) is an acute-onset autoimmune-mediated peripheral neuropathy. However, no patients of acute-onset MADD mimicking the GBS phenotype are reported previously.

Case presentation: Two patients displayed acute-onset limb weakness, areflexia, and length-dependent sensory disturbances, which clinically indicate the diagnosis of GBS, but electrophysiological and cerebrospinal fluid results threw doubtful points to the initial diagnosis. The muscle biopsy showed lipid storage disorder; and compound heterozygous mutations in the electron transfer flavoprotein dehydrogenase (ETFDH) gene were found in the two patients through targeted next generation sequencing, which provided the definite diagnostic evidences of late-onset MADD. Muscle weakness was quickly improved by riboflavin supplementation, but sensory disturbances required a long-term treatment.

Discussion: The present two cases have demonstrated that MADD can mimic GBS. Taking into consideration the significant differences of therapeutic regimen and prognosis, MADD should be included in the differential diagnosis of GBS.

Keywords: Multiple acyl-CoA dehydrogenase deficiency (MADD), Guillain-Barré syndrome (GBS), ETFDH, Phenotype, Differential diagnosis, Acute onset

Background

Guillain-Barré syndrome (GBS), also known as Landry's paralysis, is an acute or subacute polyradiculoneuropathy [1]. It has been believed that GBS may not be a single entity, but a group of immune-mediated neuropathies with pathogenesis associated with endoneurial inflammation of spinal nerve roots, distal nerve segments, and potential nerve entrapment sites [2]. The commonly recognized variants of GBS are acute inflammatory demyelinating polyneuropathy (AIDP), acute motor axonal neuropathy, acute motor sensory axonal neuropathy, and Miller-Fisher syndrome. AIDP is the most prevalent form and accounts for 70–90% of GBS cases [3]. The main clinical features of GBS include acute-onset generalized limb weakness, limb paraesthesias, and relative or complete areflexia. The typically symptomatic pattern exhibits an ascending flaccid paralysis evolving over a few days to a few weeks. In some situations, a history of antecedent respiratory or gastrointestinal infection or vaccination can be identified [4]. Respiratory failure and oropharyngeal weakness may require ventilator assistance in about one-third of hospitalized patients making it as a disease of vital importance for early management [5]. However, it is difficult to make a rapid and correct diagnosis of GBS sometimes, because some rare differential cases can mimic the clinical presentations of GBS [6–8].

Multiple acyl-CoA dehydrogenase deficiency (MADD; OMIM, 231680) is an autosomal recessive inherited metabolic disorder mainly caused by the defects of electron transfer flavoprotein ubiquinone oxidoreductase (ETF:QO) complex encoded by the ETF dehydrogenase (*ETFDH*) gene, alpha ETF (*ETFA*) gene, and beta ETF (*ETFB*) gene [9]. The phenotype of late-onset MADD is highly variable and mainly characterized by fluctuating

* Correspondence: who636@hotmail.com
[1]Department of Neurology, Peking University People's Hospital, #11 Xizhimen South Avenue, Xicheng District, Beijing 100044, China
Full list of author information is available at the end of the article

muscle weakness, vomiting, hypoglycemia, metabolic acidosis, and hepatomegaly usually preceded by metabolic stress [10]. In the recent decade, a lot of patients with late-onset MADD have been reported in Chinese population who mainly presented with proximal muscle weakness, exercise intolerance, myalgia, and dramatic riboflavin responsiveness. Therefore, this clinical phenotype is also named riboflavin responsive MADD (RR-MADD) [11].

Recently, Wang et al. reported that six patients with late-onset MADD caused by *ETFDH* mutations presented with chronic sensory disturbances besides relatively acute muscle weakness, suggesting that sensory neuropathy might be involved in the clinical spectrum of late-onset MADD [12]. However, no cases of late-onset MADD with acute-onset motor-sensory symptoms mimicking GBS were reported previously. In this report we described two Han Chinese patients initially presenting with acute-onset limb weakness, areflexia, and length-dependent sensory disturbances, which clinically pointed to the diagnosis of GBS, but a diagnosis of late-onset MADD was finally made.

Case presentation

Case 1

The patient was a 22-year-old man who came from a non-consanguineous family. Before he was referred to our department, he had a history of antecedent influenza 10 days ago. He started to have progressive limb weakness and numbness 5 days ago. He also complained of persistent soreness in both inferior calves and numbness in the distal limbs. The symptoms gradually worsen, and caused virtually bed bound. Neurological examinations revealed a length-dependent decrease of touching, temperature, pain, and vibration sensations below the knee and the wrist joints. Muscle strength was grade 2–/5 (Medical Research Council scales) in the proximal lower limbs, grade 4/5 in the distal lower limbs, grade 4–/5 in the upper limbs, and grade 3/5 in the neck flexion. The cranial nerves were intact. Deep tendon reflexes were not elicited.

Serum creatine kinase (CK) was 5809 IU/L (normal 1–171 IU/L). Blood count, blood biochemistry, inflammatory tests, thyroid hormones, serum vitamin B12 and folic acid were in normal limits. The panel of anti-ganglioside antibodies including GQ1b, GT1b, GD1b, GD1a, GM2, and GM1 was negative. Cerebrospinal fluid (CSF) results were normal at 6 days after the onset of disease. Blood acylcarnitine profile before treatment revealed a combined elevation of short-, medium-, and long-chain acylcarnitines. Urine organic acid analysis indicated an increase of multiple metabolic acids.

Motor nerve conduction velocity (MNCV) showed that a borderline decrease of compound muscle action potentials (CMAP) was recorded in the bilateral median,

bilateral ulnar, and left peroneal nerves (Table 1). Sensory NCV showed normal potentials can be recorded in both sural nerves and median nerves. The latency of H reflexes and F waves were normal in all nerves tested. Needle electromyogram showed mildly decreased motor unit action potentials (MUAP) in the right gastrocnemius muscle and anterior tibialis muscle.

Case 2

The patient was a 55-year-old man who came from a non-consanguineous family. He suddenly began to have muscle weakness in both lower limbs; meanwhile he felt numbness of the distal lower limbs. The weakness quickly ascended to upper limbs 2 days later and then progressed into difficulty of swallowing 3 days later. He also complained of tightness around the waist and abdomen, but the bladder function was normal. Muscle strength was grade 4/5 in the foot dorsiflexors, grade 5/5 in the plantar flexion, grade 2/5 in the proximal lower limbs, grade 4/5 in the hand gripping, and grade 3/5 in the proximal upper limbs. The sensations of pain, vibration, and joint position perception reduced below the knee. Deep tendon reflexes were not elicited in the lower and upper limbs.

Serum CK was 334 IU/L. Blood count, blood biochemistry, inflammatory indexes, thyroid hormones, serum vitamin B12 and folic acid were in normal limits. The panel of anti-ganglioside antibodies including GQ1b, GT1b, GD1b, GD1a, GM2, and GM1 was negative. Laboratory panels of CSF were normal at 5 days after the onset of disease. Spinal MRI was normal. Blood acylcarnitine profile before treatment revealed a multiple increase of short-, medium-, and long-chain acylcarnitines. Urine organic acid analysis showed a significant elevation of 2-hydroxyglutaric acid and 2-hydroxyadipic acid.

MNCV of the case 2 revealed decreased amplitudes of CMAP in both peroneal nerves, but other nerves were intact (Table 1). Sensory NCV showed significant impairments in nerves tested. The latency of H reflexes and F waves were normal in all nerves tested. Needle electromyogram of gastrocnemius muscle showed a little short duration and low amplitude MUAP.

Muscle biopsies were conducted at the right biceps brachii in the two patients. The muscle specimens exhibited similar pathological changes. Most myofibers were filled with numerous small vacuoles, but without significant variations of fiber diameter or proliferation of connective tissue (Fig. 1a and b). The lipid droplets were accumulated in the fibers with vacuoles (Fig. 1c and d), especially affecting the type I fibers. Nicotinamide adenine dinucleotidetetrazolium reductase (NADH-TR) stain revealed many dark particles in the fibers with numerous lipid droplets. A few fibers with negative cytochrome *c*

Table 1 Electrophysiological studies of MADD in the two patients

Motor nerve		Case 1			Case 2		
		MNCV(m/s)	dL (ms)	CMAP (mV)	MNCV(m/s)	dL (ms)	CMAP (mV)
L Median	E-W	74(≥50.0)	–	7.2(≥5.0)	54	–	13.0
	W-APB	–	3.3(≤4.2)	8.5(≥5.0)	–	3.3	13.8
R Median	E-W	67	–	5.3	56	–	16.1
	W-APB	–	3.4	5.8	–	3.0	16.9
L Ulnar	E-W	66(≥53.0)	–	7.6(≥5.5)	53	–	11.0
	W-ADM	–	2.1(≤4.2)	9.5(≥5.5)	–	2.5	12.4
R Ulnar	E-W	68	–	8.1	61	–	10.7
	W-ADM	–	2.0	8.5	–	2.2	11.0
L Peroneal	FH-A	47(≥38.0)	–	3.7(≥3.0)	43	–	2.6
	A-EBD	–	3.0(≤6.1)	5.1(≥3.0)	–	3.8	3.3
R Peroneal	FH-A	58	–	10.3	50	–	3.3
	A-EBD	–	3.7	12.5	–	4.6	3.7
L Tibial	PF-A	51(≥35.0)	–	12.0(≥3.0)	50	–	13.6
	A-AA	–	4.8(≤6.1)	13.9(≥3.0)	–	4.8	165
R Tibial	PF-A	56	–	11.4	52	–	11.5
	A-AA	–	4.4	11.2	–	5.3	12.8
Sensory nerve		SNCV (m/s)		SNAP (uV)	SNCV (m/s)		SNAP (uV)
L-Median	IIF-W	59(≥50.8)		14.4(≥8.0)	35		1.5
R-Median	IIF-W	57		11.9	48		1.1
L-Sural	A-SURA	42(≥41.9)		15.5(≥7.0)	NR		NR
R-Sural	A-SURA	45		26.3	NR		NR
F wave		F-Lat(ms)			F-Lat(ms)		
L-Median		29.5(≤32.0)			27.31		
R- Median		27.62			27.0		
H Reflex		H-Lat(ms)			H-Lat(ms)		
L Tibial		28.0(< 40.0)			32.89		
R Tibial		28.0			31.26		

MNCV motor nerve conduction velocity, *CMAP* compound motor action potential, *dL* distal motor latency, *SNCV* sensory nerve conduction velocity, *SNAP* sensory nerve action potential, *L* left, *R* right, *E* elbow, *W* wrist, *APB* abductor pollicis brevis, *ADM* abductor digiti minimi, *FH* fibula head, *A* ankle, *EDB* extensor digitorum brevis, *PF* popliteal fossa, *AA* abductor allucis, *IIF* second finger, *SURA* sural, *Lat* latency, *NR* no recorded. Normal values are given in brackets

oxidase (COX) were observed in the two cases. Neurogenic patterns such as grouping of angular atrophic fibers or target-like fibers were not observed in the acid or alkaline ATPases stain.

Genetic test was performed in the patients through targeted next generation sequencing (NGS) after informed consents were written. The NGS was conducted on selected subjects using Agilent SureDesign Panel kits for inherited myopathy and inherited peripheral neuropathy. Genetic sequencing disclosed compound heterozygous mutations: c.265-266delCA and c.1211 T > C (p.M404 T) in the case 1 (Fig. 2a); c.34G > C (p.A12P) and c.736G > A (p.E246K) in the case 2 (Fig. 2b). The variants co-segregated with their parents: c.265-266 delCA was from the mother and c.1211 T > C was from the father; c.34G > C was from the father and c.736G > A was from the mother. The variants c.736G > A and c.265-266delCA were not found in the 1000 genomes database, ExAC database, and gnomAD database, but the variants c.34G > C and c.1211 T > C had a very low allele frequency (Table 2). A homology search in different species demonstrated that the amino acid at residues 12, 246, and 404 were highly evolutionarily conserved, respectively. The variants were predicted to be damaging by several in silico tools (Table 2). The pathogenicity of variants was evaluated according to the American college medical genetics and genomics (ACMG) criteria (Table 2). No other causative mutations associated with metabolic myopathies or inherited neuropathies were found in the target gene kits including the *ETFA*, *ETFB*, flavin adenine dinucleotide synthetase 1 (*FLAD1*), and solute carrier family 25 member 32 (*SLC25A32*) genes.

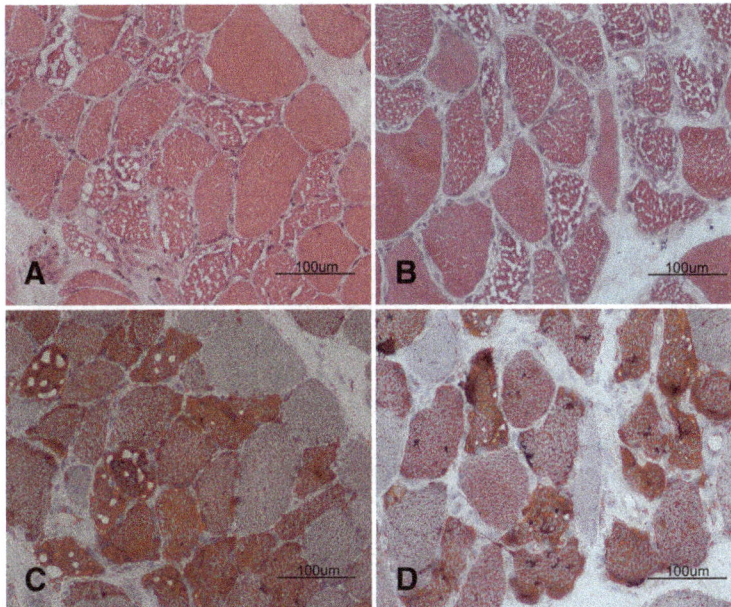

Fig. 1 Pathological changes in the muscle specimen. Hematoxylin-eosin stain revealed numerous small vacuoles appearing in most muscle fibers of case 1 (**a**) and case 2 (**b**). Oil red O stain showed massive lipid droplets depositing in the corresponding vacuoles of case 1 (**c**) and case 2 (**d**)

The two patients were initially treated with riboflavin (150 mg/d), L-camitine (2 g/d), and coenzyme Q10 (150 mg/d). One week later, limb weakness improved dramatically, and muscle strength nearly recovered 4 weeks later. The level of CK also returned to normal limits. The sensory disturbances showed no improvement; even the tightness around waist and abdomen in case 2 became worse than ever 4 weeks later. However, the patients reported significant improvement of paraesthesias after long-term administration of riboflavin (30 mg/d), CoQ10 (100 mg/d), and cobalamine (500 µg/d) for 12 months.

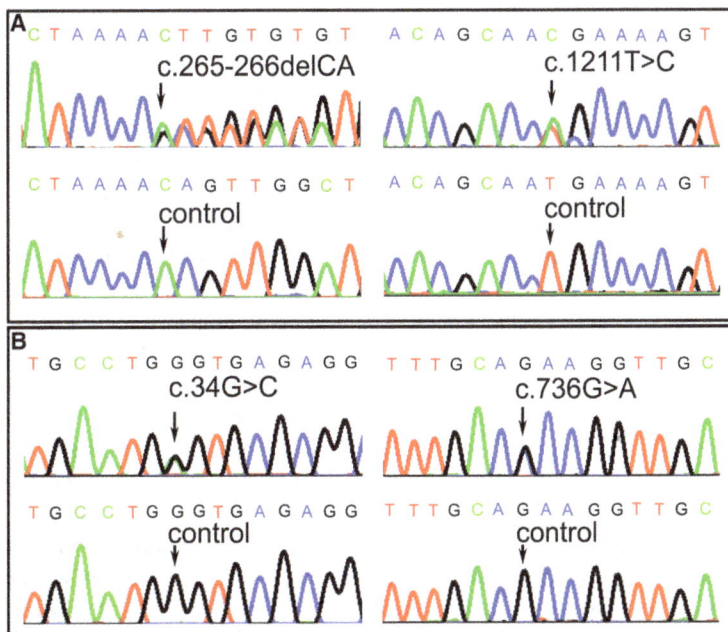

Fig. 2 The chromatogram of *ETFDH* variants. The compound heterozygous mutations c.34G > C and c.1211 T > C in case 1 (**a**), and compound heterozygous mutations c.736G > A and c.1454C > G in case 2 (**b**)

Table 2 The pathogenic analysis of variants in the *ETFDH* gene

Novel variants	Protein change	gnomAD (frequency)	PolyPhen-2	SIFT	Mutation Taster	ACMG criteria
c.34G > C	p.A12P	0.000003978	1.00	0.00	disease causing	likely pathogenic
c.265_266delCA	p.Q89Vfs*5	0	–	–	disease causing	pathogenic
c.736G > A	p.E246K	0	0.959	0.01	disease causing	pathogenic
c.1211 T > C	p.M404 T	0.00000796	0.989	0.00	disease causing	pathogenic

gnomAD Genome aggregation database, *SIFT* sorting tolerant from intolerant, *ACMG* American college medical genetics and genomics criteria
*Indicates at which codon position the new reading frame ends in a stop codon

Discussion and conclusion

The two patients clinically showed acute-onset muscle weakness and limb numbness, and the patient's condition quickly deteriorated to be bulbar paralysis or bedridden. Therefore, the patients were initially suspected as Guillain-Barre syndrome. However, when cerebrospinal fluid and electrophysiological results threw doubtful points to the initial diagnosis [4, 6], hyperCKmia gave the diagnostic clue to myopathy. Finally, muscle biopsy and genetic screening provided the definite diagnostic evidences of late-onset MADD caused by mutations in the *ETFDH* gene.

Late-onset MADD usually manifests as fluctuating weakness, but sometimes chronic or sub-acute length-dependent sensory neuropathy can be observed in MADD patients [12]. However, the patients in this report presented with acute-onset muscle weakness and limb paraesthesias resembling symptoms of GBS, because the main clinical features of GBS included monophasic disease course, symmetrical limb weakness, hypo/areflexia, and distal limb paraesthesias. Given the significant differences of therapeutic regimen and prognosis, late-onset type of MADD with acute onset should be considered as a differential diagnosis of GBS in the clinical workflow [5, 13].

MADD as a metabolic myopathy can be triggered at several days after experiencing stress conditions such as malnutrition, labored work, childbirth, and infections [14]. However, GBS usually presents with symptoms at a couple of weeks after a history of respiratory or gastrointestinal infections or vaccination [2]. Therefore, the differences of antecedent course and triggers can give valuable clues to differentiate the two diseases.

Different electrodiagnostic criteria have been proposed to diagnose GBS in the recent decades [6]. Cerebrospinal fluid analysis and electrodiagnostic testing may be normal in the early phase of GBS, but F-wave and H-reflex are the early sensitive means to detect the abnormalities of spinal nerve roots [15]. The amplitude of motor NCV showed a borderline decrease in some nerves of case 1, it might indicate a possibility that a GBS had superimposed to underlying MADD, but it might also be the consequence of inborn metabolic dysfunctions. The neurophysiological results indicated a length-dependent axonal sensory neuropathy without abnormalities of nerve roots. Cerebrospinal fluid analysis and anti-ganglioside antibodies were normal in the cases. In addition, the treatment response also rebutted the possibility of GBS superposition. Taken together, above-mentioned findings let us doubt the diagnosis of GBS, so the different neurophysiological patterns are useful to differentiate between the two diseases.

The level of serum CK can vary from normal to hundreds of times in patients with late-onset MADD, but it is only elevated to several times in a little part of GBS patients [16]. The significant hyperCKmia in the case 1 gives us an important clue to think about myopathy. Because we have the lesson from the first case, we successfully avoid a misdiagnosis of the second case, even if the level of CK is only elevated to two times. Therefore, if a patient presents with proximal muscle weakness and distal sensory disturbance, as well as hyperCKmia, MADD should be considered as one of candidate diagnosis.

Our observation indicated that riboflavin formula could quickly resolve the muscle weakness, as reported by others [17], but the symptoms of sensory disturbance had no improvement in the short-term riboflavin treatment. The therapeutic response indicated that the damage of sensory nerves might be intractable to riboflavin supplementation in the two cases. Zebrafish model with defect of ETF:QO displayed a low response to touch stimulation and a disorganized sensory axonal tract with hypomyelination [18]. Marked neurite shortening were also observed in the cells expressing the *ETFDH*-mutant, but the neurite shortening could be restored by mitochondrial cofactor supplementation with carnitine, riboflavin, or coenzyme Q10 [19]. Intriguingly, sensory disturbances in the two cases showed significant improvements after long-term administration of riboflavin, coenzyme Q10 and vitamin B12, which attested the efficiency of mitochondrial cofactor supplementation to the neurite growth impaired by *ETFDH*-mutants.

ETF-QO structurally consists of a flavin adenine dinucleotide binding region, a ubiquinones binding region, and a 4Fe4S cluster [20]. ETF:QO is an important electron transfer protein on the intra-mitochondrial membrane. Riboflavin might help the folding, assembly, and stability of defects mutant ETF-QO, and recover the catalytic activity of flavoproteins. Those can well explain the reason of lipid storage myopathy, but the detailed pathomechanism how mutant ETF-QO impairs sensory nerves is still unclear. The variants in the two patients locate in hotspot FAD binding domain, so no specific relationship of genotype-phenotype can be identified [21]. The acute-onset course may be associated with individual and environmental factors.

In conclusion, the present two cases demonstrated that *ETFDH* gene variants can cause acute-onset proximal muscle weakness and distal sensory disturbance. Taking into consideration the significant differences of therapeutic regimen and prognosis, MADD should be included in the list of differential diagnosis for GBS.

Abbreviations

AIDP: Acute inflammatory demyelinating polyneuropathy; CK: Creatine kinase; CMAP: Compound muscle action potentials; COX: Cytochrome *c* oxidase; ETF:QO: ETF ubiquinone oxidoreductase; ETFDH: Electron transfer flavoprotein dehydrogenase; GBS: Guillain-Barré syndrome; MADD: Multiple acyl-CoA dehydrogenase deficiency; MNCV: Motor nerve conduction velocity; MUAP: Motor unit action potentials; NADH-TR: Nicotinamide adenine dinucleotidetetrazolium reductase

Acknowledgements
We thank the patients and their families for cooperation. We also thank Ms. Ling Liu for pathological technician.

Funding
This study was supported by the National Natural Science Foundation of China (81460199 and 81870996). Recipient: Daojun Hong and Jun Zhang. Peking University People's Hospital Research and Development Funds (RDX2018–08). Recipient: Daojun Hong.

Authors' contributions
HD: study design, data acquisition, analysis, interpretation, drafting the manuscript, funding acquisition. YY: acquisition of data and analysis. WY: data interpretation and critical revision of the manuscript for important intellectual content. XY: data interpretation and neuroelectrophysiological research. ZJ: study concept, design, funding acquisition, and manuscript revision. All authors have read and approved the manuscript.

Competing interests
The authors declare that they have no competing interests.

Author details
¹Department of Neurology, Peking University People's Hospital, #11 Xizhimen South Avenue, Xicheng District, Beijing 100044, China. ²Department of Neurology, The first affiliated hospital of Nanchang University, Nanchang, China.

References
1. Arcila-Londono X, Lewis RA. Guillain-Barré syndrome. Semin Neurol. 2012;32: 179–86.
2. Fokke C, van den Berg B, Drenthen J, Walgaard C, van Doorn PA, Jacobs BC. Diagnosis of Guillain-Barré syndrome and validation of Brighton criteria. Brain. 2014;137:33–43.
3. Dhadke SV, Dhadke VN, Bangar SS, Korade MB. Clinical profile of Guillain Barre syndrome. J Assoc Physicians India. 2013;61:168–72.
4. Walling AD, Dickson G. Guillain-Barré syndrome. Am Fam Physician. 2013;87:191–7.
5. Sudulagunta SR, Sodalagunta MB, Sepehrar M, et al. Guillain-Barré syndrome: clinical profile and management. Ger Med Sci. 2015;13:Doc16. https://doi.org/10.3205/000220.
6. Islam MB, Islam Z, Farzana KS, et al. Guillain-Barré syndrome in Bangladesh: validation of Brighton criteria. J Peripher Nerv Syst. 2016;21:345–51.
7. Sciacca G, Nicoletti A, Fermo SL, et al. Looks can be deceiving: three cases of neurological diseases mimicking Guillain-Barrè syndrome. Neurol Sci. 2016;37:541–5.
8. Derksen A, Ritter C, Athar P, et al. Sural sparing pattern discriminates Guillain-Barré syndrome from its mimics. Muscle Nerve. 2014;50:780–4.
9. Olsen RK, Olpin SE, Andresen BS, Miedzybrodzka ZH, Pourfarzam M. ETFDH mutations as a major cause of riboflavin-responsive multiple acyl-CoA dehydrogenation deficiency. Brain. 2007;130:2045–54.
10. Zhu M, Zhu X, Qi X, et al. Riboflavin-responsive multiple acyl-CoA dehydrogenation deficiency in 13 cases, and a literature review in mainland Chinese patients. J Hum Genet. 2014;59:256–61.
11. Peng Y, Zhu M, Zheng J, et al. Bent spine syndrome as an initial manifestation of late-onset multiple acyl-CoA dehydrogenase deficiency: a case report and literature review. BMC Neurol. 2015;15:114.
12. Wang Z, Hong D, Zhang W, et al. Severe sensory neuropathy in patients with adult-onset multiple acyl-CoA dehydrogenase deficiency. Neuromuscul Disord. 2016;26:170–5.
13. Atkinson SB, Carr RL, Maybee P, Haynes D. The challenges of managing and treating Guillain-Barré syndrome during the acute phase. Dimens Crit Care Nurs. 2006;25:256–63.
14. Xi J, Wen B, Lin J, et al. Clinical features and ETFDH mutation spectrum in a cohort of 90 Chinese patients with late-onset multiple acyl-CoA dehydrogenase deficiency. J Inherit Metab Dis. 2014;37:399–404.
15. Al-Shekhlee A, Hachwi RN, Preston DC, Katirji B. New criteria for early electrodiagnosis of acute inflammatory demyelinating polyneuropathy. Muscle Nerve. 2005;32:66–72.
16. Ansar V, Valadi N. Guillain-Barré syndrome. Prim Care. 2015;42:189–93.
17. Wen B, Dai T, Li W, et al. Riboflavin-responsive lipid-storage myopathy caused by ETFDH gene mutations. J Neurol Neurosurg Psychiatry. 2010; 81:231–6.
18. Kim SH, Scott SA, Bennett MJ, et al. Multi-organ abnormalities and mTORC1 activation in zebrafish model of multiple acyl-CoA dehydrogenase deficiency. PLoS Genet. 2013;9:e1003563.
19. Liang WC, Lin YF, Liu TY, et al. Neurite growth could be impaired by ETFDH mutation but restored by mitochondrial cofactors. Muscle Nerve. 2017;56: 479–85.
20. Henriques BJ, Rodrigues JV, Olsen RK, Bross P, Gomes CM. Role of flavinylation in a mild variant of multiple acyl-CoA dehydrogenation deficiency: a molecular rationale for the effects of riboflavin supplementation. J Biol Chem. 2009;284:4222–9.
21. Olsen RK, Andresen BS, Christensen E, Bross P, Skovby F, Gregersen N. Clear relationship between ETF/ETFDH genotype and phenotype in patients with multiple acyl-CoA dehydrogenation deficiency. Hum Mutat. 2003;22:12–23.

19

Peripheral neuropathy in a case with CADASIL

Yusuke Sakiyama, Eiji Matsuura*⑩, Yoshimitsu Maki, Akiko Yoshimura, Masahiro Ando, Miwa Nomura, Kazuya Shinohara, Ryuji Saigo, Tomonori Nakamura, Akihiro Hashiguchi and Hiroshi Takashima

Abstract

Background: Cerebral autosomal dominant arteriopathy with subcortical infarcts and leukoencephalopathy (CADASIL) is characterized clinically by central nervous system dysfunctions. It is unclear whether CADASIL is involved in peripheral neuropathy.

Case presentation: A 67-year-old Japanese man with stepwise progression of sensory and motor neuropathy was admitted to our hospital. Peripheral neuropathy of the extremities was detected through electrophysiological and pathological studies, and brain magnetic resonance imaging revealed bilateral periventricular ischemic and thalamic hemorrhagic lesions. We diagnosed CADASIL after detecting granular osmiophilic material in the walls of the endoneurial vessels morphologically and identifying a heterozygous *NOTCH3* mutation p.Arg75Pro.

Conclusions: CADASIL is to be included in the work-up of not classified peripheral neuropathies.

Keywords: CADASIL, Peripheral neuropathy, Multiple mononeuropathy, *NOTCH3*, Granular osmiophilic material (GOM)

Background

Cerebral autosomal dominant arteriopathy with subcortical infarcts and leukoencephalopathy (CADASIL) is an autosomal dominant disorder. This disease caused by mutations in the Notch3 gene that encodes a transmembrane protein expressed in vascular smooth muscle cells [1]. CADASIL patients have various clinical symptoms of central nerve systems, such as migraine, recurrent stroke, progressive cognitive decline, and psychiatric disturbance. Because it is unclear whether CADASIL is involved in peripheral neuropathy, we expand the phenotype of CADASIL by reporting electrophysiological and pathological features of CADASIL patient with peripheral neuropathy.

Case presentation

A 67-year-old man had the first episode of left leg weakness at the age of 65 years and subsequently experienced numbness of the bilateral fourth and fifth fingers (Additional file 1). At the age of 66, he developed right leg weakness and difficulty in walking and was admitted to our hospital. Neurological examination revealed no abnormalities in orientation, memory, or cranial nerves. Mild weakness was noted in the distal muscle of the upper limbs, and pronator drift test was positive in the left upper limb. Lower limb muscle weakness was moderate and particularly noticeable in the left anterior tibialis muscle. Deep tendon reflexes were decreased at the triceps and brachioradialis and absent at the knees and ankles. Babinski sign was positive. Pes cavus and toe clawing were absent. There were no finger tremors. A sensory examination showed bilateral hypoesthesia in the lower leg region, below the knees and bilateral numbness of the fourth and fifth fingers. No abnormalities in the urinary tract were found. The ankle-brachial index of blood pressure was normal. The results of a blood study revealed a mild inflammatory reaction and elevated serum proteinase-3-anti-neutrophil cytoplasmic antibody (PR3-ANCA; 4.0 U/mL; normal range, < 3.5 U/mL). Complete blood count and CRP level were normal. His liver and renal function were normal. Blood sugar was 97 mg/dl and HbA1c was 6.5%. A nerve conduction study was performed at a skin temperature of approximately 30 °C (Table 1). Distal motor and sensory nerve palm latency (DL) were prolonged in the left median nerve, and a slight decrease in

* Correspondence: pine@m.kufm.kagoshima-u.ac.jp
Department of Neurology and Geriatrics, Kagoshima University Graduate School of Medical and Dental Sciences, 8-35-1 Sakuragaoka, Kagoshima City, Kagoshima 890-8520, Japan

Table 1 Summary of electrophysiological data on first admission

	Left median	Left ulnar	Left tibial
DL (ms)	4.7	3.9	3.7
CMAP (mV) dis./prox.	6.1/5.4	4.5/N.D.	12.6/8.8
MCV (m/s)	53.0		43.4
F-latency (ms)	28.4	29.7	51.8
F-frequency (%)	100	68	100
	Left median	Left ulnar	Left sural	Right ulnar
SNAP (μV)	9.3	N.D.	6.9	N.D.
SCV (m/s)	44.2		43.9	

DL distal latency, *CMAP* compound muscle action potential, *MCV* motor conduction velocity, *SNAP* sensory nerve action potential, *SCV* sensory conduction velocity. *N.D.* not detected

sensory conduction velocity (SCV) was noted. Compound muscle action potentials (CMAP) at stimulation points above the elbow and sensory nerve action potentials (SNAP) were undetectable in the left ulnar nerve. These electrophysiological abnormalities were consistent with multiple mononeuropathy. Brain magnetic resonance imaging showed asymptomatic multiple cerebral infarctions and multiple micro-bleeding lesions in the white matter (Fig. 1). His symptoms did not improve after methylprednisolone pulse therapy and oral prednisolone (30 mg/day) and azathioprine (50 mg/day) therapies.

The pathological findings of a right sural nerve showed neither inflammatory cells around vessels nor any rupture of the inner elastic plate. The loss of smaller fibers and thickening of the blood vessel wall were not observed. Electron microscopy showed granular osmiophilic material (GOM) in the wall of endoneurial small vessels, which indicated peripheral neuropathy resulting from CADASIL (Fig. 2). The heterozygous missense mutation p.Arg75Pro was detected in exon 3 of the *NOTCH3* gene in the leukocyte DNA of the patient. No family history displayed cerebrovascular diseases or peripheral neuropathies. His father was diagnosed as heart failure of unknown etiology.

There was no history of smoking or drinking.

Discussion and conclusion

We successfully diagnosed CADASIL in a Japanese case with peripheral neuropathy and the p.Arg75Pro mutation of the *NOTCH3* gene. The pathogenic mutation was previously reported as a cause of CADASIL in Japanese and Korean patients [2, 3] and most frequently found in Japanese patients with CADASIL. None of Japanese cases had peripheral neuropathy [4]. The pathophysiological mechanisms of brain lesions in CADASIL remain unclear. GOM accumulation in the small arterioles of the brain is a pathological feature of CADASIL [1].

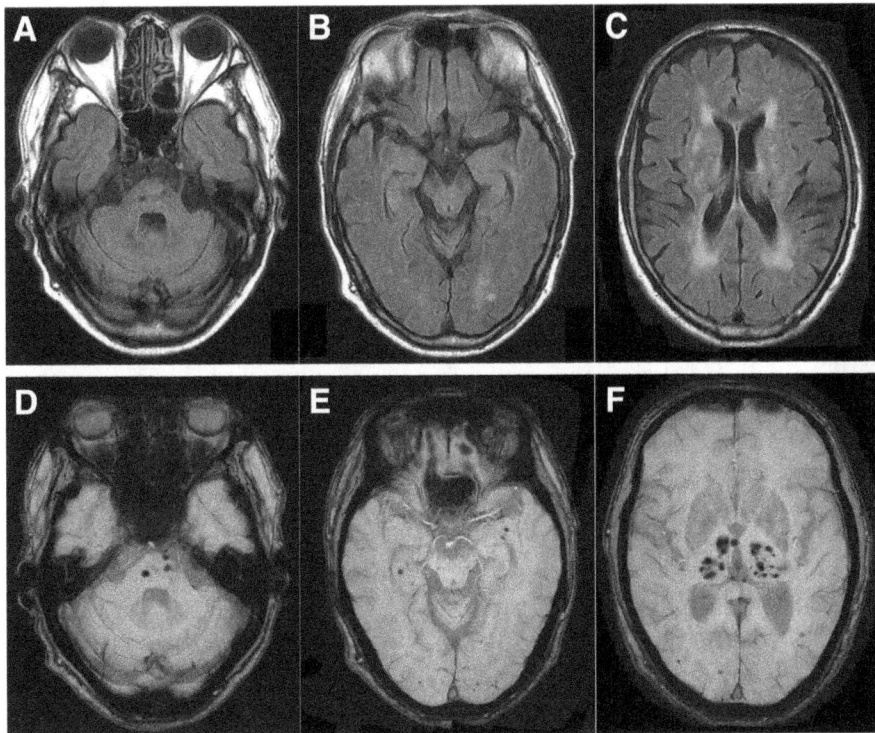

Fig. 1 Brain-MRI findings of our patient. **a–c** Axial FLAIR image showing the bilateral ischemic lesions in pons, periventricular white matter and deep white matter. **d–f**: Axial susceptibility-weighted imaging (SWI) showing multiple micro-bleeding lesions in pons, bilateral subcortical white matter and bilateral thalamus

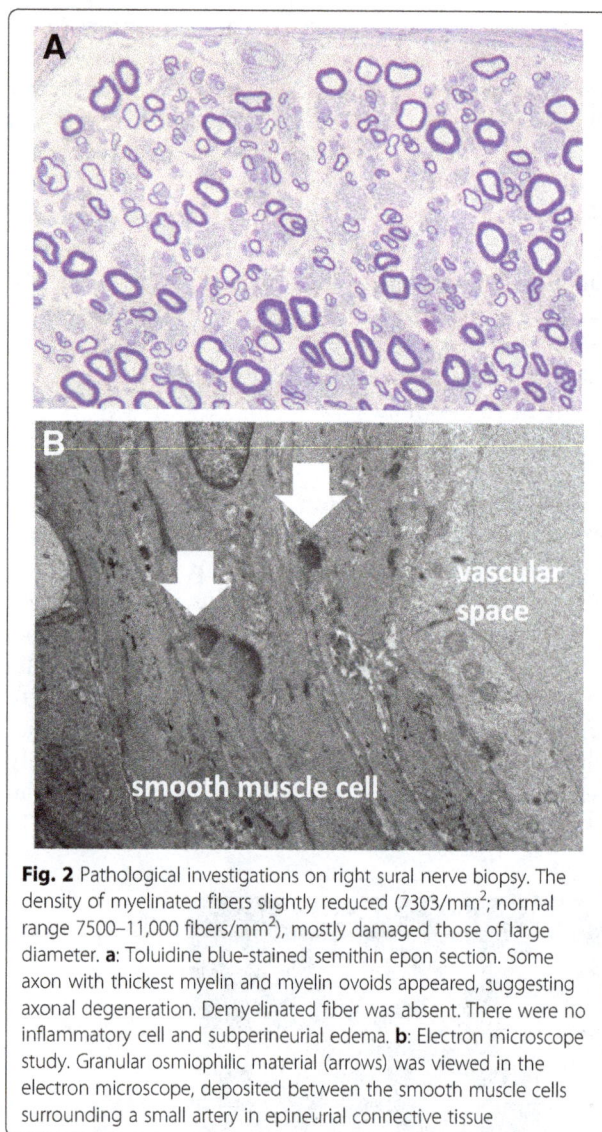

Fig. 2 Pathological investigations on right sural nerve biopsy. The density of myelinated fibers slightly reduced (7303/mm²; normal range 7500–11,000 fibers/mm²), mostly damaged those of large diameter. **a**: Toluidine blue-stained semithin epon section. Some axon with thickest myelin and myelin ovoids appeared, suggesting axonal degeneration. Demyelinated fiber was absent. There were no inflammatory cell and subperineurial edema. **b**: Electron microscope study. Granular osmiophilic material (arrows) was viewed in the electron microscope, deposited between the smooth muscle cells surrounding a small artery in epineurial connective tissue

dysfunction of blood vessels may induce hemodynamic abnormalities with low-grade chronic ischemia in peripheral nerves [5, 9]. We excluded other causes of chronic progressive axonal neuropathy, including of diabetes mellitus neuropathy, alcoholic neuropathy, ANCA–associated vasculitis, and drug or toxin.

To investigate the frequency of CADASIL in the patients with peripheral neuropathy, we performed genetic analysis of 434 patients of clinically suspected hereditary neuropathy by whole exome sequencing. However, *NOTCH3* pathogenic mutation was not found among the patients. In the previous study of CADASIL cases with peripheral neuropathy, subcortical infarcts and/or leukoencephalopathy were detected by brain MRI [5]. In other words, CADASIL cases presenting just with peripheral neuropathy have abnormal lesions in brain MRI. Although we didn't detect *NOTCH3* mutation in the patients with hereditary neuropathy, the patients with neuropathy and brain lesions have better to be analyzed for the *NOTCH3* mutation.

In conclusion, CADASIL is to be included in the work-up of not classified peripheral neuropathies. Brain MRI and *NOTCH3* gene analysis may provide a definite diagnosis for these neuropathies.

Abbreviations

CADASIL: Cerebral autosomal dominant arteriopathy with subcortical infarcts and leukoencephalopathy; CMAP: Compound muscle action potentials; CRP: C-reactive protein; DL: Distal latency; GOM: Granular osmiophilic material; PR3-ANCA: Proteinase-3-anti-neutrophil cytoplasmic antibodies; SCV: Sensory conduction velocity; SNAP: Sensory nerve action potentials

Acknowledgments

We thank Noriko Hirata for excellent technical assistance. The authors would like to thank Enago (www.enago.jp) for the English language review.

Funding

This work was supported by grants from the Nervous and Mental Disorders and Research Committee for Applying Health and Technology of the Ministry of Health, Welfare and Labour, Japan.

Authors' contributions

YS was a major contributor in writing the manuscript. EM and HT revised the manuscript for important intellectual content. EM analyzed the pathological findings. AY and MA performed the genetic examination. YM, MN, KS, RS, TN and AH gave the clinical information containing medical history, neurological findings, hematological examination, electrophysiological evaluation and treatment. All authors read and approved the final manuscript.

Competing interests

The authors declare that they have no competing interests.

Notch3 is predominantly expressed in vascular smooth muscle cells in adults [1, 5]. Previous immunoelectron microscopic examination revealed aggregated Notch3 protein in proximity to GOM deposits; however, it is unclear whether Notch3 protein is included in GOM [6–8]. While peripheral neuropathy is usually not seen in the patients with CADASIL, a few previous studies reported the association between CADASIL and peripheral neuropathy [5]. The study suggested axonal damage in peripheral nerve with clinical and electrophysiological findings. Our electron microscopic study revealed the deposition GOM in the wall of endoneurial small vessels in the peripheral nerve. Electrophysiological study showed multiple mononeuropathy, suggesting vascular dysfunction, while there was no inflammatory cell infiltration in the biopsied nerve. Novel protein–protein interactions caused by *NOTCH3* mutations has been suggested in vascular function. The

References

1. Chabriat H, Joutel A, Dichgans M, Tournier-Lasserve E, Bousser MG. Cadasil. Lancet Neurol. 2009;8(7):643–53.
2. Mizuno T, Muranishi M, Torugun T, Tango H, Nagakane Y, Kudeken T, Kawase Y, Kawabe K, Oshima F, Yaoi T, et al. Two Japanese CADASIL families exhibiting Notch3 mutation R75P not involving cysteine residue. Intern Med. 2008;47(23):2067–72.
3. Kim Y, Choi EJ, Choi CG, Kim G, Choi JH, Yoo HW, Kim JS. Characteristics of CADASIL in Korea: a novel cysteine-sparing Notch3 mutation. Neurology. 2006;66(10):1511–6.
4. Ueda A, Ueda M, Nagatoshi A, Hirano T, Ito T, Arai N, Uyama E, Mori K, Nakamura M, Shinriki S, et al. Genotypic and phenotypic spectrum of CADASIL in Japan: the experience at a referral center in Kumamoto University from 1997 to 2014. J Neurol. 2015;262(8):1828–36.
5. Sicurelli F, Dotti MT, De Stefano N, Malandrini A, Mondelli M, Bianchi S, Federico A. Peripheral neuropathy in CADASIL. J Neurol. 2005;252(10):1206–9.
6. Joutel A, Favrole P, Labauge P, Chabriat H, Lescoat C, Andreux F, Domenga V, Cecillon M, Vahedi K, Ducros A, et al. Skin biopsy immunostaining with a Notch3 monoclonal antibody for CADASIL diagnosis. Lancet. 2001; 358(9298):2049–51.
7. Joutel A, Andreux F, Gaulis S, Domenga V, Cecillon M, Battail N, Piga N, Chapon F, Godfrain C, Tournier-Lasserve E. The ectodomain of the Notch3 receptor accumulates within the cerebrovasculature of CADASIL patients. J Clin Invest. 2000;105(5):597–605.
8. Ishiko A, Shimizu A, Nagata E, Takahashi K, Tabira T, Suzuki N. Notch3 ectodomain is a major component of granular osmiophilic material (GOM) in CADASIL. Acta Neuropathol. 2006;112(3):333–9.
9. Schroder JM, Zuchner S, Dichgans M, Nagy Z, Molnar MJ. Peripheral nerve and skeletal muscle involvement in CADASIL. Acta Neuropathol. 2005;110(6):587–99.

20

Identification of a novel DNMT1 mutation in a Chinese patient with hereditary sensory and autonomic neuropathy type IE

Wenxia Zheng[1†], Zhenxing Yan[1†], Rongni He[1], Yaowei Huang[2], Aiqun Lin[1], Wei Huang[1], Yuying Su[1], Shaoyuan Li[3], Victor Wei Zhang[3,4] and Huifang Xie[1*]

Abstract

Background: DNA methyltransferase 1 (EC 2.1.1.37), encoded by DNMT1 gene, is one of key enzymes in maintaining DNA methylation patterns of the human genome. It plays a crucial role in embryonic development, imprinting and genome stability, cell differentiation. The dysfunction of this group of enzymes can lead to a variety of human genetic disorders. Until now, mutations in DNMT1 have been found to be associated with two distinct phenotypes. Mutations in exon 20 of this gene leads to hereditary sensory and autonomic neuropathy type IE, and mutations in exon 21 cause autosomal dominant cerebellar ataxia, deafness and narcolepsy.

Case presentation: Here we report a novel DNMT1 mutation in a sporadic case of a Chinese patient with cerebellar ataxia, multiple motor and sensory neuropathy, hearing loss and psychiatric manifestations. Furthermore, we elucidated its pathogenic effect through molecular genetics studies and revealed that this defective DNMT1 function is responsible for the phenotypes in this individual.

Conclusion: Our findings expand the spectrum of DNMT1-related disorders and provide a good example of precision medicine through the combination of exome sequencing and clinical testing.

Keywords: DNMT1, HSAN1E, Exome sequencing

Background

DNA methyltransferase 1 (EC 2.1.1.37), encoded by DNMT1 gene, is one of key enzymes in maintaining DNA methylation patterns of the human genome. It plays a crucial role in embryonic development, imprinting and genome stability, cell differentiation [1, 2]. The dysfunction of this group of enzymes can lead to a variety of human genetic disorders. Human DNMT1 consists of a large N-terminal region harboring multiple conserved domains and a conserved C-terminal catalytic core. The large N-terminal region is composed of the DMAP1-binding domain (DNA methyltransferase-associated protein 1), the proliferating cell nuclear antigen-binding domain (PBD), the replication focus targeting sequence (TS) 4 domains, the CXXC domain, and two bromo-adjacent homology (BAH) domains [3]. Until now, all the mutations are found to be located in TS. TS is dispensable for the selective DNA methylation activity, but it can keep DNA from gaining access to the catalytic center and undergoing methylation by inserting into the catalytic pocket stably [4, 5]. So far mutations in DNMT1 have been reported to cause two distinct neurological syndromes: hereditary sensory and autonomic neuropathy type IE with dementia and deafness (HSAN1E) related to mutations in exon 20 and autosomal dominant cerebellar ataxia, deafness and narcolepsy (ADCA-DN) with hearing loss and narcolepsy related to mutations in exon 21 [1].

Case presentation

A 38-year-old female from Guangdong province in China was admitted to Zhujiang Hospital, Southern Medical University in June 2016. At the age of 30, she developed progressive poor gait balance so that she

* Correspondence: xhffhx@126.com

†Wenxia Zheng and Zhenxing Yan contributed equally to this work.

[1]Department of Neurology, Zhujiang Hospital, Southern Medical University, 253 Industrial Avenue Middle, Guangzhou City 510282, Guangdong Province, China

Full list of author information is available at the end of the article

frequently fell down when walking. At that time, she went to a local hospital for treatment, but diagnosis was not established. She was transferred to the Second Hospital Affiliated to Guangzhou Medical Hospital for hospitalization on December in 2010, where she was clinically diagnosed as cerebellar atrophy, Type 2 Diabetes and hyperlipemia. However, the treatments prescribed did not prevent disease worsening. In 2015, she presented a slowly progressing retardation. Within the year 2016, she began to suffer from bad-response, psychiatric manifestations, bilateral hearing loss and intermittent convulsion in her upper limb during sleeping, especially the right upper limb. With such complex symptoms, she was referred to our hospital. Her parents were not consanguinity, and no neurological disorders were found in her family members except herself.

Physical examination showed that she had mild mental retardation, apathy and spoke few words. Cranial nerves were normal except for symmetric bilateral sensory hearing loss. She did not cooperate with the neurological examination and sensibility could not be tested. Her muscle strength of bilateral upper limbs was normal but was decreased in lower limbs. Muscle tone was normal, but her right upper limb had abnormal involuntary movement. The patient had no pyramidal signs. Cerebellar function examination showed mild abnormalities on finger- to- nose, heel- to-knee and rapidly alternating pronation and supination of hands. Romberg test was negative.

Electrocardiogram investigation demonstrated sinus bradycardia (44/min on average). Nerve conduction studies revealed significant deceleration of motor conduction velocity in the right peroneal nerve (25.9 m/s),

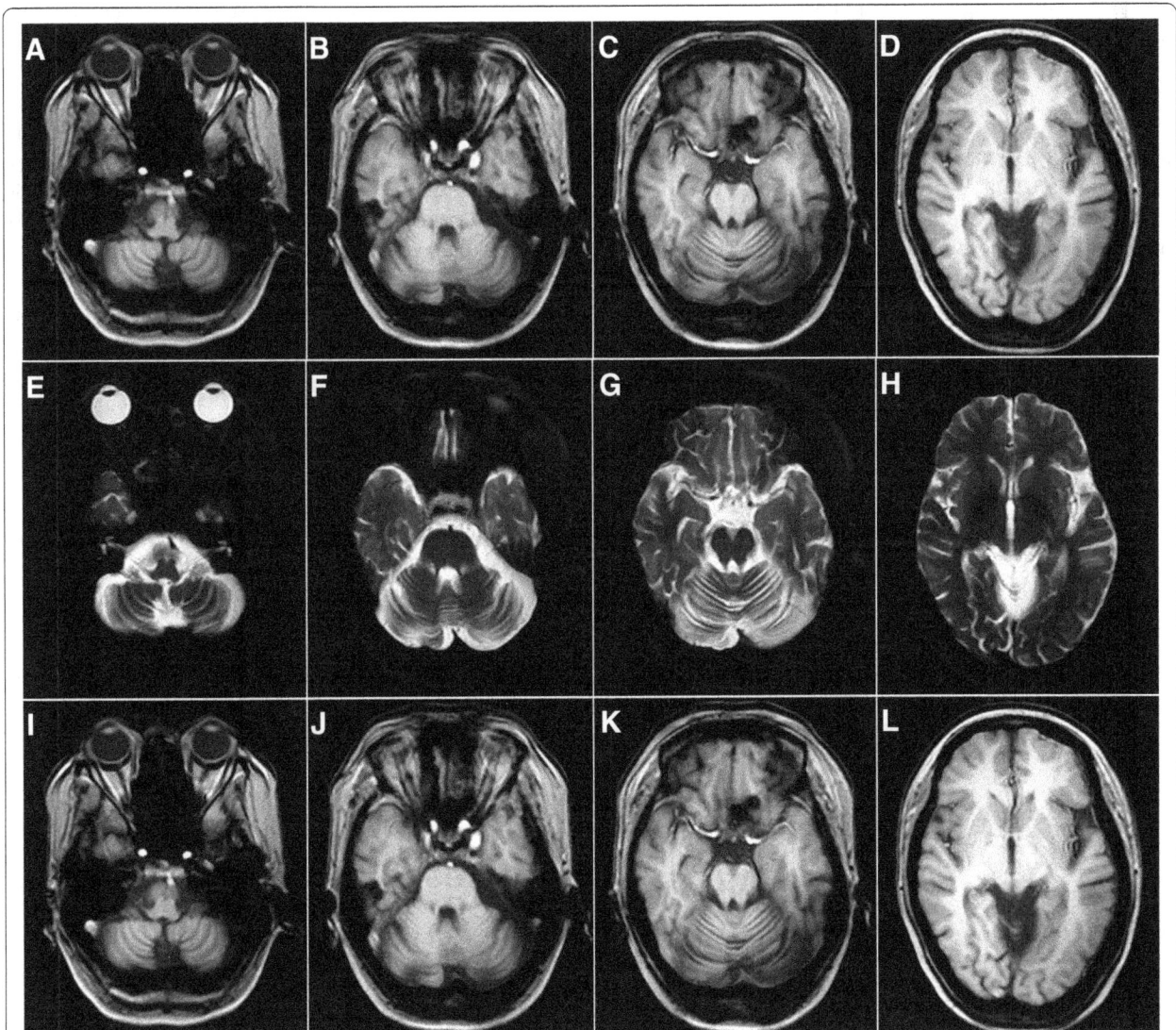

Fig. 1 Diffuse brain and cerebellar atrophy, especially the cerebellum. Sulcus inbilateral frontal, parietal, occipital lobe increases in width and depth (**a-d**: T1 weighted imaging, **e-h**: T2 weighted imaging, **i-l**: Fluid attenuated inversion recovery)

right median nerve (38.4 m/s), left ulnar nerve (45.5 m/s), right ulnar nerve (35.6 m/s) and the prolongation of F wave latency. The sensory nerve action potential could not be evoked in the bilateral peroneal nerve, sural nerve, and left median ulnar nerves. Electroencephalogram demonstrated mild to moderate abnormality and showed basic rhythms as 7.2–10 Hz and 20–40 μV slow alpha activities with low amplitude and irregular wave. Few 14–25 Hz and 20–30 μV beta waves sporadically emerged and more 4–7 Hz and 20–40 μV theta waves presented sporadically or in short-term in each lead. Visual evoked potential showed the extending of bilateral latency of P100 (Left = 101.1 mS, right = 107.0 mS) and decreased amplitude (Left = 3.24 μV, right = 1.30 μV). Brainstem auditory evoked potential showed bilateral disappearance of III-I, V-I and V-III IPL. Brain MRI revealed diffuse cerebral and cerebellar atrophy (Fig. 1).

Exome sequencing [6] (as published) performed in AmCare Genomics Lab revealed a novel heterozygous missense variant, c 1618 T > A (p. Y540N), in exon 20 of the DNMT1 (Fig. 2; Additional file 1).

Discussion and conclusions

We report a Chinese patient with suspected HSAN1E, which was finally confirmed by exome sequencing. HSAN1E is an autosomal dominant neural degenerative disorder related to the central and peripheral nervous systems characterized by sensory loss, deafness and dementia. Our patient appeared clinically normal until developing ataxic gait at hers 30s then abnormal behavioral presentations, following by hearing loss in hers 40s, It is different from the stereotypic progressive onset of hearing loss and sensory neuropathy at first and developed mental decline later. SPECT, PET image and autopsy studies in a Japanese kinship suggested the potential frontal lobe involved and abnormal behavioral presentations [7, 8]. In contrast, a previous reported study about a large American family with 11 patients clinically examined but without behavioral presentations showed that a global process without selective frontal or subcortical involvement was indicated by brain autopsy of 3 affected patients, imaging studies and multiple neuropsychometric data [7]. It is worthy to noting that although our patient appeared with abnormal behavioral presentations and mental retardation observed by neurologist, diffuse cerebral and cerebellar atrophy instead of only frontal lobe involvement. Nerve conduction studies revealed sensory involvement. Therefore, her significant cerabellar atrophy and loss of deep sensation lead to atoxic gait. All these findings were consistent with HSAN1E but different from typical HSAN1E. Additionally, recent study further supports that the extent of the phenotypic spectrum in DNMT1-related disorders is much broader and more common than currently appreciated and estimated [9].

It is noteworthy that our patient has a novel variant c 1618 T > A (p.Y540N) in DNMT1 in exon 20. Using Sanger

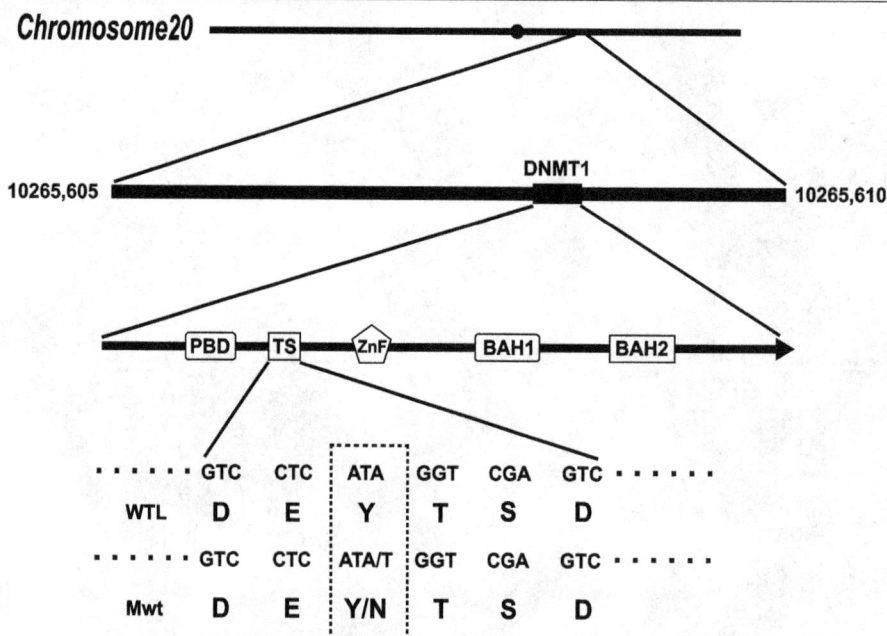

Fig. 2 Schematic representation of DNMT1 gene structure and its multiple domains in the N-terminal region. The boxes indicate PBD (the proliferating cell nuclear antigen-binding domain), TS (the replication focus targeting sequence), ZnF (zinc finger), BAH (bromo-adjacent homologydomain).The position of the mutation in the proband is indicated in the dotted box. The sequence data for mutation was deconvoluted to indicate a novel heterozygous missense variant. The tyrosine (Y) residue at amino acid position 540 is replaced with asparagine amino acid residue.

sequencing, we did not found the same variant in her mother. Unfortunately, we could not perform Sanger sequencing in her father since her father had already passed away at that time. However, although he did not appear any neurological manifestations until his death, we cannot make sure whether he carried the same mutation or not. Her siblings were not willing to accepting Sanger sequencing. But considering about her father and siblings without any neurological symptoms, we assume that her father should not have the variant. The identification heterozygous mutations in DNMT1 in patients have been published [2, 9]. Therefore, we determined that c 1618 T > A (p. Y540N) was a pathogenic variant. So far, the mutation, c 1618 T > A (p. Y540N), has not been discovered in our or other genetic database, neither published in clinical reports. Based on these results, we made a conclusion that the proband is likely to having a novel heterozygous pathogenic missense variant responsible for these symptoms.

In this study, we found a novel heterozygous missense variant, c 1618 T > A (p. Y540N) in exon 20 of the DNMT1, which is associated with HSAN1E. Meanwhile, both clinical assessment and genetic tests of this patient are quite different from the typical HSAN1E. Our findings expand the spectrum of DNMT1-related disorders and provide a good example of precision medicine through the combination of exome sequencing and clinical testing.

Abbreviations
ADCA-DN: Autosomal dominant cerebellar ataxia, deafness and narcolepsy; BAH: Bromo-adjacent homology; DMAP1-binding domain: DNA methyltransferase-associated protein 1; DNMT1: DNA methyltransferase 1; HSAN1E: Hereditary sensory and autonomic neuropathy type IE with dementia and deafness; PBD: Proliferating cell nuclear antigen-binding domain; TS: Replication focus targeting sequence

Acknowledgements
The authors thank the family and patient for their participation to this study.

Funding
This work is Major Medical Collaboration and Innovation Program of Guangzhou Science Technology and Innovation Commission (grant number 201604020020) to VWZ.

Authors' contribution
WZ and ZY drafted the manuscript. RH and YH collected the clinical data. AI,WH and YS participated in the care of the patient. SL and VWZ performed the gene panel sequencing and paper review. HX conceptualized and executed the case report. All authors read and approved the final manuscript.

Competing interests
The authors declare that they have no competing interests.

Author details
[1]Department of Neurology, Zhujiang Hospital, Southern Medical University, 253 Industrial Avenue Middle, Guangzhou City 510282, Guangdong Province, China. [2]Department of Neurology, Nanfang Hospital, Southern Medical University, 1838 Guangzhou Avenue North, Guangzhou, Guangzhou 510515, China. [3]AmCare Genomics Lab, Guangzhou, Guangzhou 510320, China. [4]Department of Molecular and Human Genetics, Baylor College of Medicine, Houston, TX 77030, USA.

References
1. Fox R, Ealing J, Murphy H, Gow DP, Gosal D. A novel DNMT1 mutation associated with early onset hereditary sensory and autonomic neuropathy, cataplexy, cerebellar atrophy, scleroderma, endocrinopathy, and common variable immune deficiency. J Peripher Nerv Syst. 2016;21(3):150–3.
2. Sun Z, Wu Y, Ordog T, Baheti S, Nie J, Duan X, Hojo K, Kocher JP, Dyck PJ, Klein CJ. Aberrant signature methylome by DNMT1 hot spot mutation in hereditary sensory and autonomic neuropathy 1E. EPIGENETICS-US. 2014;9(8):1184–93.
3. Yuan J, Higuchi Y, Nagado T, Nozuma S, Nakamura T, Matsuura E, Hashiguchi A, Sakiyama Y, Yoshimura A, Takashima H. Novel mutation in the replication focus targeting sequence domain of DNMT1 causes hereditary sensory and autonomic neuropathy IE. J Peripher Nerv Syst. 2013;18(1):89–93.
4. Maresca A, Zaffagnini M, Caporali L, Carelli V, Zanna C. DNA methyltransferase 1 mutations and mitochondrial pathology: is mtDNA methylated? Front Genet. 2015;6:90.
5. Garvilles RG, Hasegawa T, Kimura H, Sharif J, Muto M, Koseki H, Takahashi S, Suetake I, Tajima S. Dual functions of the RFTS domain of Dnmt1 in replication-coupled DNA methylation and in protection of the genome from aberrant methylation. PLoS One. 2015;10(9):e137509.
6. Barboza-Cerda MC, Wong LJ, Martinez-de-Villarreal LE, Zhang VW, Dector MA. A novel EBP c.224T>a mutation supports the existence of a male-specific disorder independent of CDPX2. Am J Med Genet A. 2014;164A(7):1642–7.
7. Klein CJ, Bird T, Ertekin-Taner N, Lincoln S, Hjorth R, Wu Y, Kwok J, Mer G, Dyck PJ, Nicholson GA. DNMT1 mutation hot spot causes varied phenotypes of HSAN1 with dementia and hearing loss. Neurology. 2013;80(9):824–8.
8. Klein CJ, Botuyan MV, Wu Y, Ward CJ, Nicholson GA, Hammans S, Hojo K, Yamanishi H, Karpf AR, Wallace DC, et al. Mutations in DNMT1 cause hereditary sensory neuropathy with dementia and hearing loss. Nat Genet. 2011;43(6):595–600.
9. Baets J, Duan X, Wu Y, Smith G, Seeley WW, Mademan I, McGrath NM, Beadell NC, Khoury J, Botuyan MV, et al. Defects of mutant DNMT1 are linked to a spectrum of neurological disorders. Brain. 2015;138(Pt 4):845–61.

21

Guillain-Barré syndrome following bacterial meningitis

Li Ding[1†], Zhongjun Chen[2†], Yan Sun[3†], Haiping Bao[4], Xiao Wu[1], Lele Zhong[1], Pei Zhang[1], Yongzhong Lin[1*] and Ying Liu[1*]®

Abstract

Background: We reported a case of an adult that presented Guillain-Barré syndrome (GBS) after bacterial meningitis which was secondary to chronic suppurative otitis media (CSOM). To our knowledge, this is the first case involving an adult presenting with GBS following bacterial meningitis.

Case presentation: A 46-year man with type 2 diabetes and otitis media (OM) suffered with fever, headache, and vomiting for 6 days. The patient's neck stiffness was obvious and the Kernig and Brudzinski signs were produced. The result of cerebrospinal fluid (CSF) analysis and cytological examination of the CSF supported the diagnose of bacterial meningitis. On day 17 the patient felt numbness in both hands and feet, which gradually progressed to weakness of the limbs. Bladder dysfunction occurred, which required catheterization. The patient showed a tetraparesis with emphasis on the legs. The deep tendon reflexes of limbs were absent. The patient had peripheral hypalgesia and deep sensory dysfunction. The symptoms were possibly a result of GBS. Nerve conduction study showed that the F wave latency of the upper and lower limbs was prolonged, particularly the lower limbs. 8 days later the repeated nerve conduction study showed a low compound muscle action potential (3.3 mV) with a normal distal motor latency (14.2 ms) and a low motor nerve conduction velocity (34.3 m/s) in the tibial nerve. The patient still required assistance when walking 3 months after onset.

Conclusions: GBS following bacterial meningitis is rare and limbs weakness in patients with bacterial meningitis was usually considered because of weakness. This case should serve as a reminder for clinical doctors that when a patient with bacterial meningitis complains about limbs numbness or weakness, GBS should be considered, especially when the patient had diabetes mellitus (DM) history.

Keywords: Guillain-Barré syndrome, Bacterial meningitis, Chronic suppurative otitis media

Background

Guillain-Barré syndrome (GBS) is an acute onset immune-mediated disorder of the peripheral nervous system. Patients with this disease usually manifest acute progressive weakness, hyporeflexia or areflexia, and elevated levels of protein in the CSF. Approximately two thirds of patients with GBS experienced a preceding infection or an antecedent event (ie. surgery or immunizations) a few weeks prior to neuropathy [1]. There are only two case reports where Guillain-Barre syndrome appeared following bacterial meningitis. One case is an 11-year-old boy who experienced Guillain-Barre syndrome following meningococcal meningitis [1] and the other case is a previously healthy 35 month old girl who had Listeria meningitis with selective spinal grey matter involvement and exhibited demyelination in the neurophysiological studies [2]. To our knowledge, this is the first case involving an adult presenting with GBS following bacterial meningitis.

* Correspondence: lin19671024@163.com; 179140376@qq.com
†Li Ding, Zhongjun Chen and Yan Sun contributed equally to this work.
[1]Department of Neurology, the Second Hospital of Dalian Medical University, No. 467 Zhongshan Road, Shahekou District, Dalian City 116027, Liaoning Province, China
Full list of author information is available at the end of the article

Case presentation

A 46-year man with type 2 diabetes (6 years) and OM (a few years) suffered with fever, headache, and vomiting for 6 days. There was purulent blood from the patient's right ear. Magnetic resonance imaging (MRI) showed turbid sulcus (Fig. 1a) and OM of the left ear (Fig. 1. arrows in b). The lower class hospital treated with Cefperazone-Sulbactam for 3 days. The symptoms did not improve so the patient was transferred to the Second Hospital of Dalian Medical University (Dalian, China). The patient's neck stiffness was obvious and the Kernig and Brudzinski signs were produced. The results of blood tests were showed in Table 1. In addition the glycosylated hemoglobin was 11.20%. The patient was diagnosed with diabetic ketoacidosis (DKA) and fluid replacement therapy was implemented. Lumbar puncture was operated on day 7 and the results of CSF analysis were showed in Table 2. The patient was diagnosed bacterial meningitis and treated with Ceftriaxone Sodium 3.0 g daily and vacocin vancomycin 1.0 g twice daily. Mannitol was used to dehydrate the cranial pressure. An otoscopy showed a bulging hyperemic tympanic membrane in the left ear and there were some bloody matter on the surface. The external auditory canal was swollen. The patient was diagnosed CSOM by an otolaryngologist and levofloxacin hydrochloride ear drops and erdosteine were prescribed. The lumbar puncture was repeated on day 14 and the results were showed in Table 2. Human albumin was added to dehydrate the cranial pressure. The blood culture was negative after cultured for 5 days. In order to reduce inflammatory reaction, dexamethasone 10 mg daily was added. On day 17 the patient felt numbness in both hands and feet, which gradually progressed to both legs and left arm. Bladder dysfunction occurred, which required catheterization. The patient showed a tetraparesis. Muscle strength in the right arm was grade 4 proximally and grade 4⁻ distally, in the left arm was grade 3 proximally and grade 2 distally, in the right leg was grade 2 proximally and grade 2⁻ distally, in the left leg was grade 0 both proximally and distally. The deep tendon reflexes of limbs were absent. The patient had distally pronounced hypalgesia and deep sensory dysfunction in arms and legs. Deep sensory dysfunction reached above wrists and was from the feet up to the knees. The symptoms were possibly a result of GBS. The blood culture was negative after an additional 5 days of culturing. IVIg was initiated at day 20. The patient's symptoms improved, but his neck stiffness remained. The lumbar puncture was repeated on day 21 and the results were showed in Table 2. On day 22 the nerve conduction study showed that the F wave latency of the upper and lower limbs was prolonged, particularly the lower limbs (Table 3). On day 30 the repeated nerve conduction study showed a low compound muscle action potential (3.3 mV) with a normal distal motor latency (14.2 ms) and a low motor nerve conduction velocity (34.3 m/s) in the tibial nerve. The F wave latency of the lower limbs was prolonged (Table 4). Both nerve conduction studies supported the diagnosis of GBS. On day 33 acoustic impedance tests showed hearing loss in the left ear. On day 35 muscle strength in the right arm was grade 5 proximally and grade 5 distally, in the left arm was grade 4 proximally and grade 3 distally, in the right leg was grade 5 proximally and grade 5 distally, in the left leg was grade 4 proximally and grade 3 distally. Deep tendon reflexes were produced in the limbs. He had peripheral deep sensory dysfunction in the lower limbs. The patient was transferred to the local rehabilitation hospital. The patient still required assistance when walking 3 months after onset.

Discussion and conclusions

GBS is a group of neuropathic diseases. Within 4 weeks of onset there are two-thirds of adult patients who have gastrointestinal tract or respiratory infection [3]. *Campylobacter jejuni* is found in 25–50% of the adult patients, and more frequently in Asian countries [4]. One

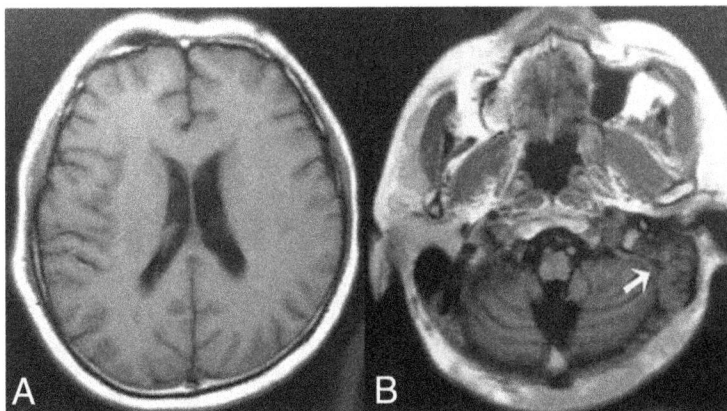

Fig. 1 MRI at the junior hospital showed turbid sulcus (**a**) and OM in the left ear (arrows in **b**)

Table 1 The results of blood tests

Characteristics	Reference range	Day 6	Day 7	Day 8	Day 14	Day 16	Day 23	Day 28
WBC	$\times 10^9$/L	23.95	21.90	12.55	11.25	10.54	6.92	
NEUT%	40.00–75.00	90.3	89.30	82.50	75.30	90.30	72.80	
Fasting blood-glucose	3.9–6.1 mmol/L	16.39	refuse	17.1	14.3	7.0	11.8	8.7
Cl⁻	98.00–107.00 mmol/L	112.00	106.46	101.66	95.40	98.89	92.08	96.68
Urinary ketone body	negative	+++	++	negative	negative	negative		
pH	7.35–7.45	7.28	7.44	7.41		7.47		
PCO₂	35–48 mmHg	15.90	27.20	25.00		34.60		
SBE	−1.5–3.0 mmol/L	−19.50	−5.10	−8.80		1.40		
cHCO₃⁻	22.5–26.9 mmol/L	−11.80	20.50	18.30		25.70		

Abbreviations: *WBC* white blood cell, *NEUT* neutrophil, *PCO₂* partial pressure of carbon dioxide, *SBE* standard base excess, *cHCO₃⁻* actual bicarbonate

study showed that *Mycoplasma pneumoniae* was found in 15% patients of GBS and was the second most common causative agent [5, 6]. Other causative agents included cytomegalovirus (CMV), Epstein-Barr virus [7], influenza A virus, *Listeria monocytogenes* [8], *Haemophilus influenza* [3], hepatitis E [9, 10], Zika and chikungunya [11]. A case report showed a case of Listeria meningitis in a previously healthy 35 month-old female with demyelination in the neurophysiological studies [2]. We reported a case of an adult that presented GBS after bacterial meningitis. Although the CSF was cultured four times and blood cultured twice, the results were all negative. The bacteria that caused this rare symptom remained unknown. The patient's bacterial meningitis was secondary to CSOM. Causative agents of chronic CSOM mainly included *Proteus mirabilis*, *Pseudomonas aeruginosa*, *Staphylococcus aureus*, or anaerobic bacteria [12]. Bacterial meningitis is the most common intracranial complication of both acute and chronic OM. The common organisms caused this complication are H. influenzae Type B, *S. pneumoniae*, and Group A streptococcus [13]. It is likely that the organism that caused the symptoms in the patient were one of these.

Acute inflammatory demyelinating polyneuropathy and acute motor axonal neuropathy are the main phenotypes of GBS spectrum. The electrophysiological results of our patient revealed a demyelinating neuropathy with reduced motor nerve conduction velocity and prolonged F wave latency, which is in line with an acute inflammatory demyelinating polyneuropathy. The patient presented GBS symptoms on day 17 following bacterial meningitis. Critical illness polyneuropathy (CIP), which manifests as distally predominant limb weakness and reduced reflexes, should be distinguished. CIP is a sensory-motor axonal polyneuropathy that commonly develops in critically ill patients [14]. The electrophysiological characteristics of this neuropathy are reduced amplitude of the compound motor and the sensory nerve action potential, the near normal motor and sensory conduction velocities, the normal F-wave latency and denervation patterns on needle electromyograms [15]. The patient was critically ill but did not meet the criteria that were required for CIP. Thus, this patient appears unique in having GBS following bacterial meningitis.

An adult that presents with bacterial meningitis and GBS is not common. A history of diabetes mellitus (DM)

Table 2 The results of analysis of CSF samples obtained by lumbar puncture

Characteristics	Reference range	Day 7	Day 14	Day 21	Day 28
Appearance		hemorrhagic cloudy	hazy yellow	yellow transparent	yellow transparent
Opening pressure (lateral decubitus)	80–180 mmH₂O	300	>330	265	250
WBC count	0–8 /μL	6400	320	92	11
L	%	5.00	19.00	46.00	
N	%	95.00	81.00	64.00	
Glucose	2.2–3.9 mmol/L	8.30	8.20	6.70	5.30
Total protein	120–600 mg/L	13,685.20	9857.70	5900.50	4545.50
Chlorides	120–132 mmol/L	119.15	107.80	112.39	117.42
CSF cultures	negative	negative	negative	negative	negative

Abbreviations: *WBC* white blood cell, *L* mononuclear cell, *N* multinuclear cell, *CSF* cerebrospinal fluid

Table 3 The results of nerve conduction study on day 22 after the onset

Nerve	Stimulation	Latency (ms)	Amp.	Velocity (m/s)	F-mean-latency	F-NO.%
Motor			(mV)			
Rt. peroneal	Ankle	3.5 (< 3.9)	6.2 (> 2.0)			
	Fibula (head)		5.1	40.2 (> 40.0)		
Lt. peroneal	Ankle	3.2 (< 3.9)	8.1 (> 2.0)			
	Fibula (head)		7.0	41.5 (> 40.0)		
Rt. tibial	Ankle	5.2 (< 5.1)	8.0 (> 4.0)		58.3 (< 53.9)	100.0 (> 70.0)
	Popliteal Fossa		8.0	43.8 (> 40.0)		
Lt. tibial	Ankle	4.3 (< 5.1)	5.1 (> 4.0)		59.9 (< 53.9)	100.0 (> 70.0)
	Popliteal Fossa		3.1	41.4 (> 40.0)		
Lt. median	Wrist	3.3 (< 4.0)	20.4 (> 7.0)		30.9(< 29.37)	100.0 (> 80.0)
	Elbow		20.1	51.0 (> 50.0)		
Lt. ulnar	Wrist	2.4 (< 3.1)	16.0 (> 7.0)		29.6 (< 29.1)	100.0 (> 80.0)
	Elbow		15.6	55.5 (> 50.0)		
Sensory			(μV)			
Rt. superficial peroneal	Lower leg	2.2	11.7 (> 5.0)	45.4 (> 40.0)		
Lt. median	Digit I	2.5	28.6(> 15.0)	52.0(> 43.4)		
	Digit III	3.0	21.9 (> 6.5)	46.6 (> 46.5)		
Lt. ulnar	Digit V	1.9	9.8 (> 7.0)	55.2(> 45.0)		
Lt. radial	Digit I	1.8	26.8(> 5.0)	52.7(> 40.0)		

Abbreviations: *Amp* amplitude, *Lt* left, *Rt* right, *F-NO.%* F wave occurrence rate

could be critical, particularly since the patient's blood glucose was not well controlled. Both DM type 1 and type 2 are associated with increased infection rates, particularly bacterial infections [16]. Infections in patients with diabetes are more likely to be severe [17]. This is likely the reason for the patient's bacterial meningitis being so severe. A recent study which involved 85 patients that had acute polyradiculoneuropathy showed that DM type 2 was present in 32% patients. The three-month prognosis was worse in patients with both GBS and diabetes [18]. This could be explained in many ways. Some patients with DM may have pre-existing nerve injuries, and the onset of the

Table 4 The results of nerve conduction study on day 30 after the onset

Nerve	Stimulation	Latency (ms)	Amp.	Velocity (m/s)	F-mean-latency	F-NO.%
Motor			(mV)			
Lt. peroneal	Ankle	3.6 (< 3.9)	7.8 (> 2.0)		59.5 (< 54.1)	56.3 (> 70.0)
	Fibula (head)		7.0	40.9 (> 40.0)		
Lt. tibial	Ankle	4.0 (< 5.1)	4.6 (> 4.0)		57.6 (< 53.9)	100.0 (> 70.0)
	Popliteal Fossa		3.3	34.3 (> 40.0)		
Lt. median	Wrist	3.3 (< 4.0)	15.5 (> 7.0)		28.7(< 29.37)	95.0 (> 80.0)
	Elbow		14.6	51.0 (> 50.0)		
Lt. ulnar	Wrist	2.4 (< 3.1)	14.8 (> 7.0)		27.9 (< 29.1)	100.0 (> 80.0)
	Elbow		14.7	58.3 (> 50.0)		
Sensory			(μV)			
Lt. superficial peroneal	Lower leg	2.6	14.6 (> 5.0)	46.1 (> 40.0)		
Lt. sural	Ankle	2.7	29.0 (> 5.0)	45.1 (> 42.0)		
Lt. median	Digit I	2.5	32.9(> 15.0)	44.0(> 43.4)		
	Digit III	2.6	27.5 (> 6.5)	50.0 (> 46.5)		
Lt. ulnar	Digit V	1.9	20.6 (> 7.0)	52.6(> 45.0)		

Abbreviations: *Amp* amplitude, *Lt* left, *Rt* right, *F-NO.%* F wave occurrence rate

GBS worsened the situation [18]. Diabetic patients have reduced rates of nerve regeneration, even before signs and symptoms of neuropathy appear. Once diabetic neuropathy appears, the capacity for nerve regeneration further decreases [19]. Diabetes could also increase the inflammation in GBS, since both diseases are associated with systemic inflammation [18].

In conclusion, GBS following bacterial meningitis is rare. However, our case shows that it should be considered in patients with bacterial meningitis suffering limb weakness and numbness, especially when the patient has DM history. Delayed diagnosis and treatment may result in poor neurological outcomes. This case should serve as a reminder for clinical doctors that when a patient with bacterial meningitis complains about limbs numbness or weakness, GBS should be considered, especially when the patient had DM history. IVIg should be started immediately after the diagnosis to prevent symptom progression.

Abbreviations
CIP: Critical illness polyneuropathy; CMV: Cytomegalovirus; CSF: Cerebrospinal fluid; CSOM: Chronic suppurative otitis media; DKA: Diabetic ketoacidosis; DM: Diabetes mellitus; GBS: Guillain-Barré syndrome; LOS: Lipooligosaccharides; Lt: Left; MRI: Magnetic resonance imaging; OM: Otitis media; Rt: Right

Acknowledgements
None.

Funding
Dr. Ying Liu was supported by Dalian Medical Science Research Project (No. 1712037). Dr. Yongzhong Lin was supported by Chinese National Natural Science Foundation (No. 81571237) and Liaoning Province Science and Technology Project (No. 2017225070). These funding were used in the design of the study and collection, analysis, and interpretation of data and in writing the manuscript.

Authors' contributions
All authors took part in the work and agree with the contents of the manuscript. YL and YZL provided concepts. HB conducted the nerve conduction study and analyzed the data. LD, ZC, and YS acquired the data. XW, LZ, and PZ did the literature review. YL drafted and submitted the initial manuscript. All authors critiqued and revised the manuscript critically for content. All authors read and approved the final manuscript.

Competing interests
The authors declare that they have no competing interests.

Author details
[1]Department of Neurology, the Second Hospital of Dalian Medical University, No. 467 Zhongshan Road, Shahekou District, Dalian City 116027, Liaoning Province, China. [2]Neuro-Interventional Ward, Dalian Municipal Central Hospital of Dalian Medical University, Dalian City, China. [3]Anesthesiology Department, Jilin University, China Japan Union Hospital, Changchun City, China. [4]Department of Nerve Electrophysiology, the Second Hospital of Dalian Medical University, Dalian City, China.

References
1. Puri V, Khalil A, Suri V. Guillain-Barre syndrome following meningococcal meningitis. Postgrad Med J. 1995;71:42–3.
2. Papandreou A, Hedrera-Fernandez A, Kaliakatsos M, Chong WK, Bhate S. An unusual presentation of paediatric listeria meningitis with selective spinal grey matter involvement and acute demyelinating polyneuropathy. Eur J Paediatr Neurol. 2016;20:196–9.
3. Jacobs BC, Rothbarth PH, van der Meche FG, Herbrink P, Schmitz PI, de Klerk MA, et al. The spectrum of antecedent infections in guillain-Barre syndrome: a case-control study. Neurology. 1998;51:1110–5.
4. Islam Z, Jacobs BC, van Belkum A, Mohammad QD, Islam MB, Herbrink P, et al. Axonal variant of guillain-Barre syndrome associated with campylobacter infection in Bangladesh. Neurology. 2010;74:581–7.
5. Sinha S, Prasad KN, Jain D, Pandey CM, Jha S, Pradhan S. Preceding infections and anti-ganglioside antibodies in patients with guillain-Barre syndrome: a single Centre prospective case-control study. Clin Microbiol Infect. 2007;13:334–7.
6. Sharma MB, Chaudhry R, Tabassum I, Ahmed NH, Sahu JK, Dhawan B, et al. The presence of mycoplasma pneumoniae infection and gm1 ganglioside antibodies in guillain-Barre syndrome. J Infect Dev Ctries. 2011;5:459–64.
7. Khatib HE, Naous A, Ghanem S, Dbaibo G, Rajab M. Case report: Guillain-Barre syndrome with pneumococcus - a new association in pediatrics. IDCases. 2018;11:36–8.
8. Vergori A, Masi G, Donati D, Ginanneschi F, Annunziata P, Cerase A, et al. Listeria meningoencephalitis and anti-gq1b antibody syndrome. Infection. 2016;44:543–6.
9. Geurtsvankessel CH, Islam Z, Mohammad QD, Jacobs BC, Endtz HP, Osterhaus AD. Hepatitis e and guillain-Barre syndrome. Clin Infect Dis. 2013; 57:1369–70.
10. van den Berg B, van der Eijk AA, Pas SD, Hunter JG, Madden RG, Tio-Gillen AP, et al. Guillain-Barre syndrome associated with preceding hepatitis e virus infection. Neurology. 2014;82:491–7.
11. Willison HJ, Jacobs BC, van Doorn PA. Guillain-barre syndrome. Lancet. 2016; 388:717–27.
12. Mittal R, Lisi CV, Gerring R, Mittal J, Mathee K, Narasimhan G, et al. Current concepts in the pathogenesis and treatment of chronic suppurative otitis media. J Med Microbiol. 2015;64:1103–16.
13. Osma U, Cureoglu S, Hosoglu S. The complications of chronic otitis media: report of 93 cases. J Laryngol Otol. 2000;114:97–100.
14. Bird SJ, Rich MM. Critical illness myopathy and polyneuropathy. Curr Neurol Neurosci Rep. 2002;2:527–33.
15. Bolton CF, Laverty DA, Brown JD, Witt NJ, Hahn AF, Sibbald WJ. Critically ill polyneuropathy: electrophysiological studies and differentiation from guillain-Barre syndrome. J Neurol Neurosurg Psychiatry. 1986;49:563–73.
16. Shah BR, Hux JE. Quantifying the risk of infectious diseases for people with diabetes. Diabetes Care. 2003;26:510–3.
17. Calvet HM, Yoshikawa TT. Infections in diabetes. Infect Dis Clin N Am. 2001; 15:407–21 viii.
18. Bae JS, Kim YJ, Kim JK. Diabetes mellitus exacerbates the clinical and electrophysiological features of guillain-Barre syndrome. Eur J Neurol. 2016; 23:439–46.
19. Polydefkis M, Hauer P, Sheth S, Sirdofsky M, Griffin JW, McArthur JC. The time course of epidermal nerve fibre regeneration: studies in normal controls and in people with diabetes, with and without neuropathy. Brain. 2004;127:1606–15.

22

Reversible reddish skin color change in a patient with compressive radial neuropathy

Jong Hyeon Ahn[1], Dae Joong Kim[2], Jung-Joon Sung[3], Yoon-Ho Hong[4], Suk-Won Ahn[5], Jeong Jin Park[6] and Byung-Nam Yoon[7*]

Abstract

Background: The motor and sensory symptoms caused by compressive radial neuropathy are well-known, but the involvement of the autonomic nervous system or the dermatologic symptoms are less well known. We report an unusual case of compressive radial neuropathy with reversible reddish skin color change.

Case presentation: A 42-year-old man was referred for left wrist drop, finger drop and a tingling sensation over the lateral dorsum of the left hand. Based on clinical information, neurologic examinations and electrophysiologic studies, he was diagnosed with compressive radial neuropathy. In addition, a reddish skin color change was observed at the area of radial sensory distribution. After two weeks of observation without specific treatment, the skin color had recovered along with a marked improvement in weakness and aberrant sensation.

Conclusions: Compressive radial neuropathy with a reversible reddish skin color change is unusual and is considered to be due to vasomotor dysfunction of the radial autonomic nerve. Compressive radial neuropathy is presented with not only motor and sensory symptoms but also autonomic symptoms; therefore, careful examination and inspection are needed at diagnosis.

Keywords: Radial neuropathy, Nerve compression syndrome, Autonomic dysreflexia, Sympathetic nervous system, Postganglionic sympathetic fibers, Red skin pigment

Background

For compressive neuropathy in the upper extremities, radial neuropathy is as frequent as median and ulnar neuropathy [1]. Compressive radial neuropathy commonly occurs at the spiral groove and results in various symptoms, such as marked wrist drop and finger drop due to denervation of extensor muscles and mild weakness of the supinator muscle. Sensory disturbance is present in the distribution of the superficial radial sensory nerve (SRN). The motor and sensory symptoms caused by compressive radial neuropathy are well known, but the involvement of the autonomic nervous system or the dermatologic

symptoms are less well known. Diverse dermatologic symptoms have been reported in carpal tunnel syndrome (CTS), including ulceration, blistering, hypohidrosis, Raynaud's phenomenon, and irritant contact dermatitis [2], but these symptoms are rare in compressive radial neuropathy. Here, we report an unusual case of compressive radial neuropathy with reversible reddish skin color change.

Case presentation

A 42-year-old male was referred for left wrist drop, finger drop and a tingling sensation over the lateral dorsum of the left hand. The patient reported that he was well until 4 days prior when he was intoxicated and awoke with the symptoms. For 4 days, slight improvement of weakness occurred. He had no history of antecedent trauma, injury, infection, or mononeuropathy. Neurologic examination revealed weakness of the left wrist and finger extension (Medical

---

* Correspondence: nrybn1230@gmail.com
[7]Department of Neurology, Seoul Paik Hospital, Inje University College of Medicine, Mareunnae-ro 9, Jung-gu, Seoul 04551, Republic of Korea
Full list of author information is available at the end of the article

Research Council grade II). Finger abduction appeared weak, but strength improved when the hand was passively extended to the neutral position. Wrist and finger flexion was intact. On sensory examination, there was a well-demarcated area of hypoesthesia and a tingling sensation over the lateral dorsum of the left hand between the thumb and index finger extending into the proximal phalanges of the 2nd finger. In addition, reddish skin color and slight edema were observed in the same area (Fig. 1). There was no definite change in skin temperature and no pain. Reflexes were normal at the biceps and triceps brachii muscles, but the left brachioradialis reflex was absent. Routine blood analysis showed white blood cell count, C-reactive protein level and uric acid level were normal. According to the clinical information and neurologic examination, he was diagnosed with compressive radial neuropathy. After approximately two weeks of observation without specific treatment, the skin color recovered along with a marked improvement of the weakness and aberrant sensation. A nerve conduction study and electromyography were performed 2 weeks after the onset of the symptoms (Table 1). On the affected left side, a normal radial compound motor action potential (CMAP) was recorded over the extensor indicis proprius muscle with the forearm and elbow stimulated. When stimulated above the spiral groove, the CMAP was reduced by 34% compared to that of

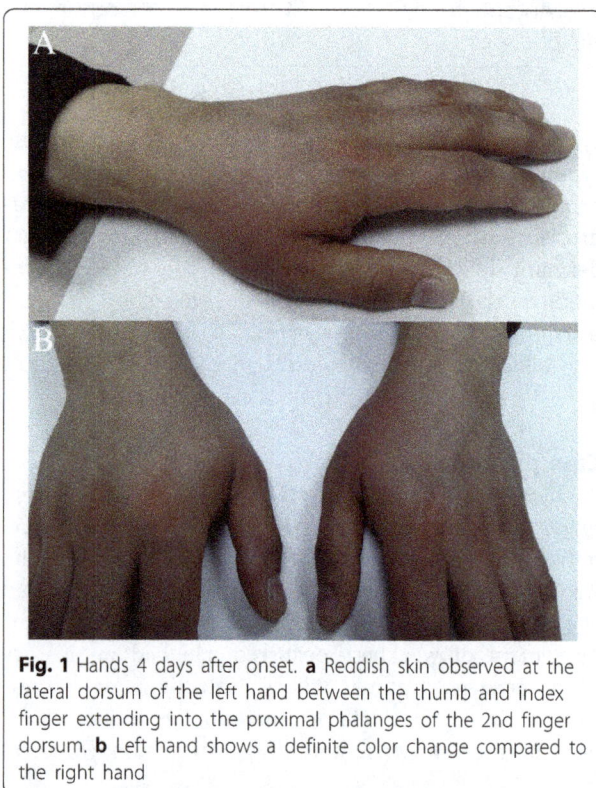

Fig. 1 Hands 4 days after onset. **a** Reddish skin observed at the lateral dorsum of the left hand between the thumb and index finger extending into the proximal phalanges of the 2nd finger dorsum. **b** Left hand shows a definite color change compared to the right hand

distal stimulations. The contralateral radial motor nerve study and sensory nerve conduction were normal. Electromyography revealed that the left extensor indicis proprius, extensor digitorum communis, extensor carpi radialis and brachioradialis showed increased insertional activity, fibrillation potentials, and positive sharp waves and reduced recruitment pattern.

Discussion and conclusion

Most peripheral nerves are mixed nerves consisting of motor, sensory and autonomic nerve fibers. The radial nerve begins as the terminal branch of the posterior cord of the brachial plexus. The radial nerve then travels distally and bifurcates into the posterior interosseous nerve (PIN) and SRN branches. Compression of the PIN presents pure motor symptoms, such as wrist and finger drop, with variable weakness of wrist extension and radial deviation of the extended wrist. SRN compression results in pain or dysesthesias on the dorsal radial forearm radiating to the thumb and index finger. Motor weakness and sensory symptoms usually occur together if the compression site is located before the bifurcation. In this case, the patient presented with a reddish skin color change, which suggested autonomic nervous system abnormality caused by vasodilation. These kinds of autonomic dysfunctions are reported in CTS but rarely reported in radial neuropathy [3]. One study reported that 54.7% of idiopathic CTS cases had autonomic dysfunction. Of the 76 cases, 59% had painful swelling of the fingers, 39% dry palms, 33% Raynaud's phenomenon, and 32% blanching of fingers. A reddish skin color change is also observed in patients with acute phase complex regional pain syndrome (CRPS). In CRPS, inhibition of sympathetic vasoconstrictor activity leads to vasodilation and skin warming [4]. In our case, similar to CRPS, sympathetic dysfunction caused by radial nerve compression may induce vasodilation and reddish skin innervated by the radial nerve. As the radial motor and sensory symptoms improve, the skin color improves. With a reddish skin color change, an elevated skin temperature could be suspected but not evident. Here, the skin thermometer test was not performed. In one cadaver study, the distribution of the sympathetic fibers of the radial nerve in the forearm was reported [5]. Studies on autonomic nerves of the radial nerve are still lacking.

Autonomic symptoms in radial neuropathy are unusual. Vasomotor innervation of skin of the radial dorsum of the hand is normally provided by the median nerve, whereas sensory and sudomotor innervation is received via the radial nerve [6]. In a study using local anesthetic nerve block, only one of 18

Table 1 The results of nerve conduction study and electromyography at 2 weeks after the onset

Nerve	Stimulation	Latency (msec)	Amp.	Velocity (m/sec)	F-latency (msec)
Motor					
Lt. radial	Forearm	1.75 (< 2.0)	5.9		
	Elbow		5.8	58.7 (> 49.0)	
Above	spiral groove		3.9*	53.5 (> 49.0)	
Rt. radial	Forearm	1.64 (< 3.6)	6.6		
	Elbow		6.4	57.9 (> 49.0)	
Above	spiral groove		6.4	58.1 (> 49.0)	
Lt. median	Wrist	2.88 (< 3.6)	11.9 (> 5.0)		26.9
	Elbow		12.3	61.3 (> 50.0)	
	Axilla		12.0	67.9 (> 56.0)	
Rt. median	Wrist	3.33 (< 3.6)	10.9 (> 5.0)		27.7
	Elbow		10.3	62.5 (> 50.0)	
	Axilla		9.8	61.3 (> 50.0)	
Sensory					
Lt. radial	Forearm	4.27	10.8 (> 8.0)	53.9 (> 50.0)	
Rt. radial	Forearm	4.19	9.4 (> 8.0)	54.9 (> 50.0)	
Lt. median	Digit 2	2.48	27.2 (> 10.0)	44.4 (> 41.3)	
Rt. median	Digit 2	2.54	21.3 (> 10.0)	43.3 (> 41.3)	

Electromyography	Spontaneous activity			Voluntary contraction		
Muscle (Left)	Insertional Activity	Fibrillation potentials	Positive sharp waves	Activation	Recruitment pattern	MUP morphology
EIP	↑	+ 1	+ 1	NL	↓	NL
EDC	↑	+ 2	+ 2	NL	↓	NL
Extensor carpi radialis	↑	+ 1	+ 2	NL	↓	NL
Brachioradialis	↑	+ 1	+ 1	NL	↓	NL
Triceps brahii	NL	0	0	NL	NL	NL
Deltoid	NL	0	0	NL	NL	NL
Biceps brachii	NL	0	0	NL	NL	NL
Abductor pollicis brevis	NL	0	0	NL	NL	NL
First dorsal interosseous	NL	0	0	NL	NL	NL
Cervical paraspinal C5-C7	NL	0	0	NL	NL	NL

* reduced 34% compared to that of distal stimulation. Latencies are in milliseconds, amplitudes of compound muscle action potentials in millivolts; amplitudes of sensory nerve action potentials in microvolts; velocities in meters/sec; Amp = amplitude; Lt = left; Rt = right; MC = musculocutaneous; EIP = extensor indicis propius; EDC = extensor digitorum communis;↑ = Increased; ↓ = reduced; NL = normal

subjects had vasomotor innervation via the radial nerve.

To the best of our knowledge, this is the first report of compressive radial neuropathy with a reversible reddish skin color change. Compressive radial neuropathy is presented with not only motor and sensory symptoms but also autonomic symptoms; therefore, careful examination and inspection are needed at diagnosis.

Abbreviations
CMAP: compound motor action potential; CRPS: complex regional pain syndrome; CTS: carpal tunnel syndrome; PIN: posterior interosseous nerve; SRN: superficial radial sensory nerve

Authors' contributions
All authors took part in the work and agree with the contents of the manuscript. JH A analyzed and interpreted the patient data and drafted the initial manuscript, DJ K provided concepts and advice for anatomy, JJ S, YH H, SW A, and JJ P critiqued and revised the manuscript critically for content, and BN Y supervised, revised the manuscript and provided important concepts. All authors read and approved the final manuscript.

Competing interests
The authors declare that they have no competing interests.

Author details
[1]Department of Neurology, Inha University Hospital, Inha University College of Medicine, Incheon, South Korea. [2]Department of Anatomy, Inha University

College of Medicine, Incheon, South Korea. [3]Department of Neurology, Seoul National University Hospital, Seoul, South Korea. [4]Department of Neurology, Seoul National University College of Medicine, Seoul National University Seoul Metropolitan Government Boramae Medical Center, Seoul, South Korea. [5]Department of Neurology, Chung-Ang University Hospital, Chung-Ang University College of Medicine, Seoul, South Korea. [6]Department of Neurology, Konkuk University Medical Center, Seoul, South Korea. [7]Department of Neurology, Seoul Paik Hospital, Inje University College of Medicine, Mareunnae-ro 9, Jung-gu, Seoul 04551, Republic of Korea.

References

1. Latinovic R, Gulliford MC, Hughes RAC. Incidence of common compressive neuropathies in primary care. J Neurol Neurosurg Psychiatry. 2006;77(2):263–5.
2. Bove D, Lupoli A, Caccavale S, Piccolo V, Ruocco E. Dermatological and immunological conditions due to nerve lesions. Funct Neurol. 2013;28(2):83–91.
3. Verghese J, Galanopoulou AS, Herskovitz S. Autonomic dysfunction in idiopathic carpal tunnel syndrome. Muscle Nerve. 2000;23(8):1209–13.
4. Wasner G, Schattschneider J, Heckmann K, Maier C, Baron R. Vascular abnormalities in reflex sympathetic dystrophy (CRPS I): mechanisms and diagnostic value. Brain. 2001;124(Pt 3):587–99.
5. Chakravarthy Marx S, Kumar P, Dhalapathy S, Anitha Marx C. Distribution of sympathetic fiber areas in the sensory nerves of forearm: an immunohistochemical study in cadavers. Romanian J Morphol Embryol. 2011;52(2):605–11.
6. Campero M, Verdugo RJ, Ochoa JL. Vasomotor innervation of the skin of the hand: a contribution to the study of human anatomy. J Anat. 1993; 182(Pt 3):361–8.

23

A novel nonsense mutation in *WNK1/HSN2* associated with sensory neuropathy and limb destruction in four siblings of a large Iranian pedigree

Behrouz Rahmani[1,2], Fatemeh Fekrmandi[3], Keivan Ahadi[4], Tannaz Ahadi[5], Afagh Alavi[6], Abolhassan Ahmadiani[2] and Sareh Asadi[2*]

Abstract

Background: Hereditary sensory and autonomic neuropathy type 2 (HSAN2) is an autosomal recessive disorder with predominant sensory dysfunction and severe complications such as limb destruction. There are different subtypes of HSAN2, including HSAN2A, which is caused by mutations in *WNK1/HSN2* gene.

Methods: An Iranian family with four siblings and autosomal recessive inheritance pattern whom initially diagnosed with HSAN2 underwent whole exome sequencing (WES) followed by segregation analysis.

Results: According to the filtering criteria of the WES data, a novel candidate variation, c.3718C > A in *WNK1/HSN2* gene that causes p.Tyr1025* was identified. This variation results in a truncated protein with 1025 amino acids instead of the wild-type product with 2645 amino acids. Sanger sequencing revealed that the mutation segregates with disease status in the pedigree.

Conclusions: The identified novel nonsense mutation in *WNK1/HSN2* in an Iranian HSAN2 pedigree presents allelic heterogeneity of this gene in different populations. The result of current study expands the spectrum of mutations of the *HSN2* gene as the genetic background of HSAN2A as well as further supports the hypothesis that *HSN2* is a causative gene for HSAN2A. However, it seems that more research is required to determine the exact effects of this product in the nervous system.

Keywords: Hereditary sensory and autonomic neuropathies, HSAN2, Nonsense mutation, Whole exome sequencing, *WNK1* gene

Background

Hereditary sensory and autonomic neuropathies (HSANs) are inherited group of neurodegenerative disorders of the peripheral nervous system associated with sensory dysfunction [1]. HSAN is characterized by the multimodal loss of sensation with or without presentation of autonomic disturbances [2]. In this group of neuropathies, motor neurons are relatively or entirely spared [3]. Based on clinical features and pattern of inheritance, HSAN has

been categorized into seven types with additional entities related to mutations in different genes [4].

HSAN type 2 (HSAN2) was first described in 1973 by Ohta M. et al. [5], but its genetic etiology was initially demonstrated from Canadian patients in 2004, and causative mutation was reported in an intron within the *WNK1* gene, referred to as *HSN2* [6]. HSAN2 occurs sporadically or with autosomal recessive inheritance pattern, which is usually diagnosed during the first two decades of life [7]. Predominantly, HSAN2 patients present sensory deficit in distal lower limbs more severely than the upper ones with possible motor involvement and variable autonomic disturbances. With the passing of time, ulcero-mutilating complications will be

---

* Correspondence: sarehasadi@gmail.com; s.asadi@sbmu.ac.ir
[2]Neuroscience Research Center, Shahid Beheshti University of Medical Sciences, Tehran, Iran
Full list of author information is available at the end of the article

revealed and, the disease can become more complicated by osteomyelitis and painless fractures [2, 8]. This disorder doesn't have a sex preference or particular ethnic distribution [9].

The recommended approach taken to the diagnosis of HSAN2 is based on detailed family history, clinical and paraclinical findings comprising neurological examinations in order to determine the extent of sensory loss and involvement of autonomic and motor nervous system, electrophysiology, histopathological evaluation of sural nerve and molecular genetic testing of candidate genes [8]. Nowadays, the genetic methods such as next-generation sequencing (NGS) based methods, are good opportunities to reduce the requirement of invasive diagnostic tests such as histological evaluation [10].

HSAN type 2 is classified into four subtypes including HSAN2A, HSAN2B, HSAN2C and HSAN2D that respectively are ascribed to genes *HSN2*, *FAM134B*, *KIF1A* and *SCN9A* in which several mutations are known to develop the diseases [11–13].

HSN2 (NM_213655) is a single-exon gene located within intron 8 of *WNK1* (WNK lysine deficient protein kinase 1). *WNK1/HSN2* appears to be expressed in satellite and Schwann cells, and sensory neurons [14]. Various *HSN2* mutations have been reported from patients with different ethnicity causing HSAN2 [1, 6, 14, 15]. Herein, we report a novel nonsense mutation in *WNK1/HSN2* associated with the clinical presentations of HSAN2 in four siblings of an Iranian family.

Subjects and methods

An HSAN2 pedigree with four affected and one unaffected sibling was recruited (Fig. 1a). The HSAN2 diagnosis was made based on clinical criteria, the results of electrophysiological evaluations, audiometry and tympanometry tests and laboratory assessments. The clinical features of the patients were recorded and summarized in Table 1.

Genetics evaluations

According to the disease inheritance pattern, patients' clinical history, and presentations, which complied with HSAN2, we initiated the molecular genetics evaluations with focused effort on this disease. Genomic DNA of all family members was extracted from blood samples using salting out protocol. The DNA fragments of genes *WNK1*, *KIF1A*, *FAM134B*, and *SCN9A* in which the prior mutations have been reported to be responsible for HSAN types 2 were respectively amplified by polymerase chain reaction (PCR). The amplicons were sequenced by Sanger method (Applied Biosystems, Foster City, CA). Afterwards, the extracted data were compared with relevant human reference sequences accessible in NCBI.

Whole exome sequencing

Whole exome sequencing (WES), Illumina HiSeq®2000 system (Illumina) was performed on the DNAs of two affected individuals HSAN- III:6 and HSAN- IV:13. Sequence alignment and variant calling were performed against human reference genome UCSC NCBI37/hg19. WANNOVAR (http://wannovar.wglab.org/) and ENSEMBL (http://asia.ensembl.org) are used to annotate the functional consequences of genetic variations. Based on the autosomal recessive inheritance of the disease and consanguinity of the parents, all heterozygous variations in father (HSAN- III:6) and homozygous variations in the proband (HSAN- IV:13) were selected. Subsequently, with the assumption that HSAN2 is a rare disease, SNPs with a reported minimal allele frequency of > 0.01 in the dbSNP database (http://www.ncbi.nlm.nih.gov/), the 1000 Genome project (http://www.internationalgenome.org/), or the NHLBI Exome Sequencing Project (http://evs.gs.washington.edu/EVS/), GnomAD (http://gnomad.broadinstitute.org/) and Iranome (http://www.iranome.com/) were removed. In the next step, variants did not affect splicing, or amino acid change (e.g. synonymous, 3UTR, 5UTR variations) were filtered out which was followed by the removal of variations with mild or moderated effect (Fig. 2).

Mutation screening

Using specific primers (fwd: 5'-ATTTCCCAGCGGCG TAAG-3' and rev: 5'-CATTGAGACGTCAGAGCCA-3'), 984 bp of the *HSN2* exon of *WNK1* containing the candidate variation -c.3718C > A- was amplified, subsequently genotyped by Sanger sequencing (Applied Biosystems, Foster City, CA). *WNK1* reference sequences used were NC_000012.12, NM_001184985, and NP_ 001171914.

Results
Clinical evaluations
HSAN2- iv: 11

A 36-year-old girl with below knee-amputated limbs and the mutilation of all distal phalanges of her upper extremities. She reported consecutive ulcers on the lower extremities from the age of six months old. Following deep ulcer infections and osteomyelitis occurrence, below knee amputations, were preceded on the left at age nine years old and on the right 13 years later (Fig. 1b).

HSAN2-iv: 12

A 32-year-old male subject, whose limb ulcerations and infections were initiated in the second year of his life. Bilateral transtibial amputations were done when he was 12 years old. The finger mutilation of his hands is shown in Fig. 1c.

HSAN2-IV: 13 and HSAN2-IV: 14

The third and fourth daughters of the family are aged 30 and 27 years old. They presented the first symptoms of

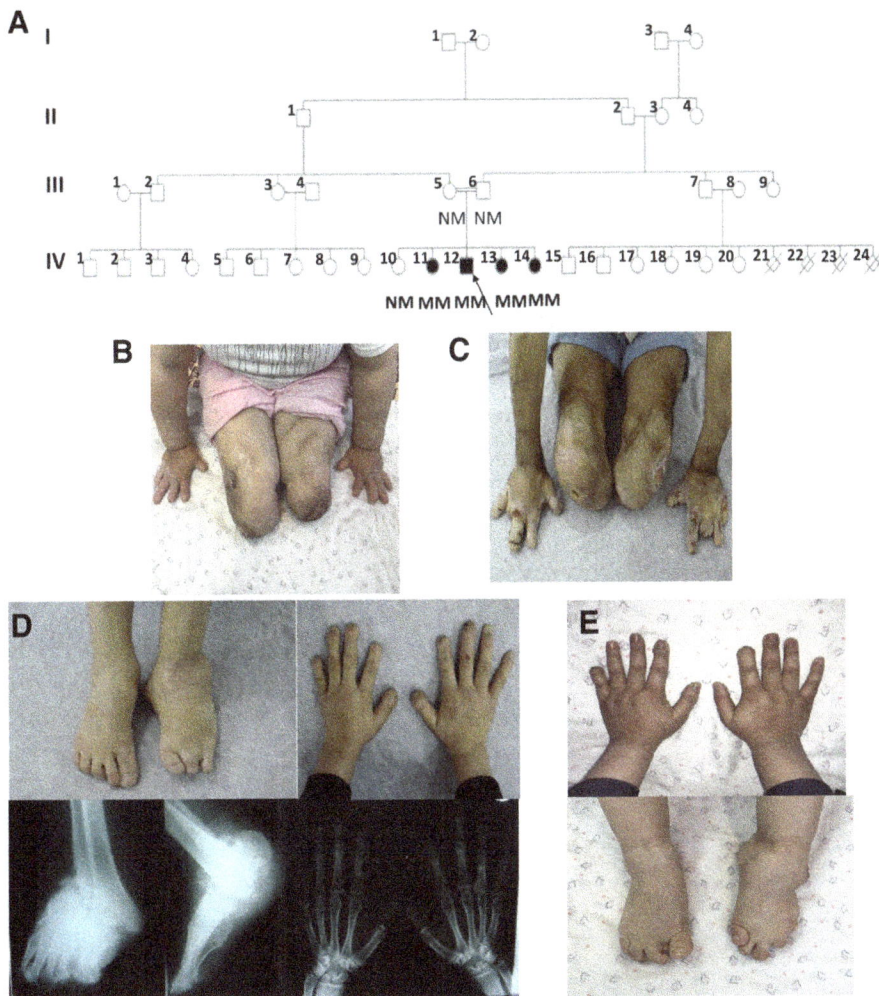

Fig. 1 The pedigree and clinical appearance of the studied family. **a** Iranian HSAN2A pedigree with a mutation in *WNK1/HSN2* gene. Genotypes of studied individuals are presented. Filled circles and squares, affected individuals; unfilled circles and squares, unaffected members; Arrow shows proband. M, mutated allele; N, normal allele; B, C. Chronic ulcers as well as the amputated and mutilated sites on upper and lower extremities of the HSAN2-IV: 11 (**b**) and HSAN2-IV: 12 (**c**). D, E. Fingers deformity and Charcot joint in the left foot of the patients HSAN2-IV: 13 (**d**) and HSAN2-IV: 14 (**e**)

consecutive limb ulcerations and infections, in seven and 10 years old, respectively. Over the time, the finger mutilation and deformity of upper and lower limbs occurred with prominent Charcot neuropathic arthropathies in their left feet (Fig. 1d and e). After profound infections around the ages between 10 and 15, the left third toe of HSAN2-IV: 13, the right second toe of HSAN2-IV: 14, and in both cases, the fifth finger of left lower extremities were amputated.

In all patients, there is a history of non-progressive symmetrical reduced multimodal sensory function in distal areas of upper and lower extremities. In the clinical examinations, pain, temperature, vibration, position, pressure, fine and crude touch perception had decreased in distal half of lower limbs in cases IV:11 and IV:12 as well as in distal one-third of lower extremities in cases

IV:13 and IV:14, with the distal end of upper limbs in all patients. The sensory impairment was more profound in pain, touch and temperature sensation with more severity in cases IV: 11 and IV: 12. Moreover, deep tendon reflexes were diminished in all patients. The clinical examinations of motor neurons, autonomic systems and cranial nerves, had no abnormal findings. All patients were in normal cognitive status. They had normal tickling sensation and sexual activity. Skin exam showed hyperkeratosis in the limbs and the lingual fungiform papillae were observed in the oral examination. Besides, there was history of neither hypertension nor recurrent fever episodes in the family (Table 1).

Electrophysiological evaluations including sensory and motor conduction studies, F wave and H reflex analysis, electromyography and the sympathetic skin response

Table 1 Clinical features and results of genetic analysis of four affected individuals with *WNK1/HSN2* mutation

	HSAN2- IV:11	HSAN2-IV:12	HSAN2-IV:13	HSAN2-IV:14
Age at onset (y)	6 months	2	7	10
Present age (y)	36	32	30	27
Sex	Female	Male	Female	Female
First symptoms	Consecutive limb ulcerations and infections	Consecutive limb ulcerations and infections	Consecutive limb ulcerations and infections	Consecutive limb ulcerations and infections
Self mutilation	Yes	Yes	Yes	Yes
Amputation	Bilateral transtibial	Bilateral transtibial	Left 3rd and 5th toes	Left 5th toe
Sensory involvement of distal extremities				
Deep tendon reflexes	Reduced	Reduced	Reduced	Reduced
Pain perception	Absent	Absent	Severely Reduced	Severely Reduced
Touch perception	Absent	Absent	Severely Reduced	Severely Reduced
Temperature sensation	Absent	Absent	Severely Reduced	Severely Reduced
Vibration sensation	Reduced	Reduced	Reduced	Reduced
Position sensation	Reduced	Reduced	Reduced	Reduced
Pressure sensation	Reduced	Reduced	Reduced	Reduced
Motor dysfunction	No	No	No	No
Autonomic involvement				
Gastroesophageal reflux	No	No	No	No
Constipation	Yes	No	No	No
Orthostatic hypotension	No	No	No	No
Episodic hypertension	No	No	No	No
Recurrent fever episodes	No	No	No	No
Hearing impairment	No	No	No	No
Skin hyperkeratosis	Yes	Yes	Yes	Yes
Lack of fungiform papillae	No	No	No	No
Mental development	Normal	Normal	Normal	Normal
Genotype	MM	MM	MM	MM

y year, *M* Mutant allele

test which have been done in cases IV: 13, 14 revealed symmetric peripheral sensory neuropathy, axonal type, with the impaired skin sympathetic response. The audiometry and tympanometry tests confirmed normal hearing. Laboratory assessments of fasting blood sugar (FBS), liver function tests (LFT), electrolytes, blood urea nitrogen, creatinine, and urine analysis were normal in all patients.

Genetics evaluations

Sanger sequencing of PCR products containing previously mutations in *WNK1*, *KIF1A*, *FAM134B*, and *SCN9A* genes showed wild type alleles; hence, we decided to perform the WES to have a better outline of genetic variations. According to the filtering criteria of the WES data a novel candidate variation, c.3718C > A in *WNK1/HSN2* gene that causes p.Tyr1025* was identified. This variation results in a truncated protein with 1025 amino acids instead of the wild-type product with 2645 amino acids; p.Tyr1025* (Fig. 3a) and segregated with disease status in the pedigree. All affected members were in the homozygous state while unaffected parents and sibling were in the heterozygous state (Fig. 3b). Also, c.3718C > A was not observed in the Iranome (http://www.iranome.ir/) and other public databases. Given that, variations in this gene have been reported as a cause of HSAN2A, so, it was assessed as the likely cause of the neurologic disorder in this family.

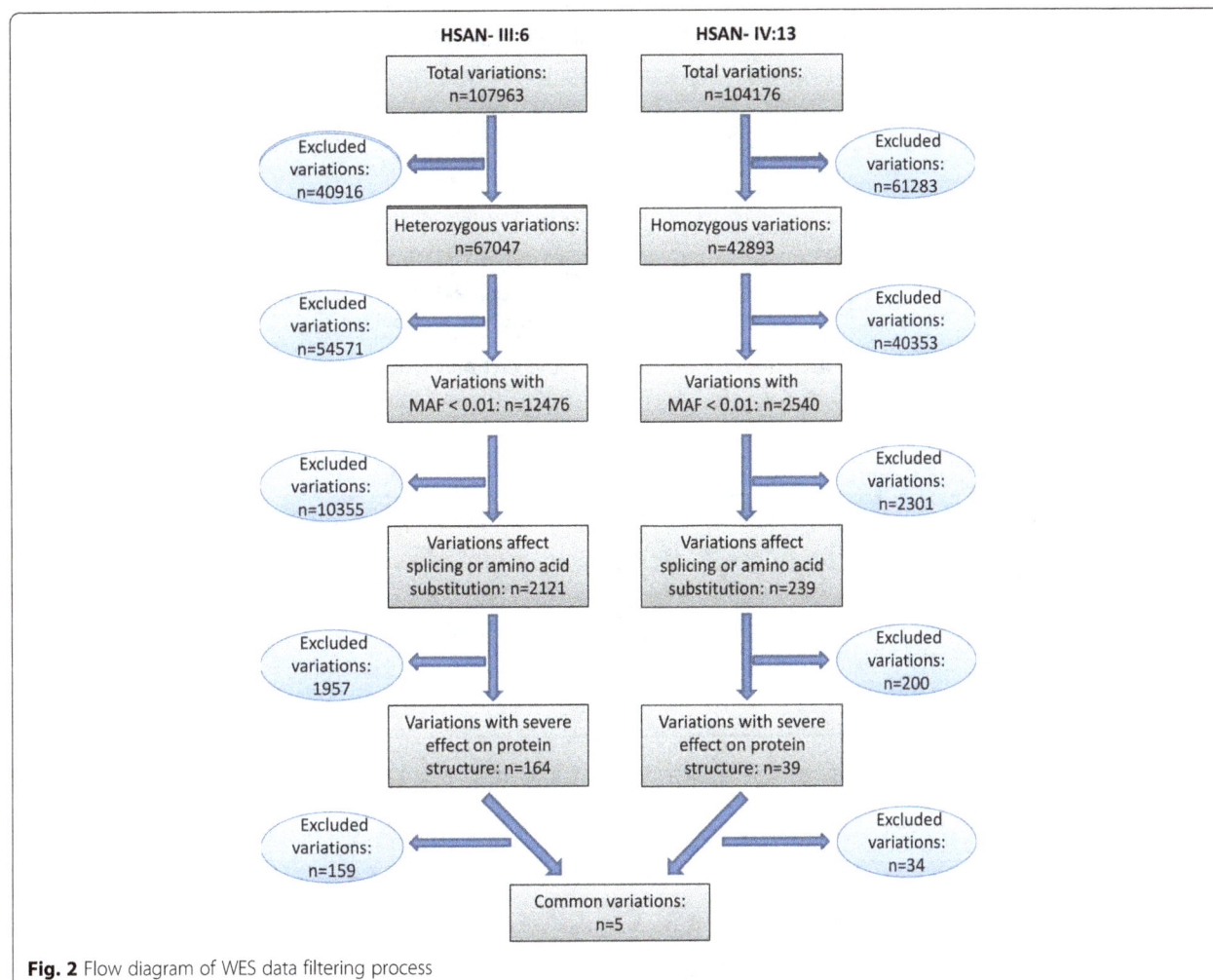

Fig. 2 Flow diagram of WES data filtering process

Discussion

With-no-lysine (K) kinase 1 (WNK1), lysine deficient protein kinase 1, a gene located on 12p13.33, consists of 28 coding exons and encodes multiple isoforms of serine/threonine-protein kinase WNK1. WNK1 proteins regulate the activity of other proteins by attaching the phosphate group to specific positions. Due to the protein kinase properties, WNK1 isoforms can control the fluxes of sodium and chloride ions and have been considered as one of the primary regulators of blood pressure. Accordingly, several mutations resulted in *WNK1* over-expression have been reported as the causative mutations of an autosomal dominant disorder, pseudohypoaldosteronism type II, which is characterized by hypertension, hyperkalemia, and renal tubular acidosis [8, 16]. In summary, it has been suggested that WNK1 proteins in cooperation with the other WNK kinases and with mediation of kinases SPAK and OSR1 have role in renal epithelial transport, maintaining cell volume homeostasis, GABA signaling, immune function and cell migration through the effect on cation-Cl⁻ co-transporters [17].

HSN2 is an alternatively spliced exon in WNK1 providing the nervous system specific isoform of WNK1 transcript, namely *WNK1/HSN2* [14]. It has been hypothesized that *WNK1/HSN2* product involves the control of neuronal ion transportation and affect membrane excitability. Furthermore, several lines of studies have been shown this protein regulates neurite extension via its effect on Nogo signaling during neuronal differentiation [18, 19]. To date, 20 homozygous mutations in *WNK1/HSN2* have been reported and almost all are in the *HSN2* exon leading to truncating and loss-of-function [15] and WNK1/HSN2 protein leads to HSAN2A disease [6, 20–23]. Analyzing the results of genetics evaluations including Sanger sequencing of previously reported mutations as well as exome sequencing showed that none of the previously reported variations for HSAN2 were present in this family, but a novel nonsense mutation c.3718C > A in *HSN2* exon of *WNK1* transcript was found that resulted in alteration of the tyrosine codon TAC to the stop codon TAA and a truncated protein

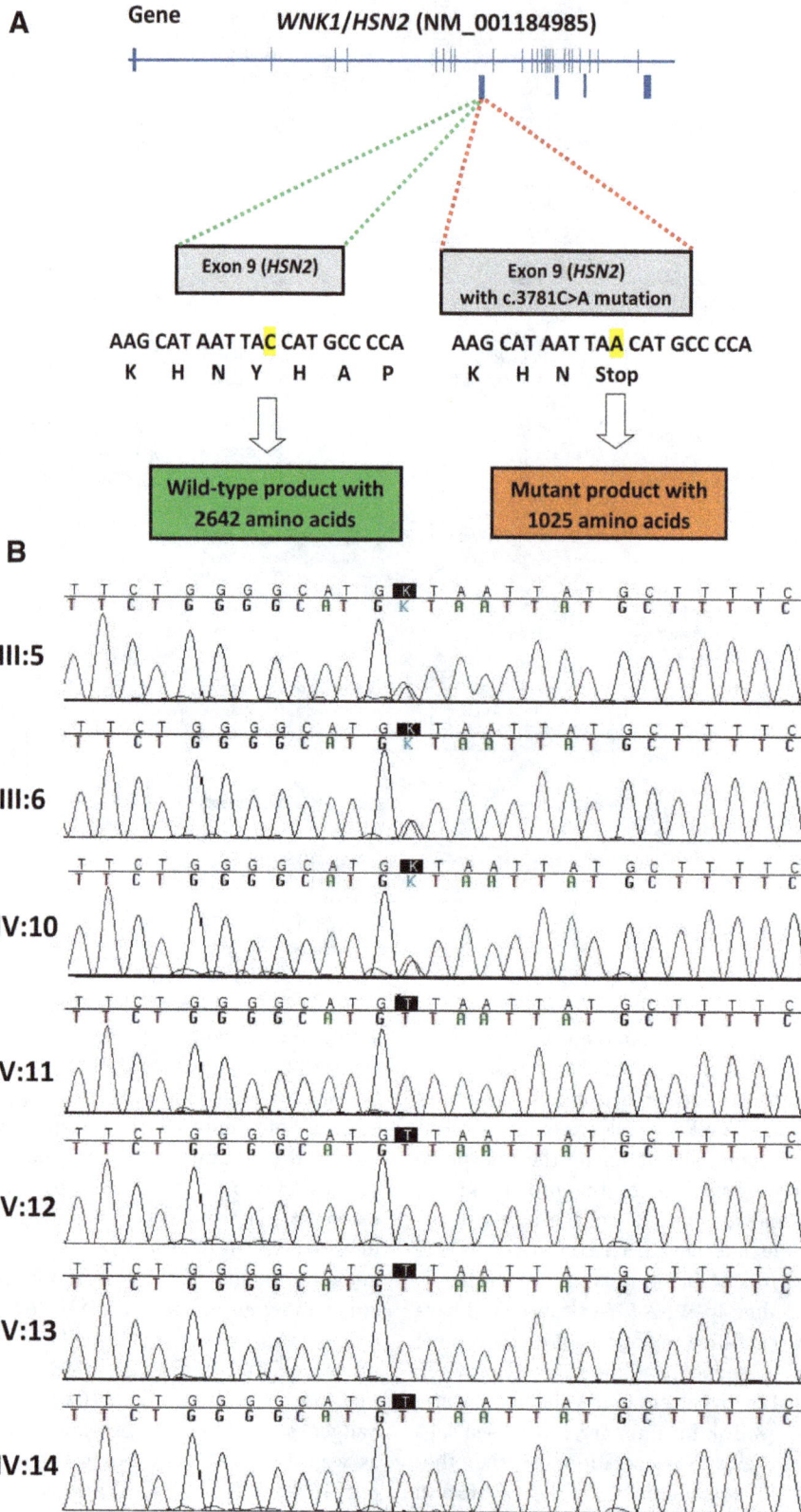

Fig. 3 (See legend on next page.)

(See figure on previous page.)

Fig. 3 a The schematic diagram of *WNK/HSN2* gene. The identified nonsense mutation c.3718C > A in HSN2 exon of WNK1 transcript alters the tyrosine codon TAC to the stop codon TAA which leads to a truncated protein. **b** Direct sequencing of the HSN2 amplicon containing the mutation in all the members of the affected family. Healthy subjects are in heterozygous status (III:5, III:6, and IV:10) but affected members (IV:11, IV:12, IV:13, and IV:14) are homozygous for this mutation

with 1025 amino acids. This result has been confirmed by subsequent segregation analysis and introduced c.3718C > A as a novel mutation for HSAN2A.

Clinical symptoms of the prior reported HSAN2A patients characterized within first two decades of life with predominant sensory polyneuropathy manifested most profound distally in a glove-stocking distribution. Sensory neuropathy was reported in lower limbs more severely than the upper limbs, although the trunk was involving in some patients. In addition, the previously reported patients presented with decreased or absent of DTRs, limb ulceration and mutilation with or without muscle weakness and variable autonomic disturbances [6, 15, 21, 23]. Our studied patients' clinical characteristics include reduced perception to pain, touch, sense of temperature, and vibration and position sensation in distal areas of upper and lower extremities with more severity in the lower limbs. They express reduced DTRs, limb mutilation and amputation, with unremarkable autonomic clinical examination without motor dysfunction (Table 1) which are consistent to the clinical presentations of previously reported data in patients with HSAN2A [8].

Clinical presentations, inheritance pattern, and genetic analyses in our reported patients confirmed the HSAN2A diagnosis by identification of a novel mutation. It is worth mentioning there are several reports of HSAN2 patients from Iran but none of them conducted genetic investigations [24–27]; thus the current study is the first report of HSAN2A in Iranian patients with complementary genetic analyses. Detection of this new mutation in *HSN2* presents allelic heterogeneity of this gene in different populations.

Consistent with previously reported mutations in *HSN2* exon, the novel mutation identified in the current Iranian HSAN2 pedigree also leads to a truncating loss-of-function mutation. Therefore, the result of present study expands the spectrum of mutations of the *HSN2* gene as the genetic background of HSAN2A as well as further support the hypothesis that *HSN2* is a causative gene for HSAN2A. However, more research is required to determine the exact effects of this mutation in the nervous system. Moreover, the relevance of WNK1/HSN2 transcript and its pathogenic mutations to HSAN needs more deciphering.

Acknowledgements
The authors thank the family members for participation in this study. We would like to thank Ms. Fatemeh Sadat Rashidi for the technical support.

Funding
This research was supported by a grant from Neuroscience Research Center, Shahid Beheshti University of Medical Sciences, Iran.

Authors' contributions
BR contributed in conception and design of the study, literature search, experimental studies, and drafting the manuscript; FF contributed in clinical data acquisition, manuscript editing and review; KA contributed in clinical data acquisition, manuscript editing and review; TA contributed in clinical data acquisition, manuscript editing and review; A Alavi contributed in exome sequencing analysis, manuscript editing and review, A Ahmadiani contributed in conception and design of the study, manuscript editing and review; SA contributed in conception and design of the study, literature search, experimental studies, manuscript editing and review. All authors read and approved the final manuscript.

Competing interests
The authors declare that they have no competing interests.

Author details
[1]Section of Physiology, Department of Basic Sciences, Faculty of Veterinary Medicine, University of Tehran, Tehran, Iran. [2]Neuroscience Research Center, Shahid Beheshti University of Medical Sciences, Tehran, Iran. [3]Department of Radiation Oncology, University Health Network, Princess Margaret Cancer Centre, Toronto, Canada. [4]Department of Orthopaedic Surgery, Milad Hospital, Tehran, Iran. [5]Neuromusculoskeletal Research Centre, Department of Physical Medicine and Rehabilitation, Iran University of Medical Sciences, Tehran, Iran. [6]Genetics Research Center, University of Social Welfare and Rehabilitation Sciences, Tehran, Iran.

References
1. Rotthier A, Baets J, Vriendt ED, Jacobs A, Auer-Grumbach M, Lévy N, et al. Genes for hereditary sensory and autonomic neuropathies: a genotype-phenotype correlation. Brain. 2009;132:2699–711.
2. Murphy SM, Davidson GL, Brandner S, Houlden H, Reilly MM. Mutation in FAM134B causing severe hereditary sensory neuropathy. J Neurol Neurosurg psychiatry. NIH public. Access. 2012;83:119–20.
3. Kurth I, Pamminger T, Hennings JC, Soehendra D, Huebner AK, Rotthier A, et al. Mutations in FAM134B, encoding a newly identified Golgi protein, cause severe sensory and autonomic neuropathy. Nat Genet. 2009;41:1179–81.
4. Axelrod FB, Kaufmann H. Hereditary sensory and autonomic neuropathies. Neuromuscul Disord Infancy, Childhood: Adolesc A Clin Approach; 2014. p. 340–52
5. Ohta M, Ellefson R, Lambert E. Hereditary sensory neuropathy, type II: clinical, electrophysiologic, histologic, and biochemical studies of a Quebec kinship. Arch. 1973.
6. Lafreniere RG, MacDonald MLE, Dube M-P, MacFarlane J, O'Driscoll M, Brais B, et al. Identification of a novel gene (HSN2) causing hereditary sensory and autonomic neuropathy type II through the study of Canadian genetic isolates. Am J Hum Genet. 2004;74:1064–73.
7. Bercier V, Brustein E, Liao M, Dion PA, Lafrenière RG, Rouleau GA, et al. WNK1/HSN2 mutation in human peripheral neuropathy deregulates KCC2 expression and posterior lateral line development in zebrafish (Danio rerio). PLoS Genet. 2013;9:e1003124.
8. Kurth I. In: Pagon RA, Adam MP, Al AHH, editors. Hereditary Sensory and Autonomic Neuropathy Type II. 2010 Nov 23 [Updated 2015 Feb 19]. Washington: GeneReviews®. Seattle Univ; 2015. p. 1993–2016.
9. Axelrod FB, Gold-von SG. Hereditary sensory and autonomic neuropathies: types II, III, and IV. Orphanet J Rare Dis. 2007;2:39.

10. Yang Y, Muzny DM, Reid JG, Bainbridge MN, Willis A, Ward PA, et al. Clinical whole-exome sequencing for the diagnosis of Mendelian disorders. N Engl J Med. 2013;369:1502–11.

11. Roddier K, Thomas T, Marleau G, Gagnon A, Dicaire M, St-Denis A, et al. Two mutations in the HSN2 gene explain the high prevalence of HSAN2 in French Canadians. Neurology. 2005;64:1762-7.

12. Rivire JB, Ramalingam S, Lavastre V, Shekarabi M, Holbert S, Lafontaine J, et al. KIF1A, an axonal transporter of synaptic vesicles, is mutated in hereditary sensory and autonomic neuropathy type 2. Am J Hum Genet. 2011;89:219–301.

13. Yuan J, Matsuura E, Higuchi Y, Hashiguchi A, Nakamura T, Nozuma S, et al. Hereditary sensory and autonomic neuropathy type IID caused by an SCN9A mutation. Neurology. 2013;80:1641–9.

14. Shekarabi M, Girard N, Rivière JB, Dion P, Houle M, Toulouse A, et al. Mutations in the nervous system-specific HSN2 exon of WNK1 cause hereditary sensory neuropathy type II. J Clin Invest. 2008;118: 2496–505.

15. Yuan J-H, Hashiguchi A, Yoshimura A, Sakai N, Takahashi MP, Ueda T, et al. WNK1/HSN2 founder mutation in patients with hereditary sensory and autonomic neuropathy: a Japanese cohort study. Clin Genet. 2017; 92:659–63.

16. Wilson FH, Disse-Nicodeme S, Choate KA, Ishikawa K, Nelson-Willams C, Desitter I, et al. Human hypertension caused by mutations in WNK kinases. Science (80-). 2001;293:1107–12.

17. Shekarabi M, Zhang J, Khanna AR, Ellison DH, Delpire E, Kahle KT. WNK Kinase Signaling in Ion Homeostasis and Human Disease. Cell Metab. 2017; 25:285–99.

18. Zhang ZH, Li JJ, Wang QJ, Zhao WQ, Hong J, Jie LS, et al. WNK1 is involved in Nogo66 inhibition of OPC differentiation. Mol Cell Neurosci. 2015;65:135–42.

19. Krueger EM, Miranpuri GS, Resnick DK. Emerging role of WNK1 in pathologic central nervous system signaling. Ann. Neurosci. 2011;18:70–5.

20. Cho H-J, Kim BJ, Suh Y-L, An J-Y, Ki C-S. Novel mutation in the HSN2 gene in a Korean patient with hereditary sensory and autonomic neuropathy type 2. J Hum Genet. 2006;51:905–8.

21. Coen K, Pareyson D, Auer-Grumbach M, Buyse G, Goemans N, Claeys KG, et al. Novel mutations in the HSN2 gene causing hereditary sensory and autonomic neuropathy type II. Neurology. 2006;66:748–51.

22. Rivière JB, Verlaan DJ, Shekarabi M, Lafrenière RG, Bénard M, Der Kaloustian VM, et al. A mutation in the HSN2 gene causes sensory neuropathy type II in a lebanese family. Ann Neurol. 2004;56:572–5.

23. Pacheco-Cuellar G, González-Huerta LM, Valdés-Miranda JM, Peláez-González H, Zenteno-Bacheron S, Cazarin-Barrientos J, et al. Hereditary sensory and autonomic neuropathy II due to novel mutation in the HSN2 gene in Mexican families. J Neurol. 2011;258:1890–2.

24. Eslami H, Fakhrzadeh V, Golizadeh N. Synchronized occurrence of two rare genetic disorders: Amelogenesis imperfect and hereditary sensory autonomic neuropathy type II. Int J Curr Res Aca Rev. 2014;2:16–20.

25. Aghaei S, Journal KP-D. Online, 2006 U. three cousins with chronic foot ulcers resulting from late-onset hereditary sensory and autonomic neuropathies type 2 (HSAN2). Dermatol Online J. 2006;12:5.

26. Gharagozlou M, Zandieh F, Tabatabaei P, Zamani G. Congenital sensory neuropathy as a differential diagnosis for phagocytic immunodeficiency. Iran J Allergy, Asthma Immunol. 2006;5:35–7.

27. Eslamian F, Soleymanpour J. Case report: two case reports of hereditary sensory autonomic neuropathy type II in a family. Med J Tabriz Uni Med Sci. 2009;31:91–4.

24

Integrated treatment for autonomic paraneoplastic syndrome improves performance status in a patient with small lung cell carcinoma

Tatsuya Ueno[1]*, Yukihiro Hasegawa[2], Rie Hagiwara[1], Tomoya Kon[1], Jin-ichi Nunomura[1] and Masahiko Tomiyama[1]

Abstract

Background: Paraneoplastic neurological syndromes (PNS) are rare disorders associated with cancer and are believed to be immune mediated. Patients with autonomic PNS suffer from variable combinations of parasympathetic and sympathetic failure. Autonomic PNS are usually associated with other PNS, such as encephalomyelitis and sensory neuropathy; however, autonomic symptoms may rarely manifest as PNS symptoms. Autonomic symptoms, therefore, may be overlooked in patients with cancer.

Case presentation: We described a 65-year-old Japanese man who was diagnosed with autonomic PNS due to small-cell lung carcinoma (SCLC) with Eastern Cooperative Oncology Group (ECOG) performance status 3, who suffered from orthostatic hypotension, and urinary retention needing a urethral balloon. Laboratory studies showed decreased levels of noradrenaline, and were positive for anti-ganglionic acetylcholine receptor antibody, type 1 antineuronal nuclear antibody, and sry-like high mobility group box 1 antibody. Nerve conduction evaluations and ^{123}I-metaiodobenzylguanidine myocardial scintigraphy showed no abnormalities. Abdominal contrast-enhanced computed tomography revealed marked colonic distention. The patient's autonomic symptoms resolved following integrated treatment (symptomatic treatment, immunotherapy, and additional chemotherapy) enabling the patient to walk, remove the urethral balloon, and endure further chemotherapy. ECOG performance status remained at 1, 10 months after admission.

Conclusions: Integrated treatment for autonomic PNS may improve autonomic symptoms and ECOG performance status of patients with cancer.

Keywords: Autonomic dysfunction, Paraneoplastic neurological syndrome, Small cell lung carcinoma, Anti-ganglionic acetylcholine receptor autoantibodies, Autonomic nervous system diseases

Background

Paraneoplastic neurological syndromes (PNS) are rare disorders associated with cancer, but are not caused directly by tumor invasion, metastasis or as a consequence of treatment. Their pathogenesis is incompletely understood, but immunological factors are believed to be important. About 3–5% of patients with small-cell lung cancer, 15–20% with thymomas, and 3–10% with B-cell or plasma-cell neoplasms develop PNS [1]. PNS are characterized by classical or non-classical neurological syndromes, and the presence of cancer and onconeural antibodies [1, 2]. Autonomic neuropathies classified as non-classical neurological syndromes of the peripheral nervous system often complicate small-cell lung carcinoma (SCLC) [1, 2], and are associated with anti-neuronal nuclear antibody type 1 (Hu) and anti-ganglionic nicotinic acetylcholine receptor (gAchR) antibody [1–3]. Autonomic failure related to anti-gAchR antibody is also known as autoimmune autonomic ganglionopathy [4]. With regard to onconeural antibodies, two main types of

* Correspondence:
lacote19thg@gmail.com; tatsuya_ueno@med.pref.aomori.jp
[1]Department of Neurology, Aomori Prefectural Central Hospital, 2-1-1 Higashi-Tsukurimichi, Aomori 030-8551, Japan
Full list of author information is available at the end of the article

antigenic targets have been described depending on their cellular location; intracellular antigens (i.e. anti-Hu antibody) and cell surface antigens (i.e. anti-gAchR antibody) [1, 5]. Patients with autonomic PNS suffer from variable combinations of parasympathetic and sympathetic failure, such as bladder and rectal disturbance, and orthostatic hypotension (OH) [6]. These autonomic symptoms result in decreased Eastern Cooperative Oncology Group (ECOG) performance status (PS) and lead to out of indication for cancer therapy. Moreover, it may be overlooked in patients with lung cancer because autonomic PNS due to lung cancer is very rare [7]. Therefore, early diagnosis of PNS, immunotherapy and appropriate treatments for PNS are essential for improving the patient's quality of life.

We herein report a case of autonomic PNS due to SCLC with anti-α3-gAchR, Hu, and Sry-like high mobility group box 1 (SOX1) antibodies, which was improved by integrated treatment (symptomatic treatment, immunotherapy and additional chemotherapy). The patient provided written informed consent for publication of this report.

Case presentation

A 65-year-old Japanese man was admitted to our department because of OH. He experienced a dry mouth 6 months before consultation. He undertook urinary catheter indwelling owing to urinary retention and noticed constipation 5 months prior to consultation. Four months previously, his primary care physician performed a screening test because he complained of appetite loss and body weight loss of 5 kg. Chest radiographs showed a tumor-like lesion. He was admitted to the Department of Respiratory Medicine in our hospital to evaluate the tumor-like lesion and was diagnosed with extensive disease-small cell lung carcinoma (ED-SCLC) 1 month before consultation. The tumor stage was stage IVA (T1cN2M1b). Following this, he noticed decreased diaphoresis, and suffered from OH. He undertook chemo-radiation therapy (carboplatin, etoposide and thoracic radiotherapy 50 Gy) for ED-SCLC 2 weeks before consultation. However, his daily living activities were restricted due to sustained OH after admission. ECOG PS decreased to 3 points. His medical history included hypertension at 40 years old, diabetes mellitus at 56 years old, and lumbar spinal stenosis at 59 years old. His family history was unremarkable. His medication included magnesium oxide, mosapride, lubiprostone, sennoside, pregabalin, voglibose and mitiglinide.

On consultation, his blood pressure and heart rate in supine position was 124/67 mmHg and 65/min. On standing, his blood pressure was decreased to 69/44 mmHg, and his heart rate was increased to 88/min. Physical examinations were normal. Neurological examination revealed no limb weakness, ataxia, and sensory disturbance. Pupil size and light reflex were normal, and the other cranial nerve examination was also normal. Deep tendon reflexes were in the normal range and plantar responses were flexor. However, he complained of autonomic nervous system impairment; dry mouth, urinary retention, constipation, decreased diaphoresis, and OH.

Laboratory evaluations showed elevated levels of fasting blood glucose (147 mg/dl) and hemoglobin A1c (7.2%). Anti-nuclear antibody, rheumatoid factor, anti-Ds-DNA antibody, anti-Sm antibody Anti-SS-A/Ro and anti-SS-B/La antibody tests were all negative. The coefficient of variation of RR interval was decreased (0.72%). 24-h urine catecholamine excretion showed normal level of adrenaline (4.5 μg/day; reference range 3.4–26.9) and dopamine (388.9 μg/day; reference range 365.0–961.5), and decreased level of noradrenaline (11.3 μg/day; reference range 48.6–168.4). Serum catecholamine levels also revealed normal levels of adrenaline and dopamine, but decreased levels of noradrenaline (30 pg/ml; reference range 100–450). Cerebrospinal fluid (CSF) analysis revealed normal cell counts (1 cells/μl), a total protein level of 34 mg/dl, and a glucose level of 94 mg/dl, with a concomitant blood glucose level of 147 mg/dl and a normal IgG index (0.65). Oligoclonal bands were negative. Motor and sensory nerve conduction evaluations showed no abnormalities and both waning and waxing were not shown by the repetitive nerve stimulation test. Abdominal contrast-enhanced computed tomography (CT) revealed marked colonic distention (Fig. 1a). Brain magnetic resonance imaging (MRI) and spinal MRI findings were unremarkable. ^{123}I-metaiodobenzylguanidine (MIBG) myocardial scintigraphy was normal (Fig. 1c). Paraneoplastic autoantibodies for Hu and SOX1 were positive. Furthermore, an anti-gAchR antibody test (anti-α3 AchR) was positive. Other paraneoplastic autoantibodies including the anti-neuronal nuclear autoantibodies type 2 (Ri), delta/notch-like epidermal growth factor-related receptor (Tr), glutamic acid decarboxylase 65 (GAD65), zinc finger protein 4 (ZIC4), titin, recoverin, paraneoplastic antigen Ma2 (PNMA2), collapsin-response mediator protein 5 (CRMP or CV2), Purkinje cell antibody type 1 (Yo) were all negative. Detection of anti-α3-gAchR and the other PNS autoantibodies was performed by radioimmunoassay methodology and immunoblot analysis, respectively. Based on these results, we diagnosed the patient with autonomic PNS due to SCLC.

We used midodrine (8 mg/day), droxidopa (900 mg/day), pyridostigmine (180 mg/day), and fludrocortisone (0.1 mg/day) to treat the OH, and intravenous immunoglobulin (IVIg) 400 mg/kg body weight daily for 5 days because of diabetes mellitus and a catheter-associated

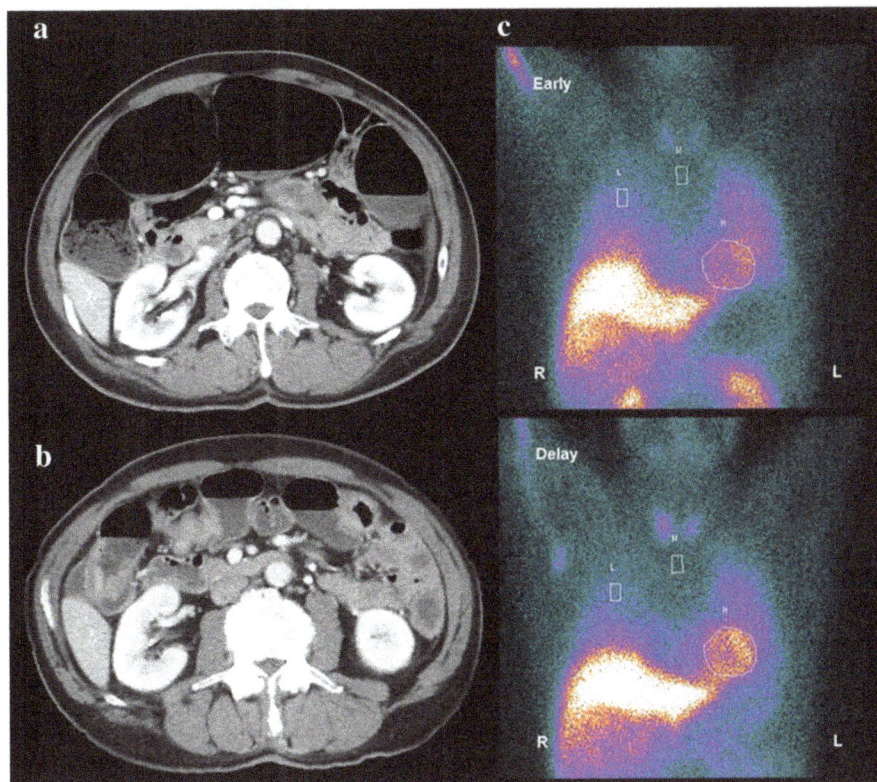

Fig. 1 Abdominal contrast-enhanced computed tomography 13 days (**a**) and 83 days (**b**) after admission and ^{123}I-metaiodobenzylguanidine (MIBG) myocardial scintigraphy 43 days after admission (**c**). Abdominal contrast-enhanced computed tomography showed marked colonic distention (**a**), and abdominal distention disappeared (**b**). The early and delayed heart/mediastinum (H/M) ratio of MIBG was 2.9 and 4.0, respectively (**c**). The washout ratio was 20.1%

urinary tract infection during admission (Fig. 2). These treatments improved his autonomic symptoms due to PNS. He was able to walk again without the symptoms of OH, and ECOG PS improved to 1 point. Amelioration of urinary retention meant that the urethral balloon could be removed. Abdominal distention disappeared, confirmed by an abdominal CT after 83 days (Fig. 1b). The patient was then able to receive the 3 remaining courses of chemotherapy as his ECOG PS improved, and he was discharged 101 days after admission. On day 43 after discharge, his blood pressure in supine and standing positions were 124/83 mmHg and 117/69 mmHg, respectively. Four-course chemotherapy for SCLC achieved a partial response. The autonomic symptoms had not recurred and his ECOG PS remained at 1 point, 10 months after admission.

Discussion

We have herein presented the autonomic PNS associated with anti-α3-gAchR, Hu and SOX1 antibodies in a patient with SCLC. This case suggests that symptomatic treatment, immunotherapy, and additional chemotherapy for autonomic PNS may improve the autonomic symptoms and performance status of patients. If patients

with cancer suffer from autonomic symptoms, oncologists and neurologists should consider the possibility of autonomic PNS even in advanced cases.

Autoantibodies involved in autonomic PNS include Hu, Yo, CV2, PCA-2, GAD-65, voltage-gated calcium channel (VGCC) and gAchR antibodies [6]. Autonomic PNS are usually associated with other PNS, such as encephalomyelitis and sensory neuropathy [6]. Patients with SCLC rarely present with chronic gastrointestinal pseudo-obstruction and OH without other neurological disturbances caused by anti-Hu antibodies [8, 9]. Autonomic symptoms, therefore, may only manifest as PNS symptoms [8, 9]. In this case, the patient had three autoantibodies for Hu, gAchR, and SOX-1. Autonomic symptoms were only detected after neurological examination and laboratory tests, and the patient had no other neurological symptoms, including sensory symptoms. With regard to autonomic symptoms, anti-Hu antibodies usually cause chronic gastrointestinal pseudo-obstruction or acute pandysautonomia as part of encephalomyelitis or subacute sensory neuropathy [6, 7, 10, 11], whereas anti-gAchR antibodies are mainly associated with subacute pandysautonomia [1, 4, 6]. Anti-SOX-1 antibodies are also detected in Lambert-Eaton

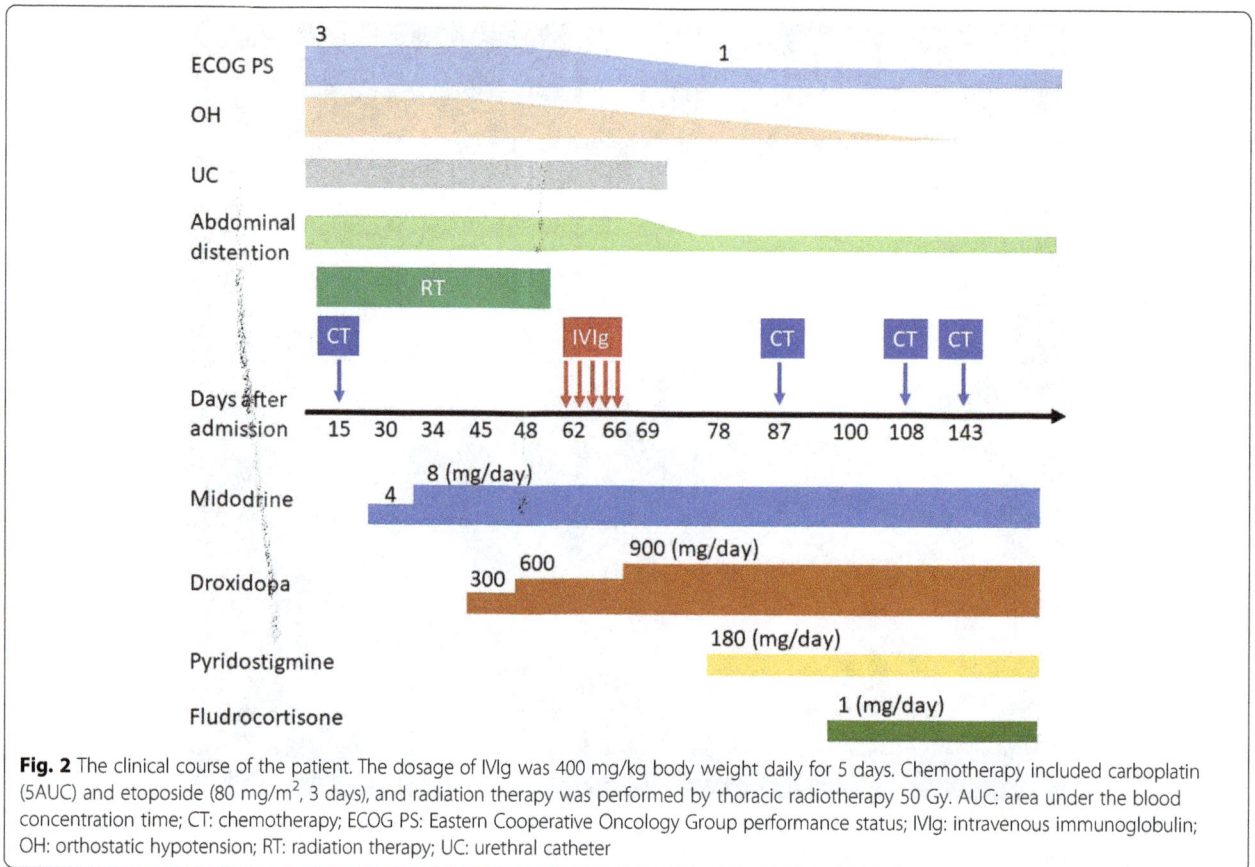

Fig. 2 The clinical course of the patient. The dosage of IVIg was 400 mg/kg body weight daily for 5 days. Chemotherapy included carboplatin (5AUC) and etoposide (80 mg/m², 3 days), and radiation therapy was performed by thoracic radiotherapy 50 Gy. AUC: area under the blood concentration time; CT: chemotherapy; ECOG PS: Eastern Cooperative Oncology Group performance status; IVIg: intravenous immunoglobulin; OH: orthostatic hypotension; RT: radiation therapy; UC: urethral catheter

syndrome with SCLC [12, 13]. SOX1 reactivity is predominantly associated with anti-Hu antibodies and SCLC [14]. Anti-Hu and SOX-1 antibodies target intracellular antigens [1, 5, 12], while anti-gAchR antibodies target cell surface antigens [1]. PNS related to antibodies for intracellular antigens respond poorly to immunotherapy; however, PNS related to antibodies for neuronal cell surface antigens usually respond well to immunotherapy [5]. The patient described herein presented with only autonomic symptoms without other PNS symptoms, along with decreased levels of 24-h urine and serum catecholamine excretion and normal MIBG scintigraphy assessing the sympathetic cardiac nerve terminals. This suggested that autonomic ganglia of the sympathetic nerve were involved. Although symptomatic treatment and chemotherapy for SCLC had an effect on the recovery of autonomic symptoms, IVIg markedly ameliorated the OH, abdominal symptoms, and urinary retention. These results demonstrate that the autonomic symptoms of this patient were caused by antibodies to cell surface antigens, especially anti-gAchR antibodies. About 15% of patients have paraneoplastic autoimmune autonomic ganglionopathy usually associated with SCLC or thymoma [15]. However, in Japanese patients with autoimmune autonomic ganglionopathy, 10% patients had ovarian

tumors, pancreas cancer, mediastinal tumors, and paranasal cancer, but not SCLC [4]. Paraneoplastic autoimmune autonomic ganglionopathy due to SCLC associated with anti-gAchR antibodies are likely overlooked in Japan.

The management of PNS requires not only immunotherapy but also oncological treatment [5]. Our patient suffered from autonomic symptoms and his ECOG PS declined. If the cause of the autonomic symptoms were not identified, the patient would have lost the opportunity to receive the additional chemotherapy. Survival from time of diagnosis is 7 month (median) in patients with anti-Hu antibodies [16]. Anti-gAchR antibodies and anti-Hu antibodies often coexist in patients with paraneoplastic autonomic neuropathy due to SCLC [17]. Our patient received the symptomatic treatment, immunotherapy, and additional chemotherapy. As a result, our patient was still alive 10 months after admission, and his ECOG PS remains 1 point. Compared with PNS due to anti-Hu antibodies, this case report highlights the improvement in ECOG PS and that ECOG PS could be maintained for 10 months because of the integrated treatment regime [16]. Furthermore, this case is unique in that the autonomic symptoms responded well to the integrated treatment, despite antibodies for intracellular antigens and neuronal cell surface antigens being simultaneously detected. Even in cases positive for anti-Hu antibodies, if neurological symptoms are only autonomic symptoms, the effects of other PNS related antibodies (i.e. anti-gAchR antibodies) should be considered, and immunotherapy ought to be performed.

Conclusion

We present a patient with autonomic PNS due to SCLC whose symptoms were improved by integrated treatment; symptomatic treatment, immunotherapy, and additional chemotherapy. Integrated treatment for autonomic PNS may improve the autonomic symptoms and ECOG PS of patients. If patients with cancer suffer from autonomic symptoms, physicians should differentiate autonomic PNS even in cases of advanced tumor stage, and integrated treatment may improve patients' survival outcome.

Abbreviations
CRMP or CV2: Collapsin-response mediator protein 5; CSF: Cerebrospinal fluid; CT: Computed tomography; ECOG: Eastern Cooperative Oncology Group; ED-SCLC: Extensive disease-small cell lung carcinoma; gAchR: ganglionic nicotinic acetylcholine receptor; GAD65: Glutamic acid decarboxylase 65; Hu: Neuronal nuclear antibody type 1; IVIg: Intravenous immunoglobulin; MIBG: 123I-metaiodobenzylguanidine; MRI: Magnetic resonance imaging; OH: Orthostatic hypotension; PNMA2: Paraneoplastic antigen Ma2; PNS: Paraneoplastic neurological syndromes; PS: Performance status; Ri: Neuronal nuclear autoantibodies type 2; SCLC: Small cell lung carcinoma; SOX-1: Sry-like high mobility group box 1; Tr: delta/notch-like epidermal growth factor-related receptor; VGCC: Voltage-gated calcium channel; Yo: Purkinje cell antibody type 1; ZIC4: Zinc finger protein 4

Acknowledgements
We thank Edanz Group (https://www.edanzediting.co.jp/) for editing a draft of this manuscript.

Funding
None.

Authors' contributions
TU, YH, RH, TK, and JN collected the clinical data and interpreted the data. TU drafted the manuscript. TU, YH, RH, TK, JN, and MT helped write and revise the manuscript. All authors read and approved the final manuscript.

Competing interests
The authors declare that they have no competing interests.

Author details
¹Department of Neurology, Aomori Prefectural Central Hospital, 2-1-1 Higashi-Tsukurimichi, Aomori 030-8551, Japan. ²Department of Respiratory Medicine, Aomori Prefectural Central Hospital, 2-1-1 Higashi-Tsukurimichi, Aomori 030-8551, Japan.

References
1. Dalmau J, Rosenfeld MR. Paraneoplastic syndromes of the CNS. Lancet Neurol. 2008;7(4):327–40.
2. Graus F, Delattre JY, Antoine JC, Dalmau J, Giometto B, Grisold W, Honnorat J, Smitt PS, Vedeler C, Verschuuren JJ, et al. Recommended diagnostic criteria for paraneoplastic neurological syndromes. J Neurol Neurosurg Psychiatry. 2004;75(8):1135–40.
3. McKeon A, Lennon VA, Lachance DH, Fealey RD, Pittock SJ. Ganglionic acetylcholine receptor autoantibody: oncological, neurological, and serological accompaniments. Arch Neurol. 2009;66(6):735–41.
4. Nakane S, Higuchi O, Koga M, Kanda T, Murata K, Suzuki T, Kurono H, Kunimoto M, Kaida K, Mukaino A, et al. Clinical features of autoimmune autonomic ganglionopathy and the detection of subunit-specific autoantibodies to the ganglionic acetylcholine receptor in Japanese patients. PLoS One. 2015;10(3):e0118312.
5. Paul NL, Kleinig TJ. Therapy of paraneoplastic disorders of the CNS. Expert Rev Neurother. 2015;15(2):187–93.
6. Lorusso L, Hart IK, Ferrari D, Ngonga GK, Gasparetto C, Ricevuti G. Autonomic paraneoplastic neurological syndromes. Autoimmun Rev. 2007;6(3):162–8.
7. Ruelle L, Bentea G, Sideris S, El Koulali M, Holbrechts S, Lafitte JJ, Grigoriu B, Sculier C, Meert AP, Durieux V, et al. Autoimmune paraneoplastic syndromes associated to lung cancer: a systematic review of the literature part 4: neurological paraneoplastic syndromes, involving the peripheral nervous system and the neuromuscular junction and muscles. Lung Cancer. 2017;111:150–63.
8. Izumi Y, Masuda T, Horimasu Y, Nakashima T, Miyamoto S, Iwamoto H, Fujitaka K, Hamada H, Hattori N. Chronic intestinal pseudo-obstruction and orthostatic hypotension associated with small cell lung Cancer that improved with tumor reduction after Chemoradiotherapy. Intern Med. 2017;56(19):2627–31.
9. Condom E, Vidal A, Rota R, Graus F, Dalmau J, Ferrer I. Paraneoplastic intestinal pseudo-obstruction associated with high titres of Hu autoantibodies. Virchows Arch A Pathol Anat Histopathol. 1993;423(6):507–11.
10. Winkler AS, Dean A, Hu M, Gregson N, Chaudhuri KR. Phenotypic and neuropathologic heterogeneity of anti-Hu antibody-related paraneoplastic syndrome presenting with progressive dysautonomia: report of two cases. Clin Auton Res. 2001;11(2):115–8.
11. Riva M, Brioschi AM, Marazzi R, Donato MF, Ferrante E. Immunological and endocrinological abnormalities in paraneoplastic disorders with involvement of the autonomic nervous system. Ital J Neurol Sci. 1997;18(3):157–61.
12. Sabater L, Titulaer M, Saiz A, Verschuuren J, Gure AO, Graus F. SOX1 antibodies are markers of paraneoplastic Lambert-Eaton myasthenic syndrome. Neurology. 2008;70(12):924–8.
13. Sculier C, Bentea G, Ruelle L, Grigoriu B, Coureau M, Gorham J, Sideris S, Holbrechts S, Lafitte JJ, Meert AP, et al. Autoimmune paraneoplastic syndromes associated to lung cancer: a systematic review of the literature: part 5: neurological auto-antibodies, discussion, flow chart, conclusions. Lung Cancer. 2017;111:164–75.
14. Stich O, Klages E, Bischler P, Jarius S, Rasiah C, Voltz R, Rauer S. SOX1 antibodies in sera from patients with paraneoplastic neurological syndromes. Acta Neurol Scand. 2012;125(5):326–31.
15. Vernino S. Autoimmune and paraneoplastic channelopathies. Neurotherapeutics. 2007;4(2):305–14.
16. Shams'ili S, Grefkens J, de Leeuw B, van den Bent M, Hooijkaas H, van der Holt B, Vecht C, Sillevis Smitt P: Paraneoplastic cerebellar degeneration associated with antineuronal antibodies: analysis of 50 patients. Brain 2003, 126(Pt 6):1409–1418.
17. Vernino S, Low PA, Fealey RD, Stewart JD, Farrugia G, Lennon VA. Autoantibodies to ganglionic acetylcholine receptors in autoimmune autonomic neuropathies. N Engl J Med. 2000;343(12):847–55.

25

The cold pressor test in interictal migraine patients – different parasympathetic pupillary response indicates dysbalance of the cranial autonomic nervous system

Ozan E. Eren[1][*] (iD), Ruth Ruscheweyh[1], Christoph Schankin[2], Florian Schöberl[1] and Andreas Straube[1]

Abstract

Background: Data on autonomic nervous system (ANS) activations in migraine patients are quite controversial, with previous studies reporting over- and underactivation of the sympathetic as well as parasympathetic nervous system. In the present study, we explicitly aimed to assess the cranial ANS in migraine patients compared to healthy controls by applying the cold pressor test to a cohort of migraine patients in the interictal phase and measuring the pupillary response.

Methods: In this prospective observational study, a strong sympathetic stimulus was applied to 20 patients with episodic migraine in the interictal phase and 20 matched controls without migraine, whereby each participant dipped the left hand into ice-cold (4 °C) water for a maximum of 5 min (cold pressor test). At baseline, 2, and 5 min during the cold pressor test, infrared monocular pupillometry was applied to quantify pupil diameter and light reflex parameters. Simultaneously, heart rate and blood pressure were measured by the external brachial RR-method at distinct time intervals to look for at least clinically relevant changes of the cardiovascular ANS.

Results: There were no significant differences between the migraine patients and controls at baseline and after 2 min of sympathetic stimulation in all the measured pupillary and cardio-vascular parameters. However, at 5 min, pupillary light reflex (PLR) constriction velocity was significantly higher in migraineurs than in controls (5.59 ± 0.73 mm/s vs. 5.16 ± 0.53 mm/s; unpaired t-test $p < 0.05$), while both cardiovascular parameters and PLR dilatation velocity were similar in both groups at this time point.

Conclusions: Our findings of an increased PLR constriction velocity after sustained sympathetic stimulation in interictal migraine patients suggest an exaggerated parasympathetic response of the cranial ANS. This indicates that brainstem parasympathetic dysregulation might play a significant role in migraine pathophysiology. More dedicated examination of the ANS in migraine patients might be of value for a deeper understanding of its pathophysiology.

Keywords: Migraine, Pupillometry, Autonomic nervous system (ANS), Parasympathetic nervous system (PSNS), Sympathetic nervous system (SNS), Cold pressor test (CPT)

* Correspondence: ozan.eren@med.uni-muenchen.de
[1]Department of Neurology, University Hospital, LMU Munich, Campus Großhadern, Marchioninistr. 15, 81377 Munich, Germany
Full list of author information is available at the end of the article

Background

A hallmark of migraine attacks is a concomitant variety of vegetative symptoms, such as loss of appetite, nausea or vomiting, with some patients even showing signs of activation of the cranial autonomic nervous system (e.g. parasympathetic system), such as lacrimation, sweating, rhinorrhea or nasal congestion [1–3]. Furthermore, there is increasing evidence that modulation of the parasympathetic nervous system might be useful in the prevention of, or the cessation of migraine attacks [4, 5]. Otherwise, previous studies of autonomic function in migraine showed inconclusive and even conflicting results regarding the role and interaction of the sympathetic and parasympathetic system.

The advantages of pupillometric testing are that it a) assesses both the sympathetic and parasympathetic innervation simultaneously concerning the pupillary reflex, and that it is b) a well-established method to evaluate autonomic function in the innervation area of the cranial nerves for various conditions [6–8]. The analyses of heart rate and blood pressure allow for at least a rough and clinically relevant evaluation of the cardiovascular autonomic nervous system (ANS). In the present study, we directly tested cranial and cardiovascular autonomic responses of migraineurs in the interictal phase during sustained sympathetic stimulation by the cold pressor test (Additional file 1). We thereby specifically tested the hypothesis whether migraine patients, when compared to age- and gender-matched controls, show different autonomic responses of the cranial ANS in the interictal phase as measured by pupillary response.

Methods

The experiments were performed at the Department of Neurology, University Hospital Munich, Campus Großhadern. The study was conducted in accordance with the Declaration of Helsinki and approved by the ethics committee of the medical faculty of the Ludwig-Maximilians-University Munich (*No. 133–13)* and all patients gave their written informed consent.

Subjects

All subjects were interviewed by a headache specialist and had a thorough, standardized neurological examination by a senior neurologist. All subjects had an unremarkable medical history except for headache in the migraine group.

Inclusion criterion was a diagnosis of episodic migraine with or without aura in accordance with the "International Classification of Headache Disorders 3 Beta" (IHCD-III beta) [1]. The migraine group consisted of 20 patients (14 women, age range 23 to 33 years, mean age 26.9 ± 2.5 years) who were tested interictally, i. e. during non-headache periods with at least 48 h

without headache before and after testing. All the 20 included migraine patients had a low to moderate attack frequency (in total 10.3 ± 10.4 in the last three months). 19 of the 20 migraineurs did not have prophylactic treatment ever; and one patient stopped his medical prophylaxis more than three months ago. Furthermore, all 20 patients did not take any acute medication in the last 14 days before autonomic testing within the study. Exclusion criteria were a past history of autonomic dysfunction such as syncope or postural orthostatic tachycardia syndrome (POTS), a history of corneal or conjunctival disease, as well as anisocoria (difference of the pupil diameter larger than 1 mm), or any other pathological findings in the neurological examination [9]. Furthermore, the subjects were tested interictally, i.e. during non-headache periods with at least 48 h without headache before and after testing.

The control group consisted of 20 subjects (10 women, age range 23 to 34 years, mean age 28.7 ± 3.5 years). No one of the healthy controls fulfilled the criteria of migraine [1] or any other primary headache. Since you only rarely find subjects, who are completely free of any headaches, at least some in the control group had a history of occasional headaches such as headache related with a flu or after alcohol exposure etc.

Psychometric measurement: Migraine Disability Assessment (MIDAS)

The MIDAS was filled in by all subjects (also the control group) and is a well-known and often used self-administered patient questionnaire to assess the impact of headache on daily life [10]. There are three scores generated: MIDAS total (impact of headache on the abilities of everyday life), MIDAS A (number of headache days in the last 3 months) and MIDAS B (average pain intensity 0–10).

Experimental measurements

Cold pressor test (CPT) / cardiovascular parameters

In general, the cold pressor test is used in clinical routine to assess the function of the ANS and the left ventricle. Temperature is a known stressor to affect heart rate (HR) and blood pressure (BP), therefore painful cold stress leads to a spike in activation of the sympathetic nervous system and consequently to the release of norepinephrine. The resulting pressor response is defined by an increase in HR and BP [11]. There is no standardized scheme to perform the cold pressor test. Traditionally, it is performed by dipping the left hand into 0–4 °C iced water (to the wrist, fingers spread) for 1–5 min. To increase sensitivity, we decided to extend the observation period up to 5 min and used 4° iced water [11–15].

To roughly assess the response of the cardiovascular autonomic nervous system we measured the HR and the

BP with the conventional external brachial RR-method on the right arm at fixed time points.

Pupillometry

Pupillary function was assessed with the monocular infrared "Compact Integrated Pupillograph (CIP)" (AMTech Pupilknowlogy GmbH, Heidelberg, Germany). Subjects were seated comfortably in front of the CIP. The pupil was automatically detected by the infrared camera and the diameter was measured continuously over 2 s at a sampling frequency of 250 Hz. The light stimulus to measure the PLR was conducted by the integrated LED with an intensity of 10,000 cd m^{-2} and a duration of 200 ms [16] and was repeated 5 times with an interval of 10 s. Measurements started after 5 min of light adaptation and subsequent 10 min of dark adaptation. The following parameters were registered automatically for the left eye:

1. **Pupillary constriction velocity in mm s^{-1}**.
2. **Pupillary dilatation velocity (slow) in mm s^{-1}**, i.e. velocity of pupillary dilatation at the end of the dilatation phase.
3. Latency time in ms, i.e. the period from the initiation of the light stimulus until the start of pupillary constriction.
4. Pupillary dilatation velocity (fast) in mm s^{-1}, i.e. velocity of pupillary dilatation at the beginning of the dilatation phase.
5. Amplitude in mm, i.e. maximum change of pupillary diameter.
6. Initial diameter in mm, i.e. pupillary diameter at the beginning of the measurement.

In order to assess the response of the ANS during the cold pressor test, we decided to analyze – in accordance with the existing literature [6–9, 16] – the pupillary constriction velocity for the parasympathetic response and slow pupillary dilatation velocity for the sympathetic response. In addition, we obtained the mean pupillary diameter for both eyes at baseline and after the cold pressor test.

Pain assessment

We obtained standardized pain ratings with a numerical rating scale (NRS), from 0 (i.e. no pain) to 10 (i.e. maximum pain), of 20 subjects (10 in each group) to evaluate whether any measured differences in the ANS are a consequence of differences in pain perception.

Statistical analysis

Data at three distinct time points were registered: T0: baseline before the cold pressor test; T1: two minutes during the cold pressor test; T2: five minutes during the cold pressor-test; T1' as additional time point only for the measurement of blood pressure; i.e. immediately after dipping the hand into the iced water. All the obtained data is given as mean ± SD. For the pupillary response, each data point was an average of at least five subsequent registrations of the pupillary light reflex (one every 10 s). For the cardiovascular parameters, mean blood pressure and heart rate were obtained once at each time point.

Statistical analysis was done using SPSS 22.1 (IBM Corp. Released 2013. IBM SPSS Statistics for Windows, Version 22.1. Armonk, NY: IBM Corp.). The data distribution was parametric as tested by the Kolmogorov-Smirnov (K-S) test. Repeated analysis of variance (ANOVA) was used to compare parameters between multiple time points within both groups (migraine, control). We performed posthoc Bonferroni-correction for multiple testing. Whenever we found a significant effect in the ANOVA, then we applied an unpaired t-Test at any timepoint(s) (T0, T1, T2) to detect the exact time point(s) (T0, T1, T2) of the statistical difference. Statistical significance was considered at $p < 0.05$.

Results

As expected, the MIDAS scores were significantly higher in the migraine group (t-test, $p < 0.01$) with a significant impact of headache on the abilities of everyday life (MIDAS total: 12.25 ± 21.39 vs. 0.40 ± 1.10), a significantly higher number of headache days in the last 3 months (MIDAS A: 10.37 ± 10.93 vs. 1.30 ± 1.49), as well as an increased pain score (MIDAS B: 6.00 ± 2.11 vs. 1.75 ± 1.80) in the migraine group. A total MIDAS score above 10 indicates moderate disability.

There were no adverse effects in the control group. In the migraine group one female suffered from a syncope shortly after T2. The data are summarized in Table 1.

Pupillary response

The pupil diameters at baseline were not different between both groups (migraineurs: 7.22 ± 0.64 mm vs. controls: 7.18 ± 0.8 mm).

Regarding pupillary constriction velocity during the light reflex (mm/s), there was a significant interaction between time and group (F = 4.26, $p < 0.05$) due to a continuous increase in pupillary constriction velocity in migraine patients, but not in controls

Table 1 Patient characteristics

Group	Migraine (n = 20)	Controls (n = 20)	p-value
Age	26.90 ± 2.45	28.7 ± 3.50	n.s.
Sex	14 female / 6 male	10 female / 10 male	n.s.
MIDAS A	10.37 ± 10.93	1.30 ± 1.49	$p < 0.05$
MIDAS B	6.00 ± 2.11	1.75 ± 1.80	$p < 0.05$
MIDAS total	12.25 ± 21.39	0.40 ± 1.10	$p < 0.05$

(Ctr) from T0 to T2: T0 (Ctr: 5.12 ± 0.46 vs. migraineurs: 5.18 ± 0.70 mm s^{-1}), T1 (Ctr: 5.13 ± 0.46 vs. migraineurs: 5.37 ± 0.66 mm s^{-1}) and T2 (Ctr: 5.16 ± 0.53 vs. migraineurs: 5.59 ± 0.73 mm s^{-1}) (Fig. 1).

Posthoc analysis by the Bonferroni-correction revealed that the migraine patients had a significantly faster constriction velocity at T2 ($p = .003$), but not at T0 or T1. We further applied an unpaired t-test to compare both groups at each time point separately. There was a significant effect for T2 ($p = 0.0042$), while T0 ($p = 0.82$) and T1 ($p = 0.33$) were not different between both groups.

For the slow pupillary dilatation velocity (mm s^{-1}) after the light reflex, there were no significant main effects for time or group and no significant interaction between time and group (F = 1.41; $p = 0.26$) from T0 to T2: T0 (Ctr: 0.72 ± 0.20 vs. migraineurs: 0.70 ± 0.16 mm s^{-1}), T1 (Ctr: 0.78 ± 0.15 vs. migraineurs: 0.73 ± 0.18 mm s^{-1}) and T2 (Ctr: 0.74 ± 0.14 vs. migraineurs: 0.77 ± 0.20 mm s^{-1}) (Fig. 1).

Cardiovascular response

There was a significant effect of time on the cardiovascular autonomic response in all three parameters ($p < 0.01$). However, there were no significant differences between groups and no significant interactions between time and group (systole F = 0.61 $p = 0.55$; diastole F = 1.02 $p = 0.37$ and heart rate F = 0.56 $p = 0.58$) (Fig. 2).

Pain ratings

We obtained ratings of maximal pain with a numerical rating scale (0–10 at T0, T1 and T2) from 20 subjects (10 from each group). There was a significant effect of time on the pain ratings ($p < 0.01$). But we did not find any significant differences between both groups and no significant interaction between time and group (F = 0.21 $p = 0.143$) (Fig. 3). Further, we did not find any significant correlation between the pain ratings and pupillary constriction velocity at any time point.

Discussion

Pupillary size and changes in pupillary size depend on many factors (e.g. time, light, environment, sleepiness, emotional state etc.), but reflect in general the balance between the sympathetic (primarily dilatation) and parasympathetic (primarily constriction) nervous system tonus.

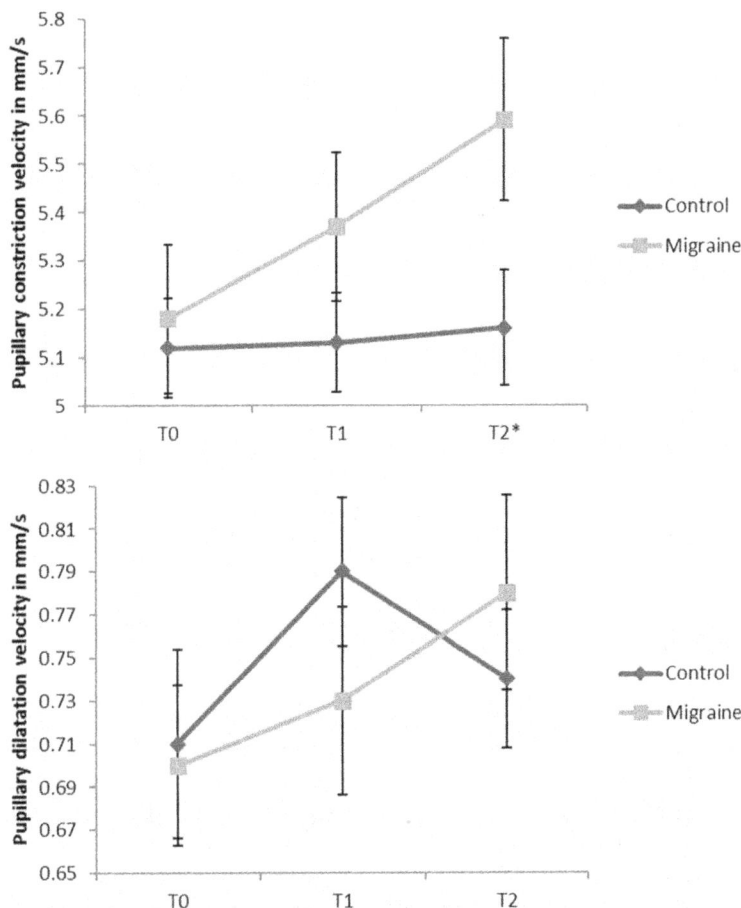

Fig. 1 Pupillary response. T0: baseline, T1: 2 min during cold pressor test, T2: 5 min during cold pressor test. Additional for cardiovascular response: T1': immediately after starting cold pressor test

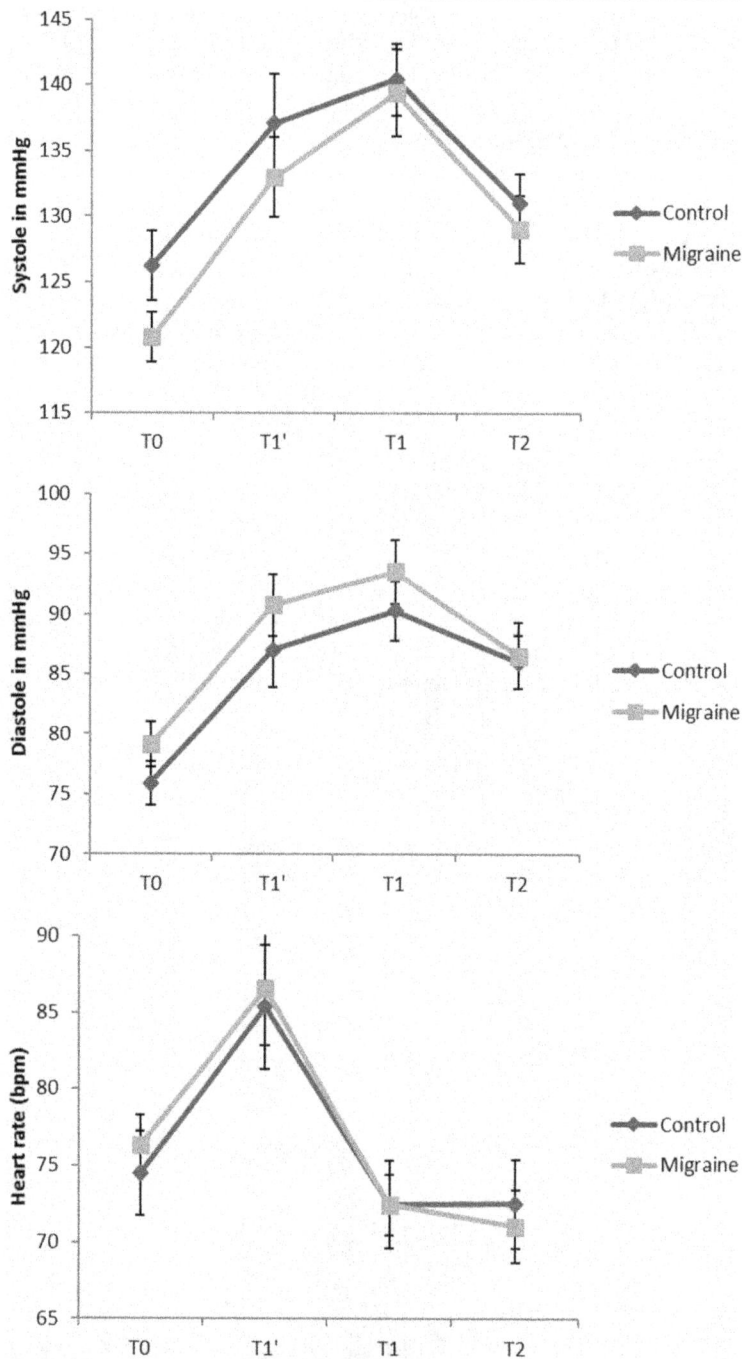

Fig. 2 Cardiovascular response. T0: baseline, T1: 2 min during cold pressor test, T2: 5 min during cold pressor test. Additional for cardiovascular response: T1': immediately after starting cold pressor test

At baseline (T0) there was no significant difference in the pupillary and cardiovascular parameters between the migraineurs and the controls, indicating that there are no profound changes in the ANS of migraine patients under normal circumstances. This is in line with a recently published study by Cambron et al., who did not find differences of pupil parameters in migraine patients, neither in the interictal phase nor during

migraine attacks [7]. However, at T2 (i.e. five minutes after sympathetic stimulation), the constriction velocity was significantly higher in the migraine patients. This might indicate that the ANS is at least slightly dysregulated in migraine patients also in the interictal, non-headache phase and that sympathetic stimulation can unravel this difference in ANS thresholds. However, the results of previous studies on the ANS

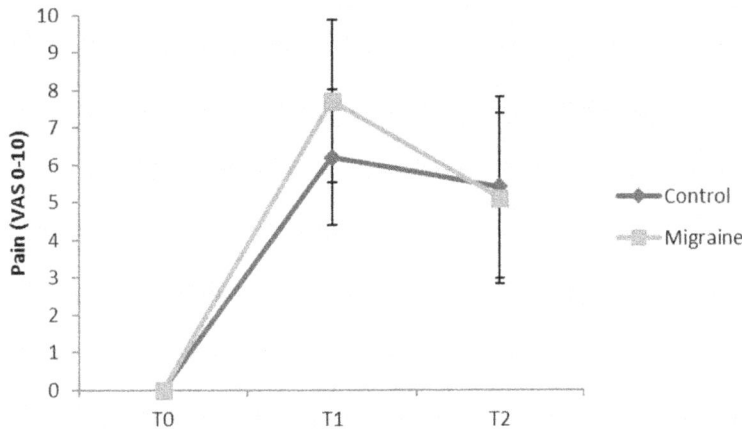

Fig. 3 Pain ratings. T0: baseline, T1: 2 min during cold pressor test, T2: 5 min during cold pressor test. Additional for cardiovascular response: T1': immediately after starting cold pressor test

thresholds and changes in migraine patients are inconclusive and partially conflictive. At first glance, in great contrast to our data, Mylius et al. showed a significantly slower constriction velocity and a smaller amplitude of pupil constriction within two days after an attack in migraine patients, thus inferring parasympathetic hypofunction [16]. However, for comparison with our data, one has to recognize that the time points of ANS-measurements were different in both studies. While they made their measurements within two days after a migraine attack, this time period was an exclusion criterion for our study, where measurements only more than two days after an attack were recorded. Thus, the data might be conclusive, since migraine patients might suffer parasympathetic dysregulation in the following way: a) lower parasympathetic thresholds under normal circumstances with activation by sympathetic stimulation, as we have shown; b) obvious parasympathetic hyperactivation during migraine attacks possibly triggered by pain in the attack, or vice versa, as a fundamental condition in the pathophysiology of migraine headache [16]; and c) parasympathetic hypofunction directly postictal after the attack, as shown by Mylius [16]. Moreover, Drummond et al. also argued for an increase of the parasympathetic tone during a migraine attack directly related to trigeminal-parasympathetic reflexes, when observing the dilatation of dermal blood vessels during attacks [17].

Corresponding to our findings, a previous study by Tassorelli et al. (15) demonstrated a miotic phase with a maximum at five minutes during the cold pressor test after an initial very short mydriasis in healthy volunteers. Our dataset implies that this physiological parasympathetic pupillary response to the cold pressor-test is more pronounced in migraine patients. This might indeed be an indirect correlate of at least slight parasympathetic dysregulation in migraine.

Pupil dilatation to baseline directly follows pupil constriction. This redilatation process can be divided into two phases: the initial and rapid redilatation phase is rather an effect of withdrawal of the parasympathetic tone than sympathetic activation, whereas the later and slower dilatation phase seems to be an active process induced by peripheral sympathetic innervation [6]. Altogether, we did not record any significant differences between the migraineurs and Ctr in this two-staged pupil dilatation process. However, analyzing the time course of the dilatation process more precisely, there was a slight delay in reaching the maximum dilatation velocity in the migraine group, while velocity itself was unchanged. The migraine group reached the highest dilatation velocity at T2, whereas the Ctr did so at T1, which may be interpreted in terms of a slight dysbalance towards the parasympathetic nervous system (PSNS) in migraine patients. Taken together our findings and the results of the previous studies, there is sufficient evidence of slight dysregulation of the parasympathetic cranial ANS in migraine patients.

Which pathophysiological mechanisms besides a primary cranial autonomic dysregulation might also contribute to the observed differences in cranial autonomic response between the migraine patients and healthy controls: First, it could be due to a difference of peripheral sensory perception and/or central pain processing. Previous studies could demonstrate cutaneous allodynia (CA) for usually not painful sensory stimuli, particularly thermal stimuli, in more than half of patients with episodic migraine during a migraine episode [18, 19]. One study even could show such changes in migraine patients prior to an episode [20]. It is generally accepted that such cutaneous allodynia is a consequence of central sensitization of pain processing pathways and an impairment of the descending pain inhibitory pathways [18, 21–23]. In fact, these mechanisms can lead to a vicious circle in that sense that recurrent migraine attacks can promote central sensitization, which in turn impairs diffuse noxious inhibitory control (DNIC) [23]. Thus, changes of central sensitization and the descending inhibitory pathways could contribute to the observed differences between migraineurs and the healthy controls by perceiving the cold stimulus during the CPT "more painful". However, comparable pain rating scores between both groups argue against that hypothesis but cannot definitely exclude it.

Secondly, habituation of sensory stimuli, which is mainly a thalamo-neocortical process, can play also a role. Previous studies have shown that migraineurs have deficits in sensory habituation after repeated stimuli of different sensory modalities (i.e. visual, somatosensory) even in the interictal phase [24, 25]. Coppola et al. [26] were able to show, that CPT can significantly change habituation of visually evoked potentials in healthy controls, but not in migraineurs indicating less plasticity of sensory cortical areas. This could result in a faster habituation of the cold stimulus by the CPT in healthy subjects as compared to the migraineurs thus successfully preventing a further continuous increase of pupillary constriction velocity, as shown by our study. However, one would expect that such a habituation deficit is not that specific affecting only constriction velocity, while dilatation velocity not.

Regarding the higher lifetime rate of syncopes (migraineurs: 46% vs. Ctr: 31%) and particularly a higher lifetime risk for repeated syncopes (migraineurs: 13% vs Ctr: 5%) in migraine patients, changes in the cardiovascular autonomic system should be expected [27]. Since we focused on the cranial ANS of migraine patients in that study, we only performed basic cardiovascular monitoring by measuring blood pressure and heart rate at different time points; however, we did not explicitly apply continuous blood pressure measurements and also did not perform analysis of the heart rate variability. The obtained basic cardiovascular responses (i.e. blood pressure and heart rate) to the cold pressor test were comparable in migraine patients and Ctr. The diastole was slightly (not significantly) increased in migraine patients compared to Ctr. Further subclassifying by headache disability by the MIDAS, we observed an only marginally higher resting state diastolic blood pressure in more disabled migraineurs. Shechter et al. explicitly compared three different groups (i.e. disabling migraine, nondisabling migraine and healthy controls) and also did not find significant differences between the three groups when comparing blood pressure response to a psychological stressor.

Cortelli et al. did not find any impairment of the autonomic control of the cardiovascular system in migraineurs interictally [28]. Domingues et al. used two different protocols to provoke a cardiovascular autonomic response, one by mental stress and one by CPT. The latter one was quite similar to our scheme and they also could not find a difference in heart rate and blood pressure after CPT in migraineurs compared to healthy controls [29]. Daluwatte et al. [30] addressed this question of coupling the cranial with cardiovascular ANS in a cohort of healthy children. They also did not find any correlation between PLR and heart rate variability (HRV), despite significant changes in HRV during the different PLR phases [30].

In our study migraine patients and Ctr did not exhibit any differences in sympathetic or parasympathetic regulation of the cardiovascular response at any timepoint (T0-T2) during the CPT. But as already mentioned, we did not apply the necessary gold standard measurements (heart rate variability and continuous blood pressure measurements) therefore to really make clear statements about that issue.

Limitations

One major limitation of this study is that as we did not have a continuous registration of blood pressure. Thus, we indeed cannot completely exclude clinically relevant fluctuations of blood pressure. We also did not analyze the power spectrum of heart rate variability by using electrocardiography (ECG), which could give further insight into ANS regulatory processes, as the extern brachial method with punctual measurement is not sensitive enough for this purpose. But we explicitly concentrated on the cranial ANS response during cold pressor-testing and only wanted to exclude major changes within the cardiovascular system such as presyncope/syncope, which in turn might affect the cranial ANS response. Furthermore, regarding the influence of emotions, food intake, and cortisol levels on the ANS, we did not explicitly randomize for these factors. Since it is very difficult to find healthy subjects, which are completely free of headaches, we also included such subjects in the control group with a history of occasional headache not fulfilling the current criteria of migraine or any other primary headache. This is also the reason, why we applied the MIDAS score in the control group and indeed found an increased total score of 0.40 ± 1.10. However, this score was really significantly different to the migraineurs and means at least only mild disability. Furthermore, the score matched with the self-rating reports of the healthy controls as not being a "headache patient".

Conclusion

In summary, our data indicate different activation thresholds of the cranial ANS in migraineurs in the interictal phase during sympathetic stimulation. Based on our findings, the role of upper brainstem parasympathetic dysregulation in the pathophysiology of migraine should be further examined and elucidated in more detail. Particularly, the underlying differences in somatosensory processing on the level of cerebral networks and neuronal ensembles might be a target for future therapy strategies.

Key findings

- There is a difference in the autonomic control of the pupillary light reflex in migraine patients outside an attack compared to healthy controls during a sympathetic stimulus.
- There is probably no such difference in the autonomic cardiovascular response, indicating anisotropy of the cranial and cardiovascular ANS in migraine patients.
- There seems to be a more selective role of parasympathetic dysregulation in the cranial innervation area in the pathophysiology of migraine.

Abbreviations

ANS: Autonomic nervous system; BP: Blood pressure; CA: Cutaneous allodynia; CIP: Compact Integrated Pupillograph; CPT: Cold Pressor Test; Ctr.: Controls; ECG: Electrocardiography; HR: Heart rate; IHCD-III beta: International Classification of Headache Disorders 3 Beta; MIDAS: Migraine Disability Assessment; NRS: Numerical rating scale; PLR: Pupillary light reflex; POTS: Postural orthostatic tachycardia syndrome; PSNS: Parasympathetic nervous system; SNS: Sympathetic nervous system; TRPM8: Transient receptor-potential M8

Funding

The authors declare that there was no financial support or funding.

Authors' contributions

OE: Conception of the work, acquisition, analysis, interpretation of data. RR: Analysis and interpretation of data, revising. FS: Analysis and interpretation of data, revising. CS: Analysis and interpretation of data, revising. AS: Conception of the work, interpretation of data, revising. All authors read and approved the final manuscript.

Competing interests

The authors declare that they have no competing interests.

Author details

[1]Department of Neurology, University Hospital, LMU Munich, Campus Großhadern, Marchioninistr. 15, 81377 Munich, Germany. [2]Department of Neurology, Inselspital, Bern University Hospital, University of Bern, Bern, Switzerland.

References

1. IHS. The international classification of headache disorders, 3rd edition (beta version). Cephalalgia. 2013;33:629–808. https://doi.org/10.1177/0333102413485658.
2. Gupta R, Bhatia MS. A report of cranial autonomic symptoms in Migraineurs. Cephalalgia. 2007;27:22–8. https://doi.org/10.1111/j.1468-2982.2006.01237.x.
3. Riesco N, Pérez-Alvarez AI, Verano L, et al. Prevalence of cranial autonomic parasympathetic symptoms in chronic migraine: usefulness of a new scale. Cephalalgia. 2016;36:346–50. https://doi.org/10.1177/0333102415593087.
4. Gaul C, Diener H-C, Solbach K, et al. gammaCore (R) use for prevention and acute treatment of chronic cluster headache: findings from the randomized phase of the PREVA study. Ann Neurol. 2014;76:S104.
5. Straube A, Ellrich J, Eren O, et al. Treatment of chronic migraine with transcutaneous stimulation of the auricular branch of the vagal nerve (auricular t-VNS): a randomized, monocentric clinical trial. J Headache Pain. 2015;16:63. https://doi.org/10.1186/s10194-015-0543-3.
6. Bremner F. Pupil evaluation as a test for autonomic disorders. Clin Auton Res. 2009;19:88–101. https://doi.org/10.1007/s10286-009-0515-2.
7. Cambron M, Maertens H, Paemeleire K, Crevits L. Autonomic function in migraine patients: ictal and Interictal Pupillometry. Headache J Head Face Pain. 2014;54:655–62. https://doi.org/10.1111/head.12139.
8. Ferrari GL, Marques JL, Gandhi RA, et al. Using dynamic pupillometry as a simple screening tool to detect autonomic neuropathy in patients with diabetes: a pilot study. Biomed Eng Online. 2010;9:26. https://doi.org/10.1186/1475-925x-9-26.
9. Takeshima T, Takao Y, Takahashi K. Pupillary sympathetic hypofunction and asymmetry in muscle contraction headache and migraine. Cephalalgia. 1987;7:257–62. https://doi.org/10.1046/j.1468-2982.1987.0704257.x.
10. Stewart WF, Lipton RB, Kolodner KB, et al. Validity of the migraine disability assessment (MIDAS) score in comparison to a diary-based measure in a population sample of migraine sufferers. Pain. 2000;88:41–52. https://doi.org/10.1016/S0304-3959(00)00305-5.
11. Silverthorn DU, Michael J. Cold stress and the cold pressor test. Adv Physiol Educ. 2013;37:93–6. https://doi.org/10.1152/advan.00002.2013.
12. Roatta S, Micieli G, Bosone D, et al. Effect of generalised sympathetic activation by cold pressor test on cerebral haemodynamics in healthy humans. J Auton Nerv Syst. 1998;71:159–66.
13. Tassorelli C, Micieli G, Osipova V, et al. Combined evaluation of pupillary and cardiovascular responses to cold pressor test in cluster headache patients. Cephalalgia. 1998;18:668–74.
14. Tassorelli C, Micieli G, Osipova V, et al. Pupillary and cardiovascular responses to the cold-pressor test. J Auton Nerv Syst. 1995;55:45–9.
15. Mitchell LA, MacDonald RAR, Brodie EE. Temperature and the cold pressor test. J Pain. 2004;5:233–7. https://doi.org/10.1016/j.jpain.2004.03.004.
16. Mylius V, Braune HJ, Schepelmann K. Dysfunction of the pupillary light reflex following migraine headache. Clin Auton Res. 2003;13:16–21. https://doi.org/10.1007/s10286-003-0065-y.
17. Drummond PD. Sweating and vascular responses in the face: normal regulation and dysfunction in migraine, cluster headache and harlequin syndrome. Clin Auton Res. 1994;4:273–85. https://doi.org/10.1007/BF01827433.
18. Bigal ME, Ashina S, Burstein R, et al. Prevalence and characteristics of allodynia in headache sufferers. Neurology. 2008;70:1525–33. https://doi.org/10.1212/01.wnl.0000310645.31020.b1.
19. Schwedt TJ, Krauss MJ, Frey K, Gereau RW. Episodic and chronic migraineurs are hypersensitive to thermal stimuli between migraine attacks. Cephalalgia Int J. Headache. 2011;31:6–12. https://doi.org/10.1177/0333102410365108.
20. Sand T, Zhitniy N, Nilsen KB, et al. Thermal pain thresholds are decreased in the migraine preattack phase. Eur J Neurol. 2008;15:1199–205. https://doi.org/10.1111/j.1468-1331.2008.02276.x.
21. Burstein R, Cutrer MF, Yarnitsky D. The development of cutaneous allodynia during a migraine attack clinical evidence for the sequential recruitment of spinal and supraspinal nociceptive neurons in migraine. Brain. 2000;123:1703–9. https://doi.org/10.1093/brain/123.8.1703.
22. Bernstein C, Burstein R. Sensitization of the Trigeminovascular pathway: perspective and implications to migraine pathophysiology. J Clin Neurol. 2012;8:89–99. https://doi.org/10.3988/jcn.2012.8.2.89.
23. Boyer N, Dallel R, Artola A, Monconduit L. General trigeminospinal central sensitization and impaired descending pain inhibitory controls contribute to migraine progression. Pain. 2014;155:1196–205.
24. Áfra J, Proietti Cecchini A, Sándor PS, Schoenen J. Comparison of visual and auditory evoked cortical potentials in migraine patients between attacks. Clin Neurophysiol. 2000;111:1124–9. https://doi.org/10.1016/S1388-2457(00)00271-6.
25. Coppola G, Lorenzo CD, Schoenen J, Pierelli F. Habituation and sensitization in primary headaches. J Headache Pain. 2013;14:65. https://doi.org/10.1186/1129-2377-14-65.
26. Coppola G, Currà A, Serrao M, et al. Lack of cold pressor test-induced effect on visual-evoked potentials in migraine. J Headache Pain. 2010;11:115–21. https://doi.org/10.1007/s10194-009-0177-4.
27. Thijs RD, Kruit MC, van Buchem MA, et al. Syncope in migraine the population-based CAMERA study. Neurology. 2006;66:1034–7. https://doi.org/10.1212/01.wnl.0000204186.43597.66.

26

Isolated optic neuritis with a concurrent abnormal trigeminal nucleus on imaging: case report of a rare complication of herpes zoster ophthalmicus

Kavin Vanikieti[1], Anuchit Poonyathalang[1], Panitha Jindahra[2], Piyaphon Cheecharoen[3], Patchalin Patputtipong[3] and Tanyatuth Padungkiatsagul[1*] ⓘ

Abstract

Background: Herpes zoster ophthalmicus (HZO) is an inflammation related to reactivation of the latent varicella zoster virus (VZV), involving the ophthalmic branch of the trigeminal nerve. Optic neuritis (ON), a rare ocular complication following HZO, has been reported in 1.9% of HZO-affected eyes. Most previous cases occurred simultaneously with other ocular complications, especially orbital apex syndrome. Moreover, detailed magnetic resonance imaging (MRI) with diffusion weighted imaging of the optic nerve and trigeminal nucleus in HZO-related ON has been rarely reported. We report a case of postherpetic isolated ON with a concurrent abnormal trigeminal nucleus on imaging.

Case presentation: A healthy 58-year-old female presented with sudden painful visual loss in her right eye for 2 days. Four weeks before the presentation, her right eye was diagnosed with HZO, and she received intravenous acyclovir for 10 days. Ophthalmic examination revealed a visual acuity of light perception and 20/20 in the right and left eyes, respectively. A relative afferent pupillary defect was present in the right eye. Neurological examination was significant for hypoesthesia in the area of the HZO. A clinical diagnosis of HZO-related right retrobulbar ON was made, and other causes of atypical ON were excluded. MRI showed enhancement and restricted diffusion of the right-sided optic nerve with linear hyperintense T2 of the right-sided spinal trigeminal nucleus and tract (STNT) along the brainstem. She received 14 days of intravenous acyclovir and 5 days of methylprednisolone. Both were switched to an oral route for 2 months. After the completion of treatment, the visual acuity was counting fingers and 20/20 in the right eye and left eye, respectively. Stable brainstem STNT abnormalities and resolution of ON were found radiologically.

Conclusions: Isolated ON is a rare ocular complication following HZO. An abnormal high signal of STNT on a T2 weighted image may be present, which may be a clue for VZV-associated complications, such as HZO-related ON, especially in cases lacking an obvious history of HZO or other concomitant ocular complications. Prompt treatment with both acyclovir and corticosteroids should be started. Restricted diffusion of the optic nerve may be a predictor for poor visual recovery.

Keywords: Herpes zoster ophthalmicus, Optic neuritis, Magnetic resonance imaging, Diffusion weighted imaging, Trigeminal nucleus

* Correspondence: Blu_c16@hotmail.com
[1]Department of Ophthalmology, Faculty of Medicine Ramathibodi Hospital, Mahidol University, 270 Rama VI Road, Bangkok 10400, Thailand
Full list of author information is available at the end of the article

Background

Herpes zoster ophthalmicus (HZO) is an inflammation related to reactivation of the latent varicella zoster virus (VZV) involving the ophthalmic branch of the trigeminal nerve [1]. Ocular complications are found in 50% of HZO patients, following the onset of a rash in 1–4 weeks [2].

Any ocular structures can be affected, although anterior uveitis and keratitis are the most common ocular complications [3]. Optic neuritis (ON), a rare ocular complication following HZO, has been reported in 1.9% of HZO-affected eyes [3]. However, HZO-related ON in many previous reports was not isolated. Most of the previous cases occurred simultaneously with other ocular complications, especially orbital apex syndrome [4, 5]. Moreover, detailed magnetic resonance imaging (MRI) with diffusion weighted imaging (DWI) of the optic nerve and trigeminal nucleus in HZO-related ON has been rarely documented. Herein, we report a case of postherpetic isolated ON with a concurrent abnormal trigeminal nucleus on imaging.

Case presentation

A previously healthy 58-year-old female presented to our clinic with a sudden painful visual loss in her right eye for 2 days. Ocular movement significantly aggravated her pain. Four weeks before the presentation, she developed a group of vesicles on the erythematous base over the right ophthalmic branch of the trigeminal nerve including the tip of her nose, which was diagnosed as HZO. At that time, she was treated with intravenous acyclovir (30 mg/kg/day) for 10 days. The group of vesicles soon disappeared and turned to hyperpigmented macules and patches (Fig. 1).

At our clinic, an ophthalmic examination revealed best-corrected visual acuity of light perception in the right eye, compared with 20/20 in the left eye. A relative afferent pupillary defect (RAPD) was present in the right eye. Intraocular pressures were 12 mmHg in both eyes. Ocular motility, anterior segment, and a fundus examination were unremarkable bilaterally. Neither proptosis nor ptosis was observed. The neurological examination was significant for hypoesthesia in the area supplied by the right ophthalmic branch of the trigeminal nerve. A clinical diagnosis of HZO-related right retrobulbar ON was made. To exclude other possible causes of atypical ON, a blood test including a complete blood count (CBC), erythrocyte sedimentation rate (ESR), c-reactive protein (CRP), Venereal Disease Research Laboratory (VDRL), *Treponema pallidum* hemagglutination (TPHA), antinuclear antibody (ANA), and aquaporin 4-antibody were performed, which all showed normal results. MRI of the brain and orbit showed enhancement and restricted diffusion of a right-sided intraorbital, intracanalicular, and prechiasmatic optic nerve (Fig. 2). Notably, linear hyperintense T2 lesions in

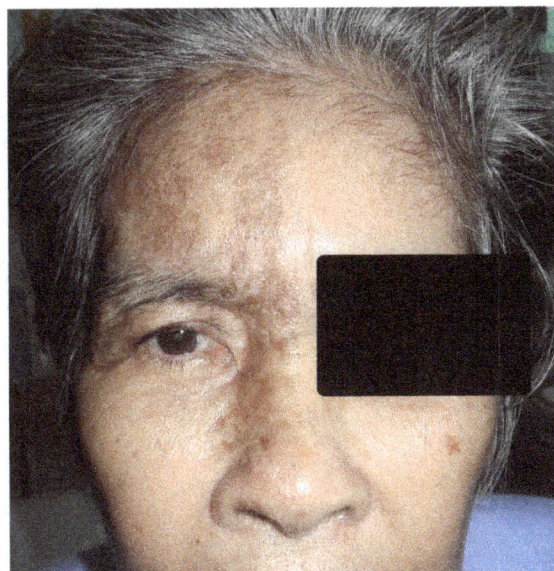

Fig. 1 External appearance. Hyperpigmented macules and patches over the right ophthalmic branch of the trigeminal nerve, including the tip of the nose

vertical orientation extending from the right dorsolateral pons down to the medulla without any enhancement or restricted diffusion were also found (Fig. 3). These vertical lesions represented the anatomical location of the spinal trigeminal nucleus and tract (STNT) along the brainstem. Lumbar puncture showed mild lymphocytic pleocytosis (22 cells, 98% lymphocytes) with normal protein and a negative polymerase chain reaction (PCR) for VZV.

Treatment was started with intravenous acyclovir (30 mg/kg/day) along with 1 g/day of intravenous methylprednisolone. Intravenous acyclovir was continued for 14 days, then reduced to 800 mg oral acyclovir daily. Acyclovir was discontinued in the third month. Oral prednisolone (1 mg/kg/day) was started after 5 days of intravenous methylprednisolone, then gradually tapered and discontinued in the third month. After the completion of the 2 month treatment, the best-corrected visual acuity was counting fingers and 20/20 in the right and left eyes, respectively. An ophthalmic examination detected a right optic disc atrophy with normal physiological cupping. MRI of the brain and orbit showed stable brainstem STNT abnormalities and resolution of the ON.

Discussion and conclusions

ON is an unusual ocular complication secondary to HZO that may present either in papillitis or retrobulbar form and occur weeks to months after the onset of the rash [6–12]. The degree of visual loss varies, ranging from mild to severe visual impairment [6–12]. Adults, especially the elderly, are more affected; however, HZO-related ON in children has also been reported [9, 13].

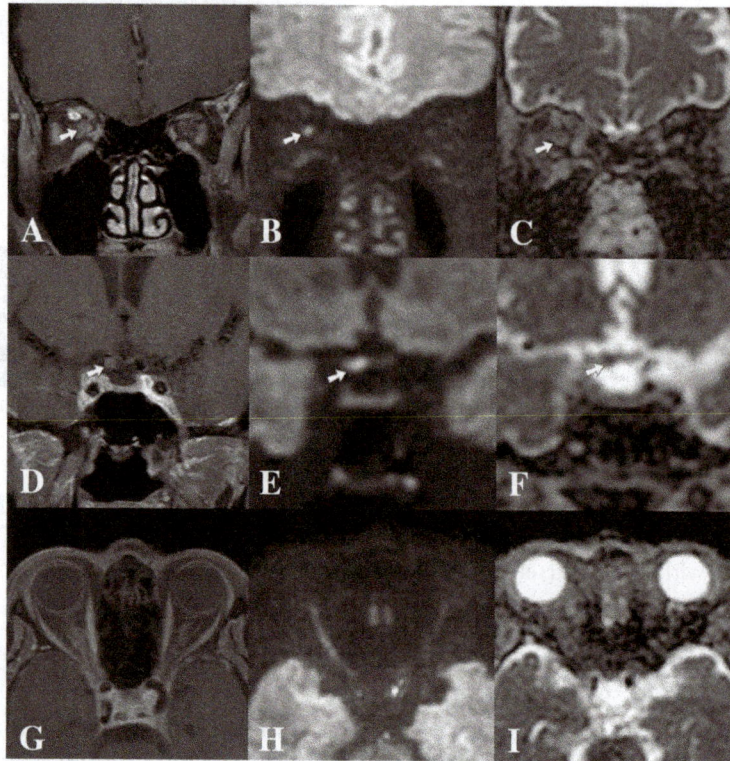

Fig. 2 Magnetic resonance imaging of the orbit with diffusion weighted imaging (DWI) and an apparent diffusion coefficient (ADC). Coronal T1 weighted with a gadolinium injection (**a**) shows enhancement of the right intraorbital optic nerve (arrow) along with restricted diffusion (arrow) on DWI (**b**), which was confirmed by the low signal (arrow) on the ADC map (**c**). Coronal T1 weighted with a gadolinium injection (**d**) shows enhancement of the right prechiasmatic optic nerve (arrow) along with restricted diffusion (arrow) on DWI (**e**), which was confirmed by the low signal (arrow) on the ADC map (**f**). Axial T1 weighted with a gadolinium injection (**g**) shows enhancement of the right optic nerve along with restricted diffusion on DWI (**h**), which was confirmed by the low signal on the ADC map (**i**)

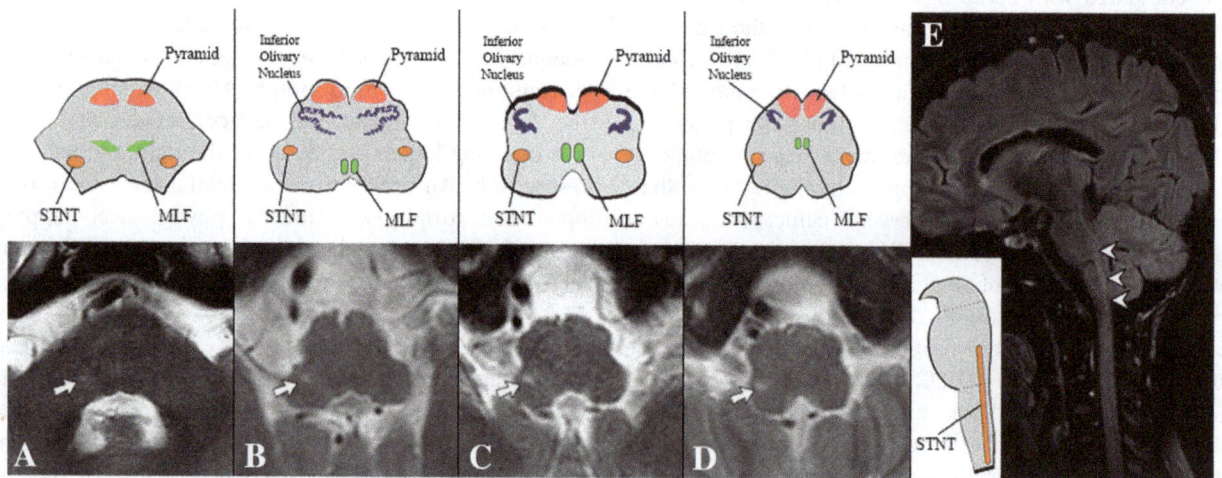

Fig. 3 Magnetic resonance imaging of the brain. Axial T2 weighted shows hyperintense T2 lesions (arrows) extending from right dorsolateral pons to the medulla (**a-d**). Sagittal fluid attenuation inversion recovery (FLAIR) shows linear, vertical-oriented hyperintense lesions (arrowheads) (**e**). These lesions represent the anatomical location of the spinal trigeminal nucleus and tract (STNT) along the brainstem. MLF, medial longitudinal fasciculus

HZO-related ON in many previous reports was found simultaneously with other ocular complications, such as anterior uveitis, keratitis, and secondary glaucoma. Moreover, it may occur as part of the orbital apex syndrome [4, 5]. Our case uniquely demonstrated an isolated HZO-related ON without any concomitant ocular complications, which has been rarely reported.

Despite the absence of VZV in the cerebrospinal fluid (CSF) using the PCR, a diagnosis of HZO-related ON was made based on the following:

(1) The concordance in laterality between the HZO and ON.
(2) Nasociliary nerve involvement of HZO based on the presence of hyperpigmented macules and patches over the tip of the nose, which was highly associated with the development of ocular complications [2].
(3) A temporal relationship between the HZO and ON.
(4) A high signal of STNT on the T2 weighted MRI.
(5) The exclusion of other possible causes of atypical ON.

The precise mechanism of ON following HZO is controversial. Viral replication in the ophthalmic branch of the trigeminal nerve, located in the cavernous sinus, spreads through the superior orbital fissure to the orbit, where it may cause direct injury to the optic nerve [14]. Extensive inflammation involving posterior ciliary arteries and nerves based on histopathology of HZO-affected eyes, which may lead to ocular ischemia and subsequent optic nerve damage, is another possible mechanism [15]. Parainfectious ON, as a consequence of a self-immune response triggered by the VZV antigen, has also been postulated [16]. These proposed mechanisms are usually difficult to differentiate from each other.

MRI findings of the optic nerve in HZO-related ON have been rarely described. Peripheral enhancement of the intraorbital optic nerve sheath has been commonly reported [4, 5, 12]. In our case, not only the optic nerve sheath, but also the axial portion of the optic nerve itself was affected. Moreover, the enhancement extended to the intracanalicular and prechiasmatic optic nerve. These results are consistent with the results of Wang et al., suggesting that these findings explained the severe visual impairment of ON and poor visual outcome in our case [12]. To our knowledge, DWI findings of the optic nerve have never been reported in HZO-related ON. However, restriction of the optic nerve on DWI, which is consistent with infarction attributed to compression or inflammation of the vessels serving the optic nerve, are rarely present in ON [17, 18]. Our case demonstrated a very long restricted diffusion of the optic nerve, including the entire intraorbital segment extending to the prechiasmatic segment. This may be a predictor for poor visual recovery in our case.

We found an unusually high signal of STNT on the T2 weighted MRI. This is thought be a result of VZV migration from the gasserian ganglion to the STNT along the brainstem [5, 19–21]. Douglas et al. reported contiguous hyperintense T2 lesions with restricted diffusion on DWI along the brainstem, which corresponded to the anatomical location of STNT in a VZV encephalitis patient [21]. Two months following complete anti-viral treatment, these lesions improved [21]. In our case, STNT failed to show any restriction on DWI. However, the restriction of the right-sided optic nerve observed in our case might be compatible with the restricted diffusion of the STNT reported by Douglas et al. [21].

Because the proposed mechanism of HZO-related ON is poorly understood and more than one mechanism can occur, it is reasonable to start the treatment with a combination of acyclovir and corticosteroids. In many previous reports, the duration of treatment varied, ranging from 10 days to 2 months [6–12]. We decided to continue the treatment up to 2 months because of the severe visual impairment of ON.

Visual recovery in ON following HZO is typically excellent [6–12]. Nevertheless, severe visual outcomes have also been reported [3]. Concomitant ocular complications, such as retinitis and secondary glaucoma may contribute to a poor visual prognosis. Based on the MRI with DWI of the optic nerve, we hypothesized that poor visual recovery in our case was due to the following:

(1) Both axial and optic nerve sheath portions were affected.
(2) A very long enhancement with restricted diffusion of the optic nerve occurred.

In summary, we report a case of isolated ON following HZO along with restricted diffusion of the optic nerve on imaging. In addition, an abnormal high signal of STNT on the T2 weighted image was found. This may be a clue of VZV-associated complications, such as HZO-related ON, especially in cases lacking an obvious history of HZO or other concomitant ocular complications. Prompt treatment with both acyclovir and corticosteroids should be started. Restricted diffusion of the optic nerve may therefore be a predictor for poor visual recovery.

Abbreviations
ANA: Antinuclear antibody; CBC: Complete blood count; CRP: C-reactive protein; CSF: Cerebrospinal fluid; DWI: Diffusion weighted imaging; ESR: Erythrocyte sedimentation rate; HZO: Herpes zoster ophthalmicus; MLF: Medial longitudinal fasciculus; MRI: Magnetic resonance imaging; ON: Optic neuritis; PCR: Polymerase chain reaction; RAPD: Relative afferent pupillary defect; STNT: Spinal trigeminal nucleus and tract; TPHA: *Treponema pallidum* hemagglutination; VDRL: Venereal Disease Research Laboratory; VZV: Varicella zoster virus

Acknowledgements

We thank Larry Takemoto, PhD, from Edanz Group (www.edanzediting.com/ac) for editing a draft of this manuscript.

Funding

None.

Authors' contributions

Substantial contributions to the conception (KV and TP) or design (KV and TP) of the work, or the acquisition (PC and TP), analysis (KV, AP, PJ, PC, PP, and TP) or interpretation (KV, PC, PP, and TP) of data. Drafting the work (KV) or revising it critically (KV). Final approval for submission (KV, AP, PJ, PC, PP, and TP).

Competing interests

The author declare that they have no competing interests.

Author details

[1]Department of Ophthalmology, Faculty of Medicine Ramathibodi Hospital, Mahidol University, 270 Rama VI Road, Bangkok 10400, Thailand.
[2]Department of Medicine, Faculty of Medicine Ramathibodi Hospital, Mahidol University, 270 Rama VI Road, Bangkok 10400, Thailand.
[3]Department of Radiology, Faculty of Medicine Ramathibodi Hospital, Mahidol University, 270 Rama VI Road, Bangkok 10400, Thailand.

References

1. Weller TH. Varicella and herpes zoster. Changing concepts of the natural history, control, and importance of a not-so-benign virus. N Engl J Med. 1983;309:1434–40.
2. Harding SP, Lipton JR, Wells JC. Natural history of herpes zoster ophthalmicus: predictors of postherpetic neuralgia and ocular involvement. Br J Ophthalmol. 1987;71:353–8.
3. Kahloun R, Attia S, Jelliti B, Attia AZ, Khochtali S, Yahia SB, Zaouali S, Khairallah M. Ocular involvement and visual outcome of herpes zoster ophthalmicus: review of 45 patients from Tunisia, North Africa. J Ophthalmic Inflamm Infect. 2014;4:25.
4. Lee CY, Tsai HC, Lee SS, Chen YS. Orbital apex syndrome: an unusual complication of herpes zoster ophthalmicus. BMC Infect Dis. 2015;15:33.
5. Paraskevas GP, Anagnostou E, Vassilopoulou S, Spengos K. Painful ophthalmoplegia with simultaneous orbital myositis, optic and oculomotor nerve inflammation and trigeminal nucleus involvement in a patient with herpes zoster ophthalmicus. BMJ Case Rep. 2012. https://doi.org/10.1136/bcr-2012-007063.
6. Deane JS, Bibby K. Bilateral optic neuritis following herpes zoster ophthalmicus. Arch Ophthalmol. 1995;113:972–3.
7. de Mello Vitor B, Foureaux EC, Porto FB. Herpes zoster optic neuritis. Int Ophthalmol. 2011;31:233–6.
8. Yalcinbayir O, Gelisken O, Yilmaz E. Unilateral optic neuritis in a case of herpes zoster ophthalmicus. Neuroophthalmology. 2009;33:339–42.
9. Hong SM, Yang YS. A case of optic neuritis complicating herpes zoster ophthalmicus in a child. Korean J Ophthalmol. 2010;24:126–30.
10. Freitas-Neto CA, Cerón O, Pacheco KD, Pereira VO, Ávila MP, Foster CS. Optic neuritis complicating herpes zoster ophthalmicus in an immunocompetent patient. Rev Bras Oftalmol. 2014;73:386–8.
11. Singh P, Karmacharya S, Rizyal A, Rijal AP. Herpes zoster ophthalmicus with retrobulbar neuritis. Nepal J Ophthalmol. 2016;8:78–81.
12. Wang AG, Liu JH, Hsu WM, Lee AF, Yen MY. Optic neuritis in herpes zoster ophthalmicus. Jpn J Ophthalmol. 2000;44:550–4.
13. Monroe LD. Optic neuritis in a child with herpes zoster. Ann Ophthalmol. 1979;11:405.
14. Gündüz K, Özdemir Ö. Bilateral retrobulbar neuritis following unilateral herpes zoster ophthalmicus. Ophthalmologica. 1994;208:61–4.
15. Naumann G, Donald J, Gass M, Font RL. Histopathology of herpes zoster ophthalmicus. Am J Ophthalmol. 1968;65:533–41.
16. Pless ML, Malik SI. Relapsing-remitting, corticosteroid-sensitive, varicella zoster virus optic neuritis. Pediatr Neurol. 2003;29:422–4.
17. Spierer O, Ben Sira L, Leibovitch I, Kesler A. MRI demonstrates restricted diffusion in distal optic nerve in atypical optic neuritis. J Neuroophthalmol. 2010;30:31–3.
18. Bender B, Heine C, Danz S, Bischof F, Reimann K, Bender M, Nägele T, Ernemann U, Korn A. Diffusion restriction of the optic nerve in patients with acute visual deficit. J Magn Reson Imaging. 2014;40:334–40.
19. Haanpää M, Dastidar P, Weinberg A, Levin M, Miettinen A, Lapinlampi A, Laippala P, Nurmikko T. CSF and MRI findings in patients with acute herpes zoster. Neurology. 1998;51:1405–11.
20. Siritho S, Pumpradit W, Suriyajakryuththana W, Pongpirul K. Severe headache with eye involvement from herpes zoster ophthalmicus, trigeminal tract, and brainstem nuclei. Case Rep Radiol. 2015. https://doi.org/10.1155/2015/402015.
21. Douglas JE, Buch VP, Mamourian AC. Varicella zoster-induced magnetic resonance imaging abnormalities of the trigeminal nucleus. J Neurol Sci. 2015;359:57–8.

27

ACUDIN – ACUpuncture and laser acupuncture for treatment of Diabetic peripheral Neuropathy

Gesa Meyer-Hamme[1], Thomas Friedemann[1], Henry Johannes Greten[2,3], Rosemarie Plaetke[4], Christian Gerloff[5] and Sven Schroeder[1*] [iD]

Abstract

Background: Diabetic peripheral neuropathy (DPN) is the most common complication of diabetes mellitus with significant clinical sequelae that can affect a patient's quality of life. Metabolic and microvascular factors are responsible for nerve damage, causing loss of nerve function, numbness, painful sensory symptoms, and muscle weakness. Therapy is limited to anti-convulsant or anti-depressant drugs for neuropathic pain and paresthesia. However, reduced sensation, balance and gait problems are insufficiently covered by this treatment. Previous data suggests that acupuncture, which has been in use in Traditional Chinese Medicine for many years, may potentially complement the treatment options for peripheral neuropathy. Nevertheless, more objective data on clinical outcome is necessary to generally recommend acupuncture to the public.

Methods: We developed a study design for a prospective, randomized (RCT), placebo-controlled, partially double-blinded trial for investigating the effect of acupuncture on DPN as determined by nerve conduction studies (NCS) with the sural sensory nerve action potential amplitude as the primary outcome. The sural sensory nerve conduction velocity, tibial motor nerve action potential amplitude, tibial motor nerve conduction velocity, the neuropathy deficit score, neuropathy symptom score, and numeric rating scale questionnaires are defined as secondary outcomes. One hundred and eighty patients with type 2 diabetes mellitus will be randomized into three groups (needle acupuncture, verum laser acupuncture, and placebo laser acupuncture). We hypothesize that needle and laser acupuncture have beneficial effects on electrophysiological parameters and clinical and subjective symptoms in relation to DPN in comparison with placebo.

Discussion: The ACUDIN trial aims at investigating whether classical needle acupuncture and/or laser acupuncture are efficacious in the treatment of DPN. For the purpose of an objective parameter, NCS were chosen as outcome measures. Acupuncture treatment may potentially improve patients' quality of life and reduce the socio-economic burden caused by DPN.

(Continued on next page)

* Correspondence: schroeder@tcm-am-uke.de
[1]HanseMerkur Center for Traditional Chinese Medicine at the University Medical Center Hamburg-Eppendorf, Martinistrasse 52, House O55, 20246 Hamburg, Germany
Full list of author information is available at the end of the article

(Continued from previous page)

Keywords: Diabetic peripheral neuropathy, Acupuncture, Laser acupuncture, Placebo-control, Randomized controlled trial, Nerve conduction studies, Neurography

Background

Diabetic peripheral neuropathy (DPN) is the most common complication of diabetes mellitus with significant clinical sequelae and impact on patients' quality of life [1, 2]. DPN manifests itself on the toes and progresses in a stocking distribution [3]. Nerve damage is related to hyperglycemia. However, various other mechanisms play a role in the pathogenesis of DPN [3]. These include elevated polyol pathway activity, advanced glycation end products (AGEs), oxidative stress, growth factors, impaired insulin/C-peptide action, and elevated protein kinase C activity. These may directly affect neuronal tissues as well as vascular structures, thus compromising nerve vascular supply [4, 5].

Clinical manifestations include paresthesia, burning sensations, and neuropathic pain as well as negative symptoms like hypesthesia, hypalgesia, and pallhypesthesia. These may contribute to balance problems and unsteady gait, leading to falls [6] and an increased risk of bone fractures and hospitalization [7]. Motor symptoms, for example muscle spasm and weakness occur less frequently [3]. DPN is associated with an increased risk of ulceration and amputation of the lower extremities as well as increased healthcare costs [8–10]. Nerve damage can occur on the myelin sheath as well as at the axonal level [11]. Differentiation is achieved by nerve conduction studies (NCS) [12]. Whilst neuropathic pain and paresthesia can be palliated by anti-convulsants, tricyclic antidepressant drugs or serotonin-noradrenalin re-uptake inhibitors [13], pharmacologic management of decreased sensation is generally ineffective, thus forming a gap in treatment strategies.

During the last decades, acupuncture has become an empirical complementary treatment option for DPN. It is recommended by the World Health Organisation [14] and the National Institute of Health [15] but treatment effectiveness is still under debate. Reviews concerning acupuncture for peripheral neuropathy (PN) have found that, despite the majority of studies reporting positive results, a reliable statement of effectiveness is not possible due to methodological limitations [16–22]. Randomized controlled, blinded clinical trials of adequate statistical power and design are still pending.

Whilst acupuncture concepts using proximal or systemic acupuncture points on upper and lower extremities failed to show efficacy [23], our pilot studies using the selection of local and distal points described here showed promising results for the treatment of DPN, chemotherapy-induced PN and PN of unknown cause(s). These studies have verified the improvement that can be found in subjective scales by means of NCS parameters [24–27]. Acupuncture has been shown to increase blood perfusion towards the periphery of the limbs following needle insertion [28]. The results of our pilot studies were potentially related to the acupuncture effect on the blood flow through vasa nervorum and dependent capillary beds supplying the neurons [26]. These findings are encouraging for setting up the framework of a clinical study of adequate sample size using strict methodological standards.

Definition of adequate controls for acupuncture

The development of appropriate designs for clinical acupuncture trials remains a methodological challenge. A major problem is the definition of placebo controls and blinding procedures, as the insertion of acupuncture needles is usually perceptible and visible.

Double-blinding of needle acupuncture has been achieved for immediate effects using invasive sham acupuncture concepts as control [29, 30]. However, this approach is problematic for long-term trials because of a possible overlap of specific as well as unspecific physiological and placebo effects. Sham acupuncture, at irrelevant or non-acupuncture points, was found to promote physiological stimuli due to an unspecific endorphin release in a range of 33–50%, exceeding the effect of a suggestive placebo therapy [31]. Hence, treatment with invasive sham acupuncture is not an inert placebo but an active treatment of unknown activity [32].

Accordingly, no reliable blinding methodology for needle acupuncture has been achieved so far for time spans of 10 weeks' intervention. Differences in verum and placebo treatment patterns could not be accurately masked from the practitioner over time, creating the risk of bias [33].

Even shallow needling showed both specific and unspecific effects [34–36], evoking physiological responses similar to classical needle acupuncture and distorting the results [37].

To overcome these obstacles we include Laserneedle® acupuncture with multichannel red laser light into the ACUDIN study design. Laser needles are not inserted into the skin but merely placed on the surface of the acupuncture points; however, the therapeutic effects are of a similar dimension to those evoked by manual needle acupuncture [38]. The initial effect of laser acupuncture is mediated by the impact of ATP release from cutaneous mast cells [39, 40], which is considered comparable to the mechanical effect of needle acupuncture [41, 42]. Patients do not feel the activation of the laser needles as the radiation intensity is optimized for this purpose [43] and they cannot distinguish between verum and placebo laser [44]. Laser acupuncture is considered an appropriate means of control for acupuncture trials for evaluating the effect of needling per se [44].

Methods/design

Trial design

The aim of the ACUDIN trial is to examine if acupuncture and laser acupuncture have beneficial effects on NCS parameters, clinical scores and patient's complaints in DPN as evaluated by standardized tests. A prospective, randomized, placebo-controlled, partially double-blinded, three-armed study design has been applied to the ACUDIN trial to compare the effects of classical needle acupuncture and laser acupuncture with those of placebo laser acupuncture.

Patients will receive 10 treatments over a period of 10 weeks. Each session will last 20 min. Neurological assessment, including NCS, is performed at baseline, week 6 and week 15 (Fig. 1).

Trial personnel

A total of four persons are involved in the ACUDIN trial procedure. The treatment is performed by the following health professionals: (i) experienced practitioners who are members of a German Physicians Society for Acupuncture. They have completed a standardized training course, undertaken formal accreditation by examination and a period of supervised medical experience required for administering the acupuncture interventions and were trained by Laserneedle® specialists for the implementation of multichannel laser acupuncture; (ii) two study nurses are involved in the treatment procedure as described below; and (iii) experienced neurologists, not involved in further study procedures, perform neurological assessments including NCS.

Study population

A total of 180 patients with DPN due to diabetes mellitus type 2 will be recruited from regional medical clinics, via the homepage of the operating institute, media reports, and advertisements.

Inclusion criteria

Participants who meet the following conditions will be included:

- Male or female aged > 18 years
- Confirmed diagnosis of diabetes mellitus type 2 (i.e., $HbA_{1c} \geq c6{,}5\%$ (48 mmol/mol)

[45] and/or on diabetes medication for more than 1 year)

- Stable levels of HbA_{1c} during the last 6 months (i.e., deviation < 1% (11 mmol/mol))
- Clinically confirmed diagnosis of DPN
- Pathologic results in NCS (i.e., sural SNAP < 10 µV, sural NLG < 42 m/s, tibial MNAP < 8 mV, tibial MNLG < 40 m/s) [46]
- Naive to laser acupuncture
- No prior acupuncture treatment for peripheral neuropathy

Exclusion criteria

Participants who present one or more of the following conditions are excluded:

- PN caused by conditions other than diabetes (e.g., alcohol abuse, chemotherapy, hereditary causes, chronic inflammatory or idiopathic PN, and others)
- History of epilepsy
- Coagulopathy or use of anticoagulants with bleeding time > 3 min, prothrombin time < 40%, platelet count < 50.000/µl, or PTT > 50 s
- Bacterial infection or other skin diseases at the lower extremities that impede acupuncture treatment
- Bone fracture of the lower extremities during the last 3 months
- Use of acupuncture during the last 3 months
- Opiate, analgesic, or drug abuse
- Psychiatric illnesses other than mild depression
- Incapacity in giving informed consent or in following the study instructions due to language disturbances, serious cognitive deficits, or lack of time
- Pregnant or breast-feeding women
- Current participation in other clinical studies

Randomization procedure

Recruited patients are randomized in a ratio of 1: 1: 1 into three parallel treatment groups of 60 participants: (i) classical needle acupuncture, (ii) verum laser acupuncture, and (iii) placebo laser acupuncture. Randomization is prepared beforehand with 180 identical closed envelopes, each.

containing one of the three possible group allocations and a randomly generated four-number pseudonym code for further data processing. Randomization is performed by envelope lottery immediately prior to the first treatment session by study nurse 1. Patients and practitioners are only informed about the patients' allocation to either

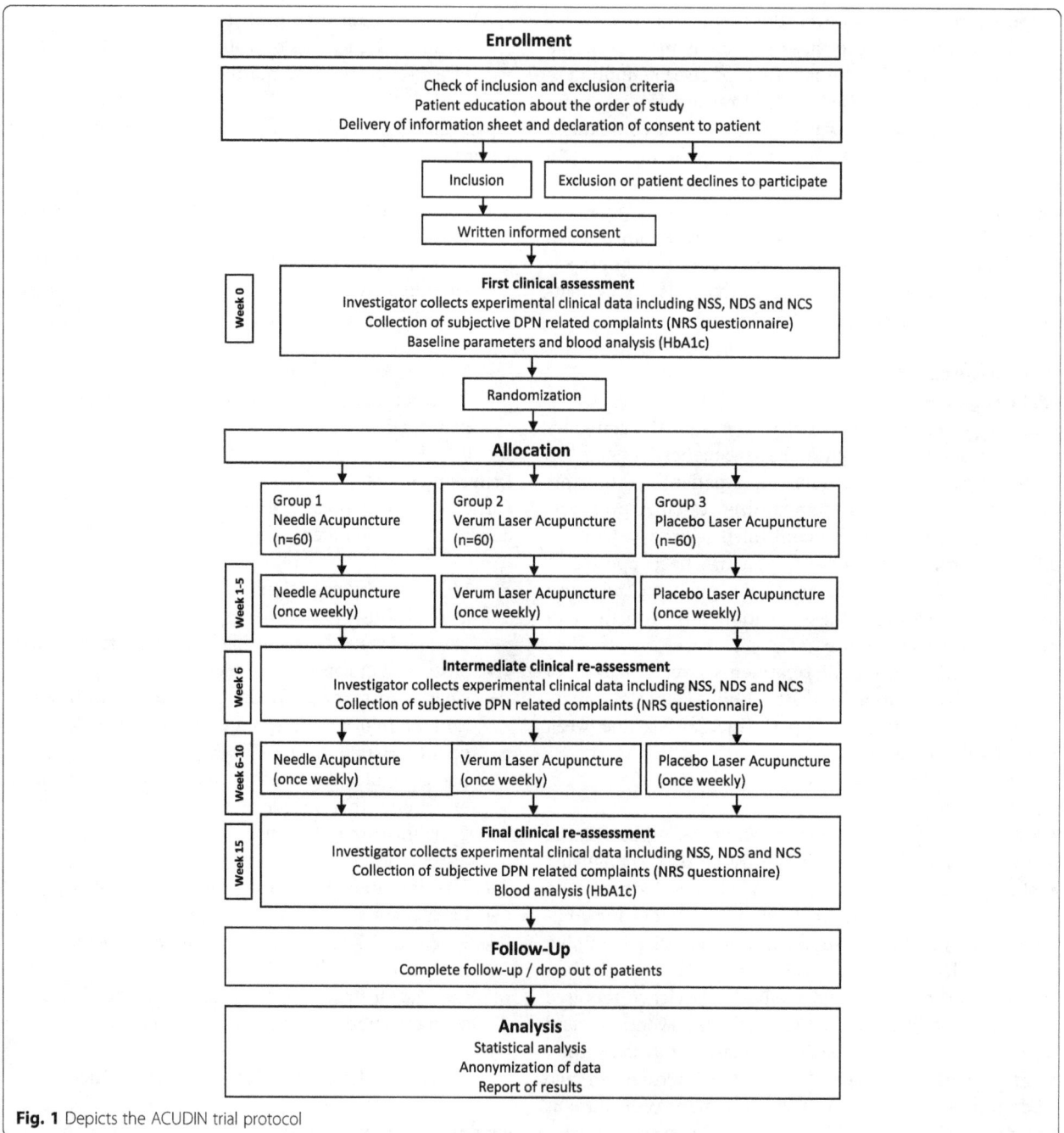

Fig. 1 Depicts the ACUDIN trial protocol

needle or laser treatment. However, patients do not know whether they will receive a true treatment or placebo. Group assignment will not be exposed until the final data analysis report is completed.

Blinding

A single-blind design is performed for needle acupuncture because of the difficulties of practitioner blinding for the needling procedure as specified above. A double-blind design is performed for laser acupuncture.

Caregiver blinding for laser acupuncture is achieved by dividing the treatment into three steps.

i. practitioner fixes the laser needles without activating them;
ii. study nurse 1 operates the laser device according to the randomization (verum or placebo);
iii. study nurse 2 removes the laser needles after treatment.

Practitioners and study nurses do not communicate concerning the patients' group allocation. Further, the investigator performing the neurological assessment and NCS does not know about the type of treatment given to the patient.

Regarding patients and the blinding procedure: the laser device is placed behind a folding screen so patients cannot see it. Patients wear laser protective glasses which make it impossible to perceive the laser light. They are informed that the laser device would emit visible and/or invisible laser beams and that the protection of the eyes is fundamental in any case because of the safety precautions as required by law. The laser needles are covered with a blanket. Acoustic functions of the laser device are deactivated prior to the study, so there is no difference between verum and placebo activation. This protocol will not be published in advance so patients cannot draw any conclusions concerning treatment allocations. Study participation is allowed only once.

For data transfer and processing, pseudonym codes are used in order to mask patient identity and treatment groups from outcome assessors and statisticians. The data is only matched after completion of statistical analysis.

ACUDIN acupuncture protocol

A total of 20 acupuncture points have been selected for the ACUDIN trial. All treatment sessions of needle and laser acupuncture are performed using the following point combination:

The 4 Bafeng points on both feet (Ex-LE-10) [47]. Needles are inserted to a depth of 3 to 5 mm and left in place without stimulation for 20 min. Laser needles are fixed with perforated plaster.

The 5 Qiduan points on both feet (Ex-LE-12) [47]. Needles are inserted to a depth of 1,5 to 2 mm and left in place without stimulation for 20 min. Laser needles are fixed with perforated plaster (Fig. 2).

The point Lianqiu on both legs (ST-34) [47]. Needles are inserted to a depth of 0,5 to 2.5 cm (depending on the diameter of the thigh) and left in place without stimulation for 20 min. Laser needles are fixed with perforated plaster.

Sterile single-use stainless steel needles size $0,2 \times 15$ mm are used for Qiduan and Bafeng points, respectively $0,3 \times 30$ mm for Lianqiu, both manufactured by Wujiang City Cloud & Dragon Medical Devise Co. Ltd, China.

Laser acupuncture device

Laser acupuncture is performed with Laserneedle® device (European patent PCT/DE 102006008774.7), a multichannel class 3B system which allows the simultaneous stimulation of individual point combinations through semiconductor laser diodes. Flexible optical

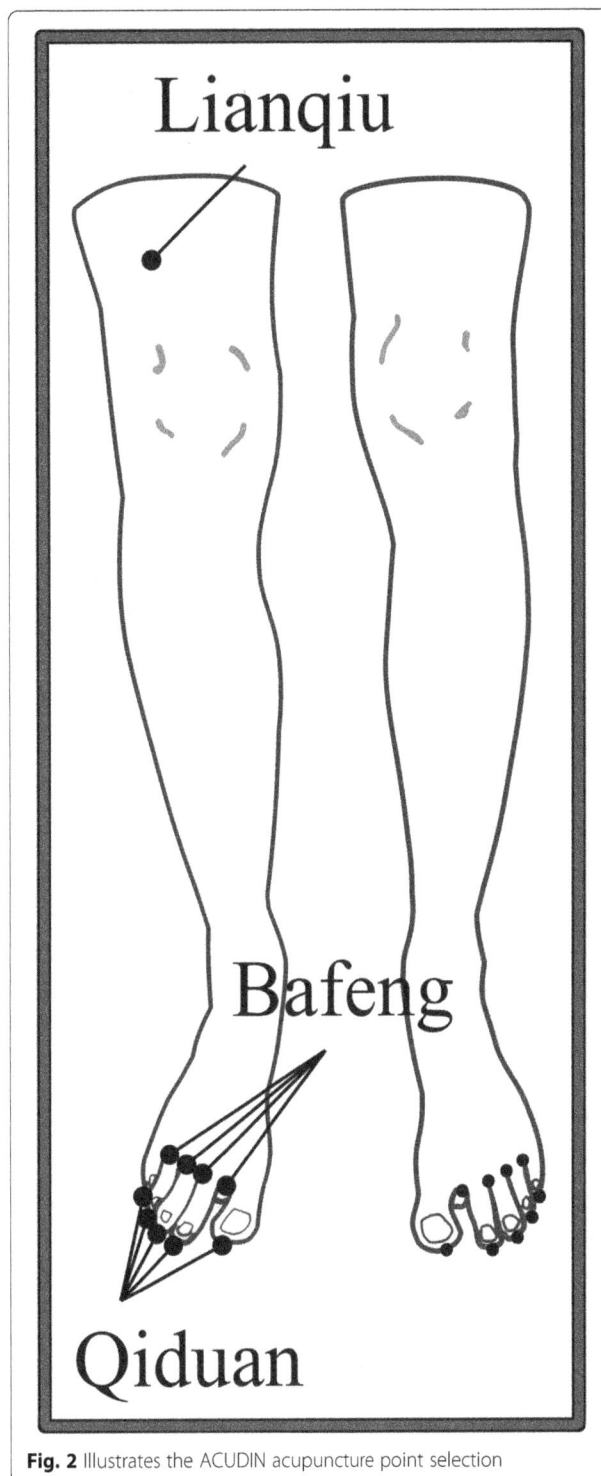

Fig. 2 Illustrates the ACUDIN acupuncture point selection

light fibers conduct the laser light without loss, providing a high optical density at the distal end [40]. Wavelengths of 685 nm (red light) are emitted in continuous mode. Each channel has an optical power of 35 mW. Power density is 2.3 kJ/cm^2 per channel. The beam diameter is 500 µm and beam divergence at the end of the laser needle is 9.5. Laser needles are placed at an angle of 90° directly on the skin, thus radiation reflection is minimized [43]. Laser needles are plugged in silicon adapters which are fixed with perforated plaster to the skin, so they stay in place without requiring the practitioner to stay with the patient. Temperature monitoring is not required because of extremely low heat development due to the weak absorption coefficient at 685 nm [48]. Previous investigations revealed no unintended side-effects of Laserneedle® treatment [40, 48]. The use of laser protection glasses is obligatory for both study nurse and patient. Two Laserneedle® machines with 10 laser needles each are used for the ACUDIN trial.

Procedures
Verum needle acupuncture
The treatment is applied according to the protocol with the patient in the supine position. The practitioner inserts the acupuncture needles after local disinfection of the skin. Needles are left in place for 20 min. They are carefully removed and disposed into a bedside sharps container at the completion of treatment by study nurse 2.

Verum laser acupuncture
The treatment is applied according to the protocol with the patient in supine position. The practitioner fixes the laser needles with perforated plaster after local disinfection of the skin. The patient's legs and feet are covered and he/she wears laser protection glasses. The practitioner then leaves the room. Study nurse 1 enters the room and activates the laser emission by pressing at the soundless touch screen of the laser device according to the randomization schedule. Laser emission stops automatically after 20 min. Laser needles are removed and cleaned after use by study nurse 2.

Placebo laser acupuncture
Placebo laser acupuncture is performed as described for verum laser acupuncture with slight modifications. Study nurse 1 provides the same steps as for the verum treatment but without activating the laser, pressing an invalid point at the soundless touch screen of the laser device. Therefore, from the patient's perspective, the procedure is identical to that used in the verum laser group.

Nerve conduction studies
The ACUDIN trial outcome measures are based on NCS parameters that are both objective and reproducible. These measures also provide quantitative data according to the Guideline for Diabetic Neuropathy [49, 50]. NCS are performed on both legs with a Neuropack-Sigma, MEB-9400, EMG/NCV/EP-System (Nihon-Khoden, Japan). Sural SNAP and tibial MNAP are measured on the first negative peak. All studies on NCS are done at room temperature (23 ± 1 °C). Sural NCS are done with standard orthodromic needle recording methods [51]. Tibial NCS are done with standard orthodromic surface electrode recording methods [51]. Skin temperatures are measured, and values of NCV are adjusted for the effect of temperature.

Clinical examination
Clinical examinations include sensory qualities such as the perception of pain and temperature, pallesthesia and two-point discrimination, patellar and Achilles reflexes, and gait qualities. The neuropathy deficit score (NDS) [52] and the neuropathy symptom score (NSS) [52] are part of the clinical assessment. Both are validated instruments for diagnosis and progress of DPN according to the Guideline for Diabetic Neuropathy [49].

Questionnaires to collect participants' opinions
Common DPN-related symptoms will be recorded weekly by questionnaires using 11-point numeric rating scales (NRS) with the terminal descriptors "no complaint" and "worst complaint possible". Whilst NRS are well validated for painful conditions [53], our questionnaires assess not only neuropathic pain but also tingling, burning pain, feeling of heat, feeling of cold, cramps, numbness, gait impairment, impairment of daily activities, sleep disturbances, and complaint frequency.

Table 1 summarizes the plan of data collection.

Outcome measures
Primary endpoint
The primary endpoint is the difference of the 15-week measurement minus baseline of the sural sensory nerve action potential amplitude (sural SNAP).

Key secondary endpoints
Secondary endpoints are the differences of the 15-week measurement minus baseline of the remaining NCS measurements:

the sural sensory nerve conduction velocity (sural SNCV),

tibial motor nerve action potential amplitude (tibial MNAP),

tibial motor nerve conduction velocity (tibial MNCV).

Additional secondary endpoints will be obtained from the questionnaires:

The differences in the 15-week measurement minus baseline of NDS, NSS, and NRS scores.

Statistical analysis
Major hypotheses tested are:

H0:

The differences of the 15-week measurements minus baseline of sural SNAP in the two groups with classical

Table 1 Baseline and outcome parameters

	Baseline parameter	Blood parameter	Neurological assessment	NCS[f] Parameter	Subjective Score
Week 0	Age Gender Weight Size Comorbidity Medication Duration of disease (Diabetes and DPN)	HbA$_{1c}$[a]	Clinical examination NSS NDS[c]	Bilateral amplitudes and NCV[b] of nn. surales and tibiales	NRS[d]
Week 6			Clinical examination NSS[e] NDS	Bilateral amplitudes and NCV of nn. surales and tibiales	NRS
Week 15	Change of medication	HbA$_{1c}$	Clinical examination NSS NDS	Bilateral amplitudes and NCV of nn. surales and tibiales	NRS Adverse events
Weekly (treatment 1–10)	Change of medication				NRS Adverse events

[a]HbA1c= glycated hemoglobin; [b]NCV = nerve conduction velocity; [c]NDS = neuropathy deficit score; [d]NRS = numeric rating scale; [e]NSS = neuropathy symptom score; [f]NCS = nerve conduction studies

needle acupuncture or laser acupuncture are the same or smaller as in the control group.

vs.

H1:

The differences of the 15-week measurement minus baseline of sural SNAP in the groups with classical needle acupuncture or laser acupuncture are larger than in the control group.

In addition, for the two types of acupuncture treatment, two-sided hypotheses will be tested.

Data analysis

Hypotheses will be tested by using one-way analysis of variance (ANOVA), followed by Tukey post-hoc tests comparing the three groups pairwise.

A reasonable approximation to a normal distribution, according to the central limit theorem, can be assumed with the calculated sample size, allowing the use of parametric analysis. Deviations of the normal distribution will be tested and appropriate transformations will be performed. Homogeneity of variance will be tested with the Levene's test.

The primary analysis will be performed with the intent-to-treat (ITT) population. Missing data will be imputed by the next-observation-carried-backwards option for initial values and last-observation-carried-forwards option for closing values. Legs with missing initial and closing data for the primary endpoint will be deleted from the analysis. The average values of both legs will be evaluated for patients with bilateral assessable measurements. For unilateral results, only the evaluable leg will be included in the analysis. The comparison between verum needle acupuncture and placebo laser acupuncture will be undertaken for validating the overall treatment effect of acupuncture. Verum laser acupuncture and placebo laser acupuncture will be compared for validating the specific treatment effect. The comparison of

needle acupuncture to verum laser acupuncture will indicate the non-specific effect of needle acupuncture. Remaining NCS outcomes will be analyzed as described for the primary outcome. Multivariate analyses of the clinical secondary outcomes (NDS, NSS, and NRS) and their correlation to NCS parameters will be performed by linear regression models.

Baseline data and clinical characteristics will be presented as mean values to assess the baseline comparability of the intervention groups. Those patients who report changes of pain medication during the study will be excluded from data analysis relating to subjective pain scales. Statistical analysis will be done with the software SPSS (IBM SPSS Statistics 22) and OriginPro 9.

Sample size calculation

An average difference of 1 µV was considered functionally relevant for sural SNAP [54]. On the basis of a pilot study [24], a pooled standard deviation of 1.83 µV was calculated. By assuming that this standard deviation represents the best estimate of the actual standard deviation for each of the three groups in a regular three-arm parallel RCT design with complete follow-up, 54 patients per arm are required to detect the above difference for sural SNAP with an alpha of 0.05 and a power of 0.8. The assumption of a conservative 10% drop-out rate for patients randomized to any of the three arms increases the sample size to 60 patient per arm or 180 patients in total.

Power evaluations were performed with statistical analysis system (SAS) 9.2 for the above described statistical analysis (one-way ANOVA) and followed by post-hoc testing for the primary outcome.

Adverse events

Any adverse event and unexpected and unintended responses to the treatment reported by the patients are recorded weekly with the NRS questionnaire. A causal relationship between treatment and adverse events will be evaluated using a six-grade-scale with the terminal descriptors 1 = definitely related and 6 = unknown. Possible adverse events related to acupuncture are hematoma, pain, nerve irritation, infection, and tiredness. An accidental irradiation of the eyes is regarded as the only relevant adverse event related to Laserneedle® treatment [40].

Timelines

Recruitment started in August 2011. Data collection started in January 2012. The ACUDIN trial is due to finish in 2017.

Discussion

DPN is a common complication of diabetes mellitus [1, 2]. Conventional medicine offers symptomatic pharmaceutical treatment for DPN masking neuropathic pain and paresthesia [13]. Unfortunately, these treatments are not always effective [3] and patients have to cope with medication side-effects [55]. Furthermore, there is no treatment for sensory loss, unsteadiness, and gait-impairment, causing a gap in medical care for diabetic patients and giving reason for extending the range of treatment options.

Acupuncture has been in use for decades for the treatment of DPN and positive results have been reported on the basis of empirical knowledge and a number of pilot studies [16–22]. However, the effectiveness of acupuncture is still under debate because of the lack of high-quality clinical research.

The peripheral nervous system has the ability of regeneration in relation to repair mechanisms and in the phenomena of spreading and sprouting [56]. In DPN, morphologic peripheral nerve regeneration is impaired and inadequate nerve regeneration contributes to the pathophysiologic mechanism of DPN [57]. However, the findings of our pilot study mention a possible improvement of NCS parameters following acupuncture treatment in DPN, indicating a certain amount of neural repair [25, 26]. Parallel to improved NCS, patients have experienced subjective improvement after acupuncture treatment compared to no specific treatment, but experienced the best medical care where positive and negative DPN-related symptoms were concerned [25]. The acupuncture protocol of the pilot studies using distal and local points on the lower extremities is taken as the basis for the ACUDIN study design because other concepts failed to show efficacy [23].

This paper presents the protocol for the prospective, randomized, placebo-controlled, partially double-blinded, three-armed clinical ACUDIN trial for testing the hypothesis that classical needle acupuncture and laser acupuncture improve objective NCS parameters, as well as clinical and subjective symptoms in DPN compared to placebo treatment. NCS has rarely been used as an objective parameter in acupuncture research [24–26, 58–62]. The ACUDIN trial is the first study using NCS as an evaluation method of acupuncture treatment of DPN of the lower extremities in the form of a randomized, partially double-blinded design type.

DPN may have a strong negative impact on patients' quality of life [13]. However, healthcare systems can encompass increased use of resources and costs which may escalate according to the severity of the disease [8–10]. Acupuncture treatment can offer a cost-effective treatment option in comparison with conventional medicine [63, 64].

The findings of the ACUDIN trial may establish the value of complementary acupuncture treatment for the potential improvement of peripheral nerve function and clinical symptoms; in addition, the findings may also lead to a reduction of the socio-economic burdens caused by DPN.

Abbreviations

ACUDIN: ACUpuncture and Laser Acupuncture for treatment of Diabetic peripheral Neuropathy; ANOVA: Analysis of Variance; DPN: Diabetic Peripheral Neuropathy; HbA$_{1c}$: Glycated Hemoglobin; HMC: HanseMerkur Center for Traditional Chinese Medicine at the University Medical Center Hamburg-Eppendorf, Germany; MNAP: Motor Nerve Action Potential; MNCV: Motor Nerve Conduction Velocity; NCS: Nerve Conduction Study; NCV: Nerve Conduction Velocity; NDS: Neuropathy DeficitScore; NRS: Numeric Rating Scale; NSS: Neuropathy Symptom Score; PN: Peripheral Neuropathy; RCT: Randomized Controlled Trial; SNAP: Sensory Nerve Action Potential; SNCV: Sensory Nerve Conduction Velocity; UKE: University Medical Center Hamburg-Eppendorf; WHO: World Health Organisation

Acknowledgments

Sarah Mirza for Fig. 2.

Funding

The ACUDIN trial is supported by the HanseMerkur Insurance Group and the Innovation Foundation, Hamburg (721.230–002) during the clinical phase. The Laserneedle GmbH (16548 Glienicke/Nordbahn) provides the laser device for the duration of the trial.

Author's contributions

SVS had the original idea for the ACUDIN trial. SVS and CG are responsible for the study design, definition of primary and secondary outcomes and preparation of the protocol. TF and RP are responsible for sample size calculation. SVS and HJG contributed to the determination of acupuncture point selection. GMH prepared the primary version of the manuscript. All authors have critically reviewed and approved the final version of the manuscript.

Authors' information

GMH is a medical doctor employed at the HMC. TF is a doctor of biology employed at the HMC. HJG is a general practitioner, head of the Heidelberg School of TCM and professor at the University of Porto. R. Plaetke is a scientist for biostatistics at the UKE. CG is the director of the department of Neurology at the UKE and vice-director of the UKE. SVS is a neurologist and director of the HMC.

Competing interests

The authors declare that they have no competing interests.

Author details

[1]HanseMerkur Center for Traditional Chinese Medicine at the University Medical Center Hamburg-Eppendorf, Martinistrasse 52, House O55, 20246 Hamburg, Germany. [2]Heidelberg School of Chinese Medicine, Karlsruher Str. 12, 69126 Heidelberg, Germany. [3]Department of Neurophysiology, Instituto di Ciencias Biomedicas Abel Salazar, University of Porto, Rua de Jorge Viterbo Ferreira n. 228, 4050, –313 Porto, Portugal. [4]Department of Medical Biometry and Epidemiology, University Medical Center Hamburg-Eppendorf, Martinistrasse 52, 20246 Hamburg, Germany. [5]Department of Neurology, University Medical Center Hamburg-Eppendorf, Martinistrasse 52, 20246 Hamburg, Germany.

References

1. Papanas N, Ziegler D. Risk Factors and Comorbidities in Diabetic Neuropathy: An Update 2015. Rev Diabet Stud. 2015 Spring-Summer;12(1–2):48–62. doi: https://doi.org/10.1900/RDS.2015.12.48. Epub 2015 Aug 10.
2. Barrett AM, Lucero MA, Le T, Robinson RL, Dworkin RH, Chappell AS. Epidemiology, public health burden, and treatment of diabetic peripheral neuropathic pain: a review. Pain Med. 2007 Sep;8(Suppl 2):S50–62.
3. Boulton ALM, Malik RA, Arezzo JC, Sosenko JM. Diabetic somatic neuropathies. Diabetes Care. 2004;27(6):1458–86.
4. Sytze Van Dam P, Cotter MA, Bravenboer B, Cameron NE. Pathogenesis of diabetic neuropathy: focus on neurovascular mechanisms. Eur J Pharmacol. 2013;719(1–3):180–6. https://doi.org/10.1016/j.ejphar.2013.07.017. Epub 2013 Jul 17
5. Cameron NE, Eaton SE, Cotter MA, Tesfaye S. Vascular factors and metabolic interactions in the pathogenesis of diabetic neuropathy. Diabetologia November. 2001;44(11):1973–88.
6. Callaghan BC, Price RS, Feldman EL. Distal symmetric polyneuropathy: a review. JAMA. 2015;314(20):2172–81. https://doi.org/10.1001/jama.2015.13611.
7. Moseley KF. Type 2 diabetes and bone fractures. Curr Opin Endocrinol Diabetes Obes. 2012;19(2):128–35. https://doi.org/10.1097/MED.0b013e328350a6e1.
8. Happich M, John J, Stamenitis S, Clouth J, Polnau D. The quality of life and economic burden of neuropathy in diabetic patients in Germany in 2002–results from the diabetic microvascular complications (DIMICO) study. Diabetes Res Clin Pract. 2008;81(2):223–30. https://doi.org/10.1016/j.diabres.2008.03.019. Epub 2008 Jul 7
9. Alleman CJ, Westerhout KY, Hensen M, Chambers C, Stoker M, Long S, van Nooten FE. Humanistic and economic burden of painful diabetic peripheral neuropathy in Europe: a review of the literature. Diabetes Res Clin Pract. 2015;109(2):215–25. https://doi.org/10.1016/j.diabres.2015.04.031. Epub 2015 May 6
10. Gordois A, Scuffham P, Shearer A, Oglesby A, Tobian JA. The health care costs of diabetic peripheral neuropathy in the U.S. Diabetes Care June. 2003;26(6):1790–5.
11. Bosch EP, Mitsumoto H. Disorders in peripheral nerves. In: Bradley WG, Daroff RB, Fenichel GM, Marsden CD, editors. Neurology in clinical practice. Boston: Butterworth-Heinemann; 1991. p. 1720–6.
12. McLeod JG. Investigation of peripheral neuropathy. J Neurol Neurosurg Psychiatry. 1995;58:274–83.
13. Ziegler D, Fonseca V. From guideline to patient: a review of recent recommendations for pharmacotherapy of painful diabetic neuropathy. J Diabetes Complications. 2015 Jan-Feb; 29(1): 146–156. Published online 2014 August 28. doi: https://doi.org/10.1016/j.jdiacomp.2014.08.008 Epub 2014 Aug 28.
14. World Health Organization. Viewpoint on Acupuncture. Geneva, Switzerland, 1979.
15. National Institutes of Health. Acupuncture. NIH Consensus Statement Online 1997 Nov 3–5; 15(5):1–34.
16. Franco LC, Souza LAF, Da Costa Pessoa AP, Pereira LV. Nonpharmacologic therapies in diabetic neuropathic pain: a review. Acta Paulista de Enfermagem. 2011;24(2):284–8.
17. Bo C, Xue Z, Yi G, Zelin C, Yang B, Zixu W, Yajun W. Assessing the quality of reports about randomized controlled trials of acupuncture treatment on diabetic peripheral neuropathy. PLoS One. 7(7):e38461. https://doi.org/10.1371/journal.pone.0038461. Epub 2012 Jul 2
18. Kowalczuk SA. Is Acupuncture An Effective Treatment For Diabetic Peripheral Neuropathy? (2012). PCOM Physician Assistant Studies Student Scholarship. Paper 74. Philadelphia College of Osteopathic Medicine, Philadelphia, Pennsylvania, USA.
19. Meyer-Hamme G, Friedemann T, Xu LW, Epplée S, Schroeder S. Structured literature review of acupuncture treatment for peripheral neuropathy. J Acupunct Tuina Science. 2012;10(4):235–42. https://doi.org/10.1155/2013/516916
20. Chen W, Yang GY, Liu B, Manheimer E, Liu JP. Manual acupuncture for treatment of diabetic peripheral neuropathy: a systematic review of randomized controlled trials. PLoS One. 2013;8(9):e73764. https://doi.org/10.1371/journal.pone.0073764. eCollection 2013
21. Franconi G, Manni L, Schröder S, Marcetti P, Robinson N. A Systematic Review of Experimental and Clinical Acupuncture in Chemotherapy-Induced Peripheral Neuropathy. Evidence-Based Complementary and Alternative Medicine, Volume 2013, Article ID 516916. doi: https://doi.org/10.1155/2013/516916. Epub 2013 Jul 24.
22. Dimitrova A, Murchison C, Oken B. Effects of Acupuncture on Neuropathic Pain: A Systematic Review and Meta-analysis (P3.306) Neurology , 2015 vol. 84 no. 14 Supplement P3.306. doi:https://doi.org/10.1089/acu.2016.29023.cpl.
23. Rostock M, Jaroslawski K, Guethlin C, Ludtke R, Schröder S, Bartsch HH. Chemotherapy-induced peripheral neuropathy in cancer patients – A four arm randomized trial on the effectiveness of electro-acupuncture. Evidence-Based Complementary and Alternative Medicine. Volume 2013 (2013), Article ID 349653. doi: https://doi.org/10.1155/2013/349653. Epub 2013 Aug 28.
24. Schröder S, Liepert J, Remppis A, Greten HJ. Acupuncture treatment improves nerve conduction in peripheral neuropathy. Eur J Neurol. 2007; 14(3):276–81.
25. Schröder S, Remppis A, Greten T, Brazkiewitz F, Morcos M, Greten HJ. Quantification of acupuncture effects of peripheral neuropathy of unknown and diabetic cause by nerve conduction studies. J Acupunct Tuina Sci. 2008;6:312–4.
26. Schroeder S, Eplée S, Bey A, Hu W, Brazkiewicz F. Adjuvant acupuncture treatment improves neuropathic pain in peripheral neuropathy and induces neural regeneration. Eur J of Pain Supplements. 2010;4:47–146,130.
27. Schroeder S, Meyer-Hamme G, Eplée S. Acupuncture for chemotherapy-induced peripheral neuropathy (CIPN): a pilot study using neurography. Acupunct Med. 2012;30(1):4–7. https://doi.org/10.1136/acupmed-2011-010034. Epub 2011 Dec 5
28. Litscher G, Wang L, Huber E, Nilsson G. Changed skin blood perfusion in the fingertip following acupuncture needle introduction as evaluated by laser Doppler perfusion imaging. Lasers Med Sci. 2002;17(1):19–25.
29. Hauer K, Wendt I, Schwenk M, Rohr C, Oster P, Greten J. Stimulation of acupoint ST-34 acutely improves gait performance in geriatric patients during rehabilitation: a randomized controlled trial. Arch Phys Med Rehabil. 2011;92(1):7–14. https://doi.org/10.1016/j.apmr.2010.09.023.
30. Karner M, Brazkiewicz F, Remppis A, Fischer J, Gerlach O, Stremmel W, Subramanian SV, Greten HJ. Objectifying specific and nonspecific effects of acupuncture: a double-blinded randomized trial in osteoarthritis of the knee. Evid Based Complement Alternat Med. 2013;2013:427265. https://doi.org/10.1155/2013/427265. Epub 2013 Jan 10
31. Pomeranz B, Bermann B. Scientific basis of acupuncture. Basics of acupuncture; 2003. p. 7–86.
32. Birch, S. A Review and Analysis of Placebo Treatments, Placebo Effects, and Placebo Controls in Trials of Medical Procedures When Sham Is Not Inert. The Journal of Alternative and Complementary Medicine. doi: https://doi.org/10.1089/acm.2006.12.303
33. Linde K, Niemann K, Schneider A, Meissner K. How large are the nonspecific effects of acupuncture? A meta-analysis of randomized controlled trials. BMC Med. 2010;8:75. https://doi.org/10.1186/1741-7015-8-75.
34. Brinkhaus B, Witt CM, Jena S, Linde K, Streng A, Wagenpfeil S, Irnich D, Walther HU, Melchart D, Willich SN. Acupuncture in patients with chronic low back pain: a randomized controlled trial. Arch Intern Med. 2006;166: 450–7.

35. Nabeta T, Kawakita K. Relief of chronic neck and shoulder pain by manual acupuncture to tender points: a sham-controlled randomized trial. Complement Ther Med. 2002;10:217–22.
36. Miyazaki S, Hagihara A, Kanda R, Mukaino Y, Nobutomo K. Applicability of press needles to a double-blind trial: a randomized, double-blind. Placebo-controlled Trial The Clinical Journal of Pain Issue: Volume. 2009;25(5):438–44. https://doi.org/10.1097/AJP.0b013e318193a6e1.
37. Lund I, Naeslund J, Lundeberg T. Minimal acupuncture is not a valid placebo control in randomized controlled trials of acupuncture: a physiologist's perspective. Chin Med. 2009;4:1. https://doi.org/10.1186/1749-8546-4-1.
38. Litscher G, Wang L, Schikora D, Rachbauer D, Schwarz G, Schöpfer A, Ropele S, Huber E. Biological effects of painless laser needle acupuncture. Medical Acupuncture. 2004;16(1):24–9.
39. Chen K, Shen XY, Ding GH, Wu F. Relationship between laser acupuncture analgesia and the function of mast cells. Zhogguo Zhen Jiu. 2009;29(6):478–83.
40. Litscher G, Schikora D. Laserneedle – acupuncture: science and practice. Pabst Science Publishers, Lengerich, Berlin, Bremen, 2007.
41. Zhang D, Spielmann A, Wang L, Ding G, Huang F, Gu Q, Schwarz W. Mast-cell degranulation induced by physicsl stimuli involves the activation of transient-receptor-potential channel TRPV2. Physiol Res. 2012;61:113–24. Epub 2011 May 16
42. Wang L, Sikora J, Hu L, Shen X, Grygorczyk R, Schwarz W. ATP release from mast cells by physical stimulation: a putative early step in activation of acupuncture points. Evid Based Complement Alternat Med. 2013;2013: 350949. https://doi.org/10.1155/2013/350949. Epub 2013 Jun 4
43. Litscher G, Schikora D. Cerebral vascular effects of non-invasive laserneedles measured by transorbital and transtemporal Doppler sonography. Lasers Med Sci. 2002;17(4):289–95.
44. Irnich D, Norbert S, Offenbächer M, Fleckenstein J. Is Sham Laser a Valid Control for Acupuncture Trials? Evidence-Based Complementary and Alternative Medicine 2011, Article ID 485945. https://doi.org/10.1093/ecam/neq009
45. American Diabetes Association. Diagnosis and classification of diabetes mellitus. Diabetes Care. 2010;33(Suppl 1):S62–9. https://doi.org/10.2337/dc10-S062
46. Conrad B, Bischoff C, Benecke R. Das EMG-Buch. 1998 Georg Thieme Verlag Stuttgart. Stuttgart, ISBN-13: 978–3131103413.
47. Focks C. atlas of Acupuncture (2008). London: Elsevier Churchill Livingstone; ISBN-13: 978–0443100284.
48. Litscher G, Nemetz W, Smolle J, Schwarz G, Schikora D, Uranüs S. Histological investigation of micro-morphological effects of the application of a laserneedle – results of an animal experiment. Biomed Tech. 2004; 49(1–2):2–5.
49. Haslbeck M, Luft D, Neundörfer B, Stracke H, Ziegler D. Diagnosis, Treatment and Follow-up of Diabetic Neuropathy. http://www.deutsche-diabetes-gesellschaft.de/fileadmin/Redakteur/Leitlinien/Englische_Leitlinien/GUIDELINE_DIABETIC_NEUROPATHY_05_2004_DDG_01_2006.pdf. Visited 2016–01–05 21:43 +01.00.
50. Dyck PJ, Carter RE, Litchy WJ. Modeling nerve conduction criteria for diagnosis of diabetic polyneuropathy. Muscle Nerve. 2011 Sep;44(3):340–5. https://doi.org/10.1002/mus.22074.
51. Neundörfer B, Heuß D. (Editors). Polyneuropathien. Referenz-Reihe Neurologie: Klinische Neurologie.Thieme Stuttgart, 1. Auflage, 2007. ISBN 978-3-13-139511-5. http://d-nb.info/980675502.
52. Dyck PJ, Karnes JL, PC O'B, Litchy WJ, Low PA, Melton LJ III. The Rochester diabetic neuropathy study. Reassessment of tests and criteria for diagnosis and staged severity. Neurology. 1992;42(6):1164. https://doi.org/10.1212/WNL.42.6.1164.
53. Farrar JT, Young JP Jr, LaMoreaux L, Werth JL, Poole RM. Clinical importance of changes in chronic pain intensity measured on an 11-point numerical pain rating scale. Pain. 2001;94(2):149–58.
54. Sural nerve myelinated fiber density differences associated with meaningful changes in clinical and electrophysiological measurements. J Neurol Sci 1996; 135:114–117.
55. Rosenberg CJ, Watson JC. Treatment of painful diabetic peripheral neuropathy. Prosthetics Orthot Int. 2015;39(1):17–28. https://doi.org/10.1177/0309364614542266.
56. van Niekerk EA, Tuszynski MH, Lu P, Dulin JN. Molecular and Cellular Mechanisms of Axonal Regeneration After Spinal Cord Injury. Mol Cell Proteomics. 2015 Dec 22. pii: mcp.R115.053751. [Epub ahead of print]. Visited 2016–01–08 13:33 +01:00.
57. Yasuda H, Terada M, Maeda K, Kogawa S, Sanada M, Haneda M, Kashiwagi A, Kikkawa R. Diabetic neuropathy and nerve regeneration. Prog Neurobiol. 2003;69:229–85.
58. Schroeder S, Eplée S. Effective adjuvant treatment of neuropathic pain in peripheral neuropathy by acupuncture. International Proceedings of the 3rd international Congress of Neuropathic Pain. Medimond (ISBN 978–88–7587–567–1) 161–166, 2010.
59. Tong Y, Guo H, Han B. Fifteen-day acupuncture treatment relieves diabetic peripheral neuropathy. J Acupunct Meridian Stud. 2010;3(2):95–103. https://doi.org/10.1016/S2005–2901(10)60018–0.
60. Jin Z, Zhang BF, Shang LX, Wang LN, Wang YL, Chen J, Jiang SS. Clinical observation on diabetic peripheral neuropathy treated with electroacupuncture and acupoint injection. Zhongguo Zhen Jiu. 2011;31(7):613–6. https://doi.org/10.1186/1745–6215–14–254.
61. Khosrawi S, Moghtaderi A, Haghighat S. Acupuncture in treatment of carpal tunnel syndrome. A randomized controlled trial study. J Res Med Sci. 2012 Jan;17(1):1–7.
62. Xia Q, Liu XW, Wang XL, Tao Y. Efficacy observation of carpal tunnel syndrome treated with electroacupuncture. Zhongguo Zhen Jiu. 2013 Aug; 33(8):700–2.
63. Herman PM, Craig BM, Caspi O. Is complementary and alternative medicine (CAM) cost-effective? A systematic review BMC Complement Altern Med. 2005 Jun 2;5:11.
64. Jabbour M, Sapko MT, Miller DW, Weiss LM, Gross M. Economic evaluation in acupuncture: past and future. The American Acupuncturist. 2009;49:11–7.

28

The cubital tunnel syndrome caused by intraneural ganglion cyst of the ulnar nerve at the elbow

Pengfei Li[1], Danfeng Lou[2] and Hui Lu[3*]

Abstract

Background: Cubital tunnel syndrome is common nerve compression syndrome among peripheral nerve compression diseases. However, the syndrome caused by intraneural ganglion cysts has been rarely reported. Medical approaches, like ultrasound-guided aspiration and open surgical treatment remain to be discussed.

Case presentation: A 57-year-old woman presented with occasional pain, numbness and paralysis in her left hand and a palpable, painless mass in the ulnar side of her left elbow. Ultrasound-guided aspiration of the mass was performed to decompress the ulnar nerve. The patient experienced an evident release of pain in her hand, but symptoms of numbness and paralysis recurred 3 months later which greatly bothered the patient's daily life. After evaluation, we had to perform an open surgery to excise the cyst. External neurolysis and anterior subcutaneous transposition were done. The patient was followed up for 2 years, and she made a complete recovery with no functional limitation.

Conclusions: The symptoms caused by intraneural ganglion cyst can be alleviated by accurate puncture. But puncture may be not complete and symptoms could recur. Complete external neurolysis can be counted as a complete and reliable treatment. Therefore, early diagnosis, careful preoperative imaging assessment and full decompression can be expected to receive a good rehabilitation.

Keywords: Cubital tunnel syndrome, Intraneural ganglion cyst, Ultrasound-guided aspiration

Background

Cubital tunnel syndrome is known as the second most common upper extremity compressive neuropathy, which may cause chronic ulnar nerve dysfunction, like permanent loss of sensation, muscle weakness, and joint contractures [1, 2]. However, cubital tunnel syndrome caused by intraneural ganglion cysts has been rarely reported [3–6]. Their pathogenesis has been controversial. Different treatments have been recommended [7, 8]. We reported a case of cubital tunnel syndrome caused by intraneural ganglion cyst of the ulnar nerve at the elbow. We first tried aspiration of the cyst. But there was a recurrence 3 months later. We then fully excised the cyst and externally relaxed the ulnar nerve which gave the

patient a complete recovery. The advantages and disadvantages of these two treatments were discussed.

Case presentation

A 57-year-old female patient presented in our clinic with complaints of occasional pain, numbness and paralysis in her left hand and a palpable, painless mass in the ulnar side of her left elbow for the last 2 months. There was no history of trauma. Besides the discomfort in the left elbow, the patient had a history of lumbar disc protrusion and hypertension, which was well controlled with medication. No other medical related history could be traced. Physical examination showed a painless mass (about 1 cm*2 cm) in the ulnar side of her left elbow with no inflammation. Neurologic examination revealed light numbness on the ulnar side of her left hand and fingers. No pathological sign was detected positive. Electromyography (EMG) showed the ulnar nerve across the elbow was injured. Magnetic resonance imaging (MRI)

* Correspondence: huilu@zju.edu.cn
[3]Department of Hand Surgery, The First Affiliated Hospital, College of Medicine, Zhejiang University, #79 Qingchun Road, Hangzhou, Zhejiang Province 310003, People's Republic of China
Full list of author information is available at the end of the article

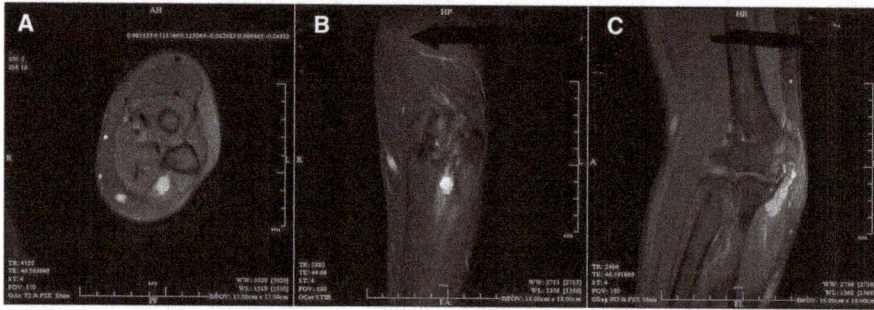

Fig. 1 Display of magnetic resonance imaging before medical intervention. **a** Hyperintense lesion in ulnar nerve at cubital tunnel on T2-weighted image in transverse section. **b** Hyperintense lesion in ulnar nerve at cubital tunnel on T2-weighted image in coronal section. **c** Hyperintense beaded lesion in ulnar nerve at distal elbow on T2-weighted image in median sagittal section

disclosed a subcutaneous irregular abnormal signal in the upper ulnar side of left forearm, hyperintense on T1 and T2-weighted image which was considered to be a benign lesion, and joint effusion in the left elbow (Fig. 1). X-ray showed degenerated change in the left elbow joint. Laboratory studies revealed the routine blood test, tumor markers, erythrocyte sedimentation rate (ESR), and high-sensitivity C-reactive protein were all within normal range. The mass was considered to be a cystic form disease which compressed the ulnar nerve. With the guidance of ultrasound, we first located the cyst. Precise puncture and aspiration were made with a 18G biopsy needle (Gallini, Italy) to evacuate mucinous material inside the cyst. The mass deflated mostly and the patient experienced an evident release of the pain with no significant improvement in other symptoms.

Three months later, the patient came to the clinic complaining the recurrence of symptoms of numbness and paralysis which still tremendously affected her daily life. Further evaluation indicated that open surgery was inevitable. The ulnar nerve was then surgically explored along its trajectory with a curve incision. The ulnar epineurium at cubital tunnel was thickened and the tunnel was constricted. After careful dissection, ruptured cystic wall was disclosed within nerve fibers (Fig. 2). Full excision of the cystic wall was performed and a sample of the lesion was sent for frozen section. Distal constriction of the ulnar nerve by fat and vascular tissue was discovered and complete decompression was operated. External neurolysis of the ulnar nerve was carefully done together with anterior subcutaneous transposition to relocate ulnar nerve on the soft tissue bed.

Histopathology revealed that the sample was fiber tissues in cystic wall (Fig. 3). Reporting diagnosis was intraneural ganglion cyst. The patient was evaluated 2 weeks after the surgery with improvement in motor function and some minor alleviation in dysesthesia. Follow-up of 2 years showed complete release in the symptoms and the latest MRI imaging revealed no sign of recurrence.

Discussion and conclusions

Cubital tunnel syndrome is a commonly seen neuropathy of the upper extremity caused by entrapment of the ulnar nerve in the elbow [1, 2]. One rare cause of the syndrome is intraneural ganglion cysts which are benign, mucinous, non-neoplastic lesions of the peripheral

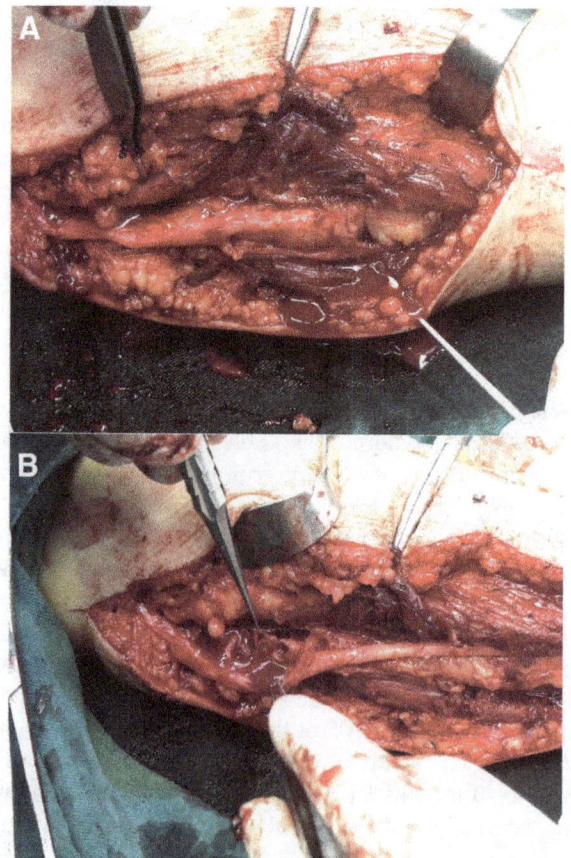

Fig. 2 Intraoperative findings: **a** Initial exposure revealed thickened epineurium of the ulnar nerve in the elbow and compression of fat and vascular tissue in the distal side of the ulnar nerve. **b** Further dissection disclosed ruptured cystic wall within nerve fibers

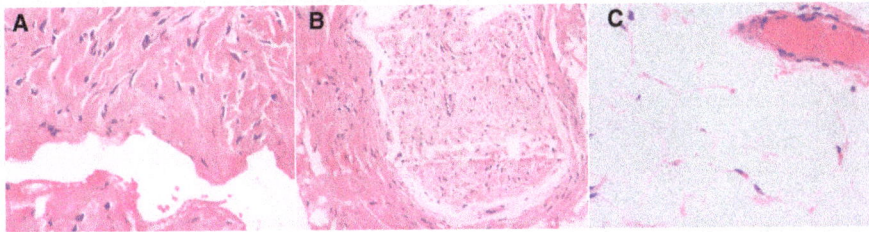

Fig. 3 Histopathology of the lesion demonstrating features of an intraneural ganglion cyst. **a** Fibrous tissues of cystiform (40*10 H&E). **b** Nerve tissue (20*10 H&E). **c** Fat and vascular tissue in the distal of the ulnar nerve (40*10 H&E)

nerves [3–5]. Mild to severe symptoms, ranging from discomfort, numbness, pain to disability, loss of function in the affected hand, can be felt in afflicted patients due to nerve compression [1, 9, 10]. The pathogenesis of intraneural ganglion cysts remains unclear. Though trauma was proposed to be the possible reason for the lesion [11, 12], the theory of articular unification which was proved by evidences was mainly accepted [3]. In our case, the latter was considered to be the cause.

Decompression of the enlarged nerves and resection of the articular branch are the pertinent treatments for intraneural ganglion cysts [3, 13]. Choice of interventions is generally based on severity of nerve compression, surgeons' preference, and patients' specific situations [14, 15]. Though there are a wide range of treatments to choose from, they do not allow the same results. Desy [13] et al. showed an increased rate of recurrence after primary surgery in his literature analysis. Thus, careful evaluation and cautious selection of treatment are of significance.

In this case, the patient suffered moderate pain, numbness and paralysis in her left hand which is applicable for ultrasound-guide diagnosis puncture [8, 16]. We tried ultrasound-guided aspiration first which achieved an obvious alleviation of the pain in the hand and deflated the palpable mass about the elbow. With a minimal invasion, the aspiration could deflate the cyst to decompress the constriction allowing reinnervation and recovery. While guided by ultrasound, it is highly possible that the aspiration would injure the nerve which was adjacent to the cyst. Although no sample could be collected for pathological examination, the cyst was initially considered to be intraneural, instead of extraneural. In addition, the numbness and paralysis in her left hand remained 3 months later which indicated that there were still some compressions unhandled inside. Combined with the discovery from the open surgery, there were two problems retained. First, while the cyst was released, the epineurium was waiting to be decompressed. Second, complete dissection couldn't be done to discover the distal entrapment by fat and vascular tissue of the ulnar nerve which was barely reported before.

The trajectory of the ulnar nerve was thoroughly explored surgically. Besides full excision of the cystic wall, another compression in the distal side of the ulnar nerve was relaxed. The patient experienced a full rehabilitation afterwards with no recurrence in the 2 years of follow-up.

From this case, it is indicated that there might be more anatomic factors that caused compression along the ulnar nerve which resulted in the cubital tunnel syndrome. Simply deflating the intraneural ganglion cyst could relieve the symptoms, but complete decompression demands for open surgery and external neurolysis.

The cubital tunnel syndrome caused by intraneural ganglion cyst needs to be treated seriously.

Aspiration may be not complete and symptoms could recur. Complete external neurolysis in open surgeries is a more effective and reliable method than ultrasound-guided aspiration. Early diagnosis, careful preoperative imaging assessment and full decompression can be expected to achieve a good rehabilitation.

Abbreviations
EMG: Electromyography; ESR: Erythrocyte sedimentation rate; MRI: Magnetic resonance imaging

Acknowledgements
First, I'd like to show my sincere gratitude to my colleagues Dr. JW and ZS who provided me with invaluable help and support in carrying out the study. Also, I really appreciate all the funding programs for sponsoring our research. Last but not least, I want to thank all my families and friends, especially my mother who backed me all the way to where I am.

Funding
The National Natural Science Foundation of China (grant number 81702135) funded in the design of the study; Zhejiang Traditional Chinese Medicine Research Program (grant numbers 2016ZA124, 2017ZB057) sponsored in the collection, analysis, and interpretation of data; Zhejiang Medicine and Hygiene Research Program (grant numbers 2016KYB101, 2015KYA100), and Zhejiang Medical Association Clinical Scientific Research Program (grant numbers 2013ZYC-A19, 2015ZYC-A12) funded the study in the writing part.

Authors' contributions
PL drafted the manuscript and participated in the analysis of the study. DL took part in the analysis of the case and helped revise the manuscript. HL participated in the design and coordination of the study, performed the analysis, and helped revise the manuscript. All authors read and approved the final manuscript.

Competing interests
The authors declare that they have no competing interests.

Author details
[1]Department of Plastic and Aesthetic Center, The First Affiliated Hospital, College of Medicine, Zhejiang University, #79 Qingchun Road, Hangzhou, Zhejiang Province 310003, People's Republic of China. [2]Department of Infectious Diseases, Shulan(Hangzhou) Hospital, #848 Dongxin Road, Hangzhou, Zhejiang Province 310000, People's Republic of China. [3]Department of Hand Surgery, The First Affiliated Hospital, College of Medicine, Zhejiang University, #79 Qingchun Road, Hangzhou, Zhejiang Province 310003, People's Republic of China.

References
1. Staples JR, Calfee R. Cubital tunnel syndrome: current concepts. J Am Acad Orthop Surg. 2017;25(10):e215-24.
2. An TW, Evanoff BA, Boyer MI, Osei DA. The prevalence of cubital tunnel syndrome: a cross-sectional study in a U.S. metropolitan cohort. J Bone Joint Surg Am. 2017;99(5):408-16.
3. Desy NM, Wang H, Elshiekh MA, Tanaka S, Choi TW, Howe BM, Spinner RJ. Intraneural ganglion cysts: a systematic review and reinterpretation of the world's literature. J Neurosurg. 2016;125(3):615-30.
4. Mobbs RJ, Phan K, Maharaj MM, Chaganti J, Simon N. Intraneural ganglion cyst of the ulnar nerve at the elbow masquerading as a malignant peripheral nerve sheath tumor. World Neurosurg. 2016;96:613.e5-8.
5. Colbert SH, Le MH. Case report: intraneural ganglion cyst of the ulnar nerve at the wrist. Hand. 2011;6(3):317–20.
6. Öztürk U, Salduz A, Demirel M, Pehlivanoğlu T, Sivacioğlu S. Intraneural ganglion cyst of the ulnar nerve in an unusual location: a case report. Int J Surg Case Rep. 2017;31:61–4.
7. Yahya A, Malarkey AR, Eschbaugh RL, Bamberger HB. Trends in the surgical treatment for cubital tunnel syndrome: a survey of members of the American Society for Surgery of the Hand. Hand. 2018;13(5):516-21.
8. Jose J, Fourzali R, Lesniak B, Kaplan L. Ultrasound-guided aspiration of symptomatic intraneural ganglion cyst within the tibial nerve. Skelet Radiol. 2011;40(11):1473–8.
9. Palmer BA, Hughes TB. Cubital Tunnel Syndrome. Neurology. 2010;35(1):153–63.
10. Lu H, Chen Q, Shen H. Pigmented villonodular synovitis of the elbow with rdial, median and ulnar nerve compression. Int J Clin Exp Pathol. 2014;8(11):14045–9.
11. Lu H, Chen LF, Jiang S, Shen H. A rapidly progressive foot drop caused by the posttraumatic Intraneural ganglion cyst of the deep peroneal nerve. BMC Musculoskelet Disord. 2018;19:298.
12. Spinner RJ, Crnkovich F, Ahmed IKM, Amrami KK. Can trauma cause tibial intraneural ganglion cysts at the superior tibiofibular joint? Clin Anat. 2012; 25(6):785–7.
13. Desy NM, Lipinski LJ, Tanaka S, Amrami KK, Rock MG, Spinner RJJCA. Recurrent intraneural ganglion cysts: Pathoanatomic patterns and treatment implications. Clin Anat. 2015;28(8):1058–69.
14. Novak CB, Mackinnon SE. Selection of operative procedures for cubital tunnel syndrome. Hand. 2009;4(1):50-4.
15. Bartels RHMA, Menovsky T, Overbeeke JJV, Verhagen WIM. Surgical management of ulnar nerve compression at the elbow: An analysis of the literature. J Neurosurg. 1998;89(5):722-7.
16. Liang T, Panu A, Crowther S, Low G, Lambert R. Ultrasound-guided aspiration and injection of an intraneural ganglion cyst of the common peroneal nerve. HSS J. 2013;9(3):270–4.

29

Rebound of relapses after discontinuation of rituximab in a patient with MOG-IgG1 positive highly relapsing optic neuritis

Seok-Jin Choi[1], Boram Kim[2], Haeng-Jin Lee[3], Seong-Joon Kim[3], Sung-Min Kim[2*] and Jung-Joon Sung[2]

Abstract

Background: Myelin oligodendrocyte glycoprotein immunoglobulin G1 (MOG-IgG1)-associated disease is suggested as a separate disease entity distinct from multiple sclerosis and neuromyelitis optica spectrum disorder. Nonetheless, the optimal treatment regimen for preventing relapses in MOG-IgG1-associated disease remains unclear.

Case presentation: We describe the case of a 45-year-old man with MOG-IgG1-positive highly relapsing optic neuritis who had experienced 5 attacks over 21 months and had monocular blindness despite prednisolone and azathioprine therapy. He began treatment with rituximab, which reduced the rate of relapse markedly. Following discontinuation of rituximab, however, the patient experienced two successive optic neuritis attacks 2 and 4 months after B-lymphocyte restoration.

Conclusions: Highly relapsing MOG-IgG1-associated disease can be prevented with rituximab even when the MOG-IgG1 titers are relatively stationary. Discontinuation of rituximab and restoration of B-lymphocytes may be associated with the rebound of disease activity.

Keywords: MOG-IgG1, Optic neuritis, Highly relapsing, Rituximab

Background

Myelin oligodendrocyte glycoprotein immunoglobulin G1 (MOG-IgG1)-associated disease is suggested as a separate disease entity distinct from multiple sclerosis and neuromyelitis optica spectrum disorder (NMOSD) with anti-aquaporin-4 IgG (AQP4-IgG); it has a predilection for the optic nerve rather than spinal cord, perineural enhancement extending to adjacent soft tissues on magnetic resonance imaging (MRI), and a less unfavorable prognosis than NMOSD [1]. Recent studies with a sufficient number of patients and duration of follow-up have indicated that a considerable number of patients with MOG-IgG1 have relapsing attacks in the central nervous system followed by neurological deficits [2, 3]. Nonetheless, the optimal treatment regimen for preventing relapses in patients with MOG-IgG1-associated disease has only recently begun to be studied [4]. Here, we describe a patient with highly relapsing optic neuritis (ON) associated with MOG-IgG1, whose ON attacks were relatively well-prevented with rituximab (RTX) treatment. However, the patient experienced rebounds of repeated ON attacks shortly after the restoration of B-cells following discontinuation of RTX.

Case presentation

A 45-year-old man presented with decreased right visual acuity (VA) accompanied by periocular pain lasting for 1 week. Ophthalmological examination revealed that the patient's right eye was only able to perceive light (best-corrected VA, light perception/0.9 in decimals, measured using a Snellen chart) and had relative afferent pupillary defect of grade 3, diffuse disc swelling, and inferior disc hemorrhage. Neurological examination showed normal muscle strength in all extremities, no sensory deficits,

* Correspondence: sueh916@gmail.com
[2]Department of Neurology, Seoul National University Hospital, 101, Daehak-Ro Jongno-Gu, Seoul 03080, Republic of Korea
Full list of author information is available at the end of the article

normoactive deep tendon reflexes, and no signs of bladder or bowel dysfunction. Orbit MRI revealed T2 high signal intensities and diffuse contrast enhancement along the right anterior and posterior optic nerve, as well as perineural enhancement [1] (Fig. 1-a and b). The results of cerebrospinal fluid (CSF) analysis showed a red blood cell count of 0/μL, a white blood cell count of 1/μL, and a protein level of 27 mg/dL. CSF oligoclonal band measured by isoelectric focusing was negative and IgG index was 0.64. The result of a serum AQP4-IgG flow cytometry assay using AQP4-M23-expressing live cells was negative [5]. Right ON was suspected, and intravenous methylprednisolone (1000 mg pulse therapy) for 5 days followed by oral prednisolone (60 mg daily) were prescribed. The right VA of the patient was improved to 0.5 (visual Functional System score improved to 2 from 5).

The second right ON attack (0.15/1.0) occurred 4 months after the first ON when the prednisolone dose had been tapered to 10 mg daily. Thus, azathioprine 50 mg twice per day was started in a remission state between the second and third ON (4 months prior to the third ON). The average thickness of a retinal nerve fiber layer measured by spectral-domain optical coherence tomography was decreased in the right eye (right 51 μm and left 105 μm) (Fig. 2-a). The third (hand movement/0.9) and fourth (finger count/1.2) right ON attacks occurred 6 and 10 months after the second ON, respectively, while the prednisolone dose was maintained at 5 mg daily and azathioprine was 75 mg twice per day. Following these attacks, the patient developed left central serous chorioretinopathy (0.15/0.9) associated with long-term steroid use. The 25 mg dose of prednisolone was thus tapered out at this point. Nevertheless, right ON recurred 2 months later for a fifth time (hand movement/0.9) when the patient was under azathioprine treatment only. At this time, the patient developed

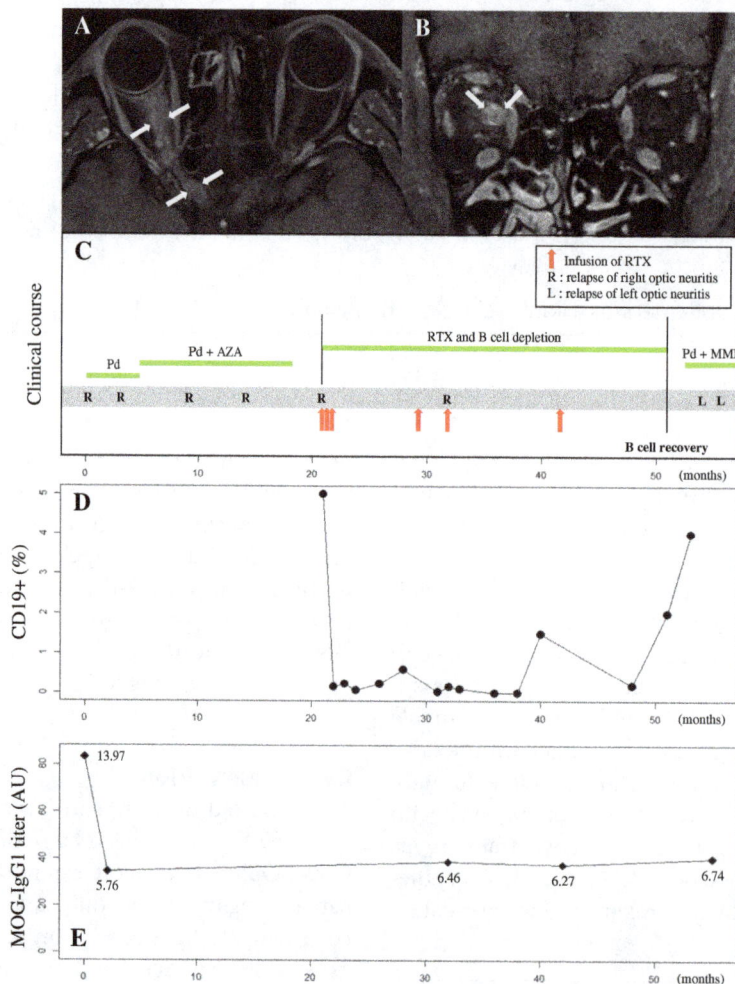

Fig. 1 (a) Axial and (b) coronal T1-weighted magnetic resonance images demonstrating diffuse gadolinium enhancement and swelling along the right anterior and posterior optic nerve. c Longitudinal clinical course of recurrent optic neuritis. d Change of CD19+ B-lymphocytes (%) during rituximab treatment. e Change of MOG-IgG1 titers measured by a geometric mean fluorescence (G-mean) ratio of the MOG-expressing cells that bound to IgG1 using in-house flow cytometry (G-mean ratio = G-mean values of the patient's sera / G-mean values of the healthy control)

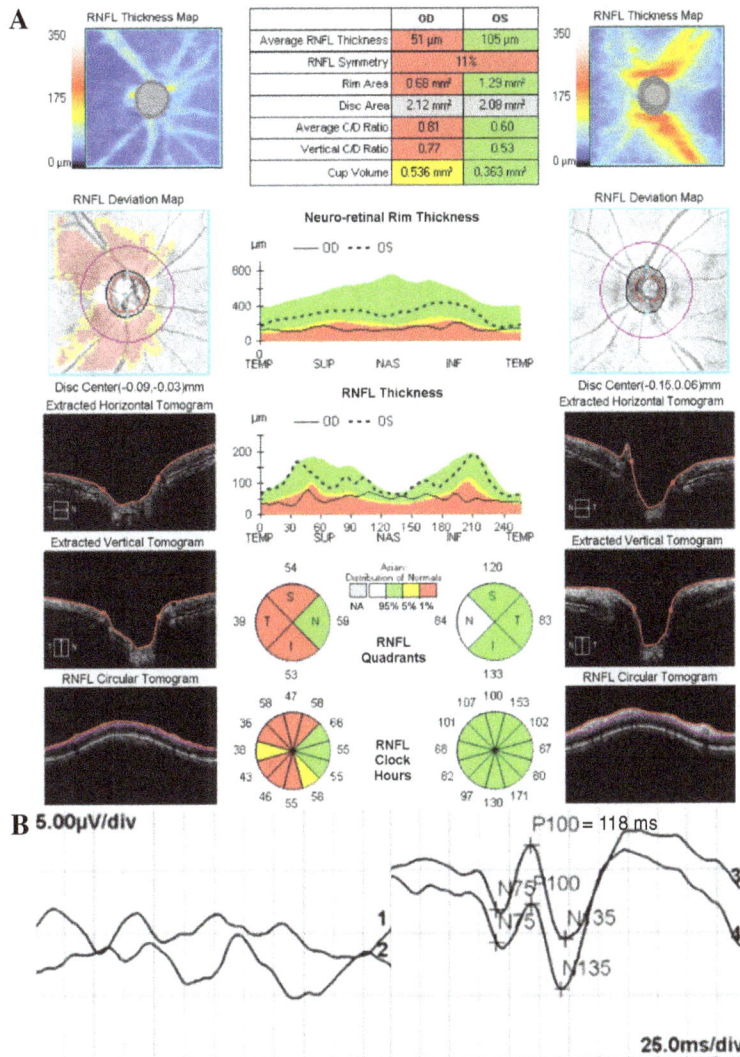

Fig. 2 a (Remission state after the second optic neuritis) the average retinal nerve fiber layer thickness measured by spectral-domain optical coherence tomography was decreased in the right eye (right 51 μm and left 105 μm), with preferential thinning of the superior, temporal, and inferior quadrants. **b** (During fifth optic neuritis) the pattern-reversal visual evoked potential showed an abnormal waveform in the right eye with diminished amplitude. The left eye presented a relatively preserved response with prolonged P100 latency (118 ms)

monocular blindness. The pattern-reversal visual evoked potential showed an abnormal waveform in the right eye with diminished amplitude. The left eye presented a relatively preserved response with prolonged P100 latency (118 ms) (Fig. 2-b). Serum from the patient sampled at the time of the fifth ON attack was tested for MOG-IgG1 using a cell-based assay utilizing full-length human MOG (Radcliffe Hospital, Oxford, UK) [6]. The result of this test was positive.

Despite continued immunosuppressive treatment and due to the repeated ON attacks and the side effect of the steroid (chorioretinopathy), the patient was administered RTX (375 mg/m², 3 weekly infusion for induction and 3 maintenance doses under CD19+ B-cell monitoring over 29 months). Although one mild ON attack (no light

perception/1.2) occurred in the patient's right eye during RTX treatment, the rate of relapse decreased markedly and the patient's visual function was well-maintained. However, 32 months after the initiation of RTX treatment, we became unable to maintain RTX treatment due to insurance issues (denial for reimbursement). As a result, the treatment was switched to mycophenolate mofetil (250 mg twice per day) combined with oral prednisolone (5 mg every other day). The patient's CD19+ B-lymphocyte level was restored to 2 and 4% at 9 and 11 months after the last RTX infusion, respectively. Subsequently, 2 more left ON attacks (hand movement/1.0 and hand movement/0.15) occurred within a one-month interval (Fig. 1-c and 1-D). The titer of MOG-IgG1 was measured by a geometric mean fluorescence (G-mean) ratio of the MOG-expressing cells bound to IgG1 using in-house flow cytometry. The G-mean ratio was calculated for each sera as followings: G-mean values of the patient's sera / G-mean values of the healthy control. The titer was not associated with the continuation or cessation of the RTX treatment (Fig. 1-e).

Discussion and conclusions

Here, we describe the longitudinal clinical course and treatment response to RTX therapy in a patient with MOG-IgG1-positive highly relapsing ON. We found that 1) highly relapsing MOG-IgG1-associated disease can be prevented with RTX even when the MOG-IgG1 titers are relatively preserved, and 2) discontinuation of RTX in patients with this condition can cause rebound of disease activity with restoration of B-lymphocytes.

Initial reports regarding MOG-IgG1-associated disease indicated that it typically has a monophasic and benign disease course [7]. However, recent multicenter studies have shown that a considerable proportion of patients have a relapsing course of disease, and some have significant neurological deficits [2, 3]. More recently, RTX was reported to reduce the rate of relapse in some cases of MOG-IgG1-associated disease [4]. Nevertheless, the results of studies comparing the patient's condition before vs. after the treatment should be interpreted with caution because the disease may have a naturally decreasing relapse rate in the later stages, as in NMOSD [8], and also the statistical phenomenon of regression towards the mean. In this regard, the present case, wherein we observed a restoration of B-lymphocytes and a subsequent rebound of relapses after discontinuation of RTX treatment, implies that long-term RTX maintenance therapy may be helpful in patients with highly relapsing MOG-IgG1-associated disease.

Despite initial treatment with azathioprine and prednisolone, the patient had a high relapse rate of 0.238/year (5 attacks over 21 months) and subsequent unilateral visual loss in the right eye. After initiating RTX treatment, his relapse rate markedly decreased to 0.031/year (1 attack over 32 months). However, the patient experienced 2 ON attacks over 4 months following cessation of RTX treatment and restoration of B-lymphocytes.

In summary, the case described here illustrates that RTX can be a good treatment option for preventing relapses in MOG-IgG1-associated disease. The treatment effect was observed despite the relatively unchanged MOG-IgG1 titers during the treatment period. Finally, cessation of RTX treatment and restoration of B-lymphocytes may be associated with the rebound of disease activity. RTX may serve as an effective treatment regimen in MOG-IgG1-associated disease, especially in patients with high relapse rates.

Abbreviations

AQP4: anti-aquaporin-4; CSF: cerebrospinal fluid; IgG: immunoglobulin G; MOG: myelin oligodendrocyte glycoprotein; MRI: magnetic resonance imaging; NMOSD: neuromyelitis optica spectrum disorder; ON: optic neuritis; RTX: rituximab; VA: visual acuity

Acknowledgements

None.

Funding

This work was supported by grant no. HI17C0335 and HI17C0789 from the Korea Health Industry Development Institute Research fund. The funders had no role in the design of the study, interpretation of data and in writing the manuscript. They had contributed to the data collection and analysis of AQP4-IgG and MOG-IgG1 antibodies.

Authors' contributions

S-MK conceived of the study. S-JC and S-MK analyzed and interpreted the data, and involved in drafting and revising the manuscript. BK contributed to acquisition and analysis of the data, and involved in revising the manuscript critically. J-JS contributed to interpretation of the data, and involved in revising the manuscript critically. H-JL and S-JK made substantial contributions to interpretation of ophthalmological data and also involved in revising the manuscript critically; as a result, this manuscript came to have more intellectual content on ophthalmology. All listed authors have participated sufficiently in the work to take public responsibility for appropriate portions of the content, and agreed to be accountable for all aspects of the work in ensuring that questions related to the accuracy or integrity of any part of the work are appropriately investigated and resolved.

Competing interests

The authors declare that they have no competing interests.

Author details

[1]Department of Neurology, Inha University Hospital, Incheon, Republic of Korea. [2]Department of Neurology, Seoul National University Hospital, 101, Daehak-Ro Jongno-Gu, Seoul 03080, Republic of Korea. [3]Department of Ophthalmology, Seoul National University Hospital, Seoul, Republic of Korea.

References

1. Kim SM, Woodhall MR, Kim JS, Kim SJ, Park KS, Vincent A, Lee KW, Waters P. Antibodies to MOG in adults with inflammatory demyelinating disease of the CNS. Neurol Neuroimmunol Neuroinflamm. 2015;2(6):e163.
2. Jurynczyk M, Messina S, Woodhall MR, Raza N, Everett R, Roca-Fernandez A, Tackley G, Hamid S, Sheard A, Reynolds G, et al. Clinical presentation and prognosis in MOG-antibody disease: a UK study. Brain. 2017;140(12):3128-38.
3. Cobo-Calvo A, Ruiz A, Maillart E, Audoin B, Zephir H, Bourre B, Ciron J, Collongues N, Brassat D, Cotton F, et al. Clinical spectrum and prognostic value of CNS MOG autoimmunity in adults: The MOGADOR study. Neurology. 2018;90(21):e1858-e1869.
4. Ramanathan S, Mohammad S, Tantsis E, Nguyen TK, Merheb V, Fung VSC, White OB, Broadley S, Lechner-Scott J, Vucic S, et al. Clinical course, therapeutic responses and outcomes in relapsing MOG antibody-associated demyelination. J Neurol Neurosurg Psychiatry. 2018;89(2):127-137.
5. Yang J, Kim SM, Kim YJ, Cheon SY, Kim B, Jung KC, Park KS. Accuracy of the Fluorescence-Activated Cell Sorting Assay for the Aquaporin-4 Antibody (AQP4-Ab): Comparison with the Commercial AQP4-Ab Assay Kit. PLoS One. 2016;11(9):e0162900.
6. Waters P, Woodhall M, O'Connor KC, Reindl M, Lang B, Sato DK, Jurynczyk M, Tackley G, Rocha J, Takahashi T, et al. MOG cell-based assay detects non-MS patients with inflammatory neurologic disease. Neurol Neuroimmunol Neuroinflamm. 2015;2(3):e89.
7. Kitley J, Woodhall M, Waters P, Leite MI, Devenney E, Craig J, Palace J, Vincent A. Myelin-oligodendrocyteglycoprotein antibodies in adults with a neuromyelitis optica phenotype. Neurology. 2012;79(12):1273-1277.
8. Kim SM, Park J, Kim SH, Park SY, Kim JY, Sung JJ, Park KS, Lee KW. Factors associated with the time to next attack in neuromyelitis optica: accelerated failure time models with random effects. PLoS One. 2013;8(12):e82325.

Permissions

The contributors of this book come from diverse backgrounds, making this book a truly international effort. This book will bring forth new frontiers with its revolutionizing research information and detailed analysis of the nascent developments around the world.

We would like to thank all the contributing authors for lending their expertise to make the book truly unique. They have played a crucial role in the development of this book. Without their invaluable contributions this book wouldn't have been possible. They have made vital efforts to compile up to date information on the varied aspects of this subject to make this book a valuable addition to the collection of many professionals and students.

This book was conceptualized with the vision of imparting up-to-date information and advanced data in this field. To ensure the same, a matchless editorial board was set up. Every individual on the board went through rigorous rounds of assessment to prove their worth. After which they invested a large part of their time researching and compiling the most relevant data for our readers.

The editorial board has been involved in producing this book since its inception. They have spent rigorous hours researching and exploring the diverse topics which have resulted in the successful publishing of this book. They have passed on their knowledge of decades through this book. To expedite this challenging task, the publisher supported the team at every step. A small team of assistant editors was also appointed to further simplify the editing procedure and attain best results for the readers.

Apart from the editorial board, the designing team has also invested a significant amount of their time in understanding the subject and creating the most relevant covers. They scrutinized every image to scout for the most suitable representation of the subject and create an appropriate cover for the book.

The publishing team has been an ardent support to the editorial, designing and production team. Their endless efforts to recruit the best for this project, has resulted in the accomplishment of this book. They are a veteran in the field of academics and their pool of knowledge is as vast as their experience in printing. Their expertise and guidance has proved useful at every step. Their uncompromising quality standards have made this book an exceptional effort. Their encouragement from time to time has been an inspiration for everyone.

The publisher and the editorial board hope that this book will prove to be a valuable piece of knowledge for researchers, students, practitioners and scholars across the globe.

List of Contributors

Kostas Athanasakis, Ioannis Petrakis, Eleftheria Karampli and John Kyriopoulos
Department of Health Economics, National School of Public Health, Athens, Greece

Elli Vitsou and Leonidas Lyras
Pfizer Hellas, Athens, Greece

M. Staudt, J. M. Diederich, A. Meisel and J. Klehmet
Department of Neurology, Charité University Medicine, Charitéplatz 1, 10117 Berlin, Germany

C. Meisel
Department of Clinical Immunology, Charité University Medicine, Charitéplatz 1, Berlin, Germany

Hui Qing Hou, Xue Dan Feng, Xiu Juan Song and Li Guo
Department of Neurology, the Second Hospital of Hebei Medical University, Key laboratory of Hebei Neurology, Shi jia zhuang, Hebei 050000, China

Jun Miao
Department of Neurosurgery, the General Hospital of North China Petroleum Administration Bureau, Ren qiu, HeBei 062550, China

Mei Han
Emergency Department, the Second Hospital of Hebei Medical University, Shi jia zhuang, Hebei 050000, China

Sonali Sihindi Chapa Gunatilake, Rohitha Gamlath and Harith Wimalaratna
Teaching Hospital, Kandy, Sri Lanka

Aaron I. Vinik and Etta J. Vinik
Eastern Virginia Medical School, Strelitz Diabetes Center, 855 W Brambleton Avenue, Room 2018, Norfolk, VA 23510, USA

Serge Perrot
Hôpital Hôtel Dieu, Paris Descartes University, Paris, France

Ladislav Pazdera
Vestra Clinics - Dedicated Research Clinics, Rychnov nad Kneznou, Czech Republic

Hélène Jacobs, Malcolm Stoker, Robert J. Snijder and Marjolijne van der Stoep
Astellas Pharma Europe B. V, Leiden, The Netherlands

Enrique Ortega
Hospital Rio Hortega, Valladolid, Spain

Nathaniel Katz
Analgesic Solutions, Natick, MA, USA
Tufts University School of Medicine, Boston, MA, USA

Stephen K. Long
Eastern Virginia Medical School, Strelitz Diabetes Center, 855 W Brambleton Avenue, Room 2018, Norfolk, VA 23510, USA
INC Research, Camberley, UK

Jagar Jasem
School of Medicine/ Faculty of Medical Sciences/ University of Duhok, Nakhoshkhana Street, Duhok, Kurdistan Region, Iraq
Internal Medicine, Ohio State University, Columbus, Ohio, USA

Sirwan Aswad and Kawa Marof
Directorate of Preventive Health Affairs, Directorate General of Health, Mazi Street, Duhok, Kurdistan Region, Iraq

Adnan Nawar
National Communicable Disease Control, Ministry of Health, Bab Al Mudam Area, Baghdad, Iraq

Yosra Khalaf and Faisal Hamdani
AFP Surveillance Laboratory, Ministry of Health, Bab Al Mudam Area, Baghdad, Iraq

Monirul Islam
College of Public Health, University of Nebraska Medical Center, Omaha, Nebraska, USA

Andre Kalil
Division of Infectious Diseases/Department of Internal Medicine, University of Nebraska Medical Center, Omaha, Nebraska, USA

Angelo Maurizio Clerici, Marco Mauri, Federico Sergio Squellati and Giorgio Giovanni Bono
Neurology Unit, Circolo & Macchi Foundation Hospital - Insubria University – DBSV, Viale L. Borri 57, 21100 Varese, Italy

Eduardo Nobile-Orazio
2nd Neurology, Humanitas Clinical and Research Institute, Department of Medical Biotechnology and Translational Medicine (BIOMETRA), Milan University, Rozzano, Milan, Italy

Keiko Yamada
Center for Pain Management, Osaka University Hospital, 2-15 Yamadaoka, Suita-shi, Osaka 565-0871, Japan
Public Health, Department of Social Medicine, Osaka University Graduate School of Medicine, 2-2 Yamadaoka, Suita-shi, Osaka 565-0871, Japan

Junhui Yuan and Hiroshi Takashima
Department of Neurology and Geriatrics, Kagoshima University Graduate School of Medical and Dental Sciences, 8-35-1 Sakuragaoka, Kagoshima 890-8520, Japan

Tomoo Mano
Department of Neuromodulation, Osaka University Graduate School of Medicine, 2-2 Yamadaoka, Suita-shi, Osaka 565-0871, Japan

Masahiko Shibata
Center for Pain Management, Osaka University Hospital, 2-15 Yamadaoka, Suita-shi, Osaka 565-0871, Japan
Department of Pain Medicine, Osaka University Graduate School of Medicine, 2-2 Yamadaoka, Suita-shi, Osaka 565-0871, Japan

Xiaowen Li, Jinting Xiao, Yanan Ding, Jing Xu, Yating He, Hui Zhai, Bingdi Xie and Junwei Hao
Department of Neurology and Tianjin Neurological Institute, Tianjin Medical University General Hospital, Tianjin 300052, China

Chuanxia Li
Department of Neurology, Tianjin Haihe Hospital, Tianjin 300060, China

Ins Brs Marques, Gavin Giovannoni and Monica Marta
Queen Mary University London, Blizard Institute, 4 Newark Street, London E1 1AT, UK

Inés González-Suárez, Irene Sanz-Gallego, Francisco Javier Rodríguez de Rivera and Javier Arpa
Section of Neuromuscular diseases, Department of Neurology, La Paz University Hospital, Paseo de la Castellana, Madrid 261.28046, Spain

Ling-Yu Pang, Yang-Yang Wang and Li-Ying Liu
Department of Pediatrics, Chinese PLA General Hospital, Beijing 100853, China

Chang-Hong Ding
Department of Neurology, Beijing Children's Hospital, The Capital Medical University, Beijing, China

Qiao-Jun Li
Department of Pediatrics, First Affiliated Hospital of the People's Liberation Army General Hospital, Beijing 100048, China

Li-Ping Zou
Department of Pediatrics, Chinese PLA General Hospital, Beijing 100853, China
Center of Epilepsy, Beijing Institute for Brain Disorders, Beijing 100069, China

Mirza Jusufovic and Anne Hege Aamodt
Dept of Neurology, Oslo University Hospital, Oslo, Norway

Bård Nedregaard
Dept of Radiology, Oslo University Hospital, Oslo, Norway

Emilia Kerty
Dept of Neurology, Oslo University Hospital, Oslo, Norway
Institute of Clinical Medicine, University of Oslo, Oslo, Norway

Astrid Lygren
Dept of Neurology, Oslo University Hospital, Oslo, Norway
Dept of Psychiatry, Akershus University Hospital, Lørenskog, Norway

Richard J Bright
Faculty of Health Sciences, School of Dentistry, University of Adelaide, Adelaide, Australia
School of Biomedical Sciences, Charles Sturt University, Wagga Wagga, Australia
Faculty of Health Sciences, Immunotherapy Research Laboratory, Royal Adelaide Hospital, Adelaide, Australia

Jenny Wilkinson
School of Biomedical Sciences, Charles Sturt University, Wagga Wagga, Australia

Brendon J Coventry
Faculty of Health Sciences, Immunotherapy Research Laboratory, Royal Adelaide Hospital, Adelaide, Australia

Colette Mankowski, Chris D. Poole, Cecil Treadwell and Isaac Odeyemi
Astellas Pharma Europe Ltd, 2000 Hillswood Drive, Chertsey KT16 0PS, UK

Etienne Ernault
Astellas Pharma Europe B.V., Leiden, The Netherlands

Roger Thomas and Ellen Berni
Pharmatelligence, Cardiff, UK

Craig J. Currie
Cardiff University, Cardiff, UK

José I. Calvo
Complejo Hospitalario de Navarra, Pamplona, Spain

Christina Plastira and Eirini Zafeiropoulou
Evangelismos General Hospital, Athens, Greece

Sonali Sihindi Chapa Gunatilake and Harith Wimalaratna
Teaching Hospital, Kandy, Sri Lanka

David Adams
CHU Hôpital Bicêtre, Le Kremlin-Bicêtre CEDEX, Paris, France

Ole B. Suhr
Department of Public Health and Clinical Medicine, Umeå University Hospital, Umeå, Sweden

Peter J. Dyck and William J. Litchy
Department of Neurology, Mayo Clinic, Rochester, MN, USA

Jihong Chen, Jared Gollob and Raina G. Leahy
Alnylam Pharmaceuticals, Cambridge, MA, USA

Teresa Coelho
Hospital Santo António, Centro Hospitalar do Porto, Porto, Portugal

Daojun Hong, Yan Xu and Jun Zhang
Department of Neurology, Peking University People's Hospital, #11 Xizhimen South Avenue, Xicheng District, Beijing 100044, China

Yanyan Yu and Yuyao Wang
Department of Neurology, The first affiliated hospital of Nanchang University, Nanchang, China

Yusuke Sakiyama, Eiji Matsuura, Yoshimitsu Maki, Akiko Yoshimura, Masahiro Ando, Miwa Nomura, Kazuya Shinohara, Ryuji Saigo, Tomonori Nakamura, Akihiro Hashiguchi and Hiroshi Takashima
Department of Neurology and Geriatrics, Kagoshima University Graduate School of Medical and Dental Sciences, 8-35-1 Sakuragaoka, Kagoshima City, Kagoshima 890-8520, Japan

Wenxia Zheng, Zhenxing Yan, Rongni He, Aiqun Lin, Wei Huang, Yuying Su and Huifang Xie
Department of Neurology, Zhujiang Hospital, Southern Medical University, 253 Industrial Avenue Middle, Guangzhou City 510282, Guangdong Province, China

Yaowei Huang
Department of Neurology, Nanfang Hospital, Southern Medical University, 1838 Guangzhou Avenue North, Guangzhou, Guangzhou 510515, China

Shaoyuan Li
AmCare Genomics Lab, Guangzhou, Guangzhou 510320, China

Victor Wei Zhang
AmCare Genomics Lab, Guangzhou, Guangzhou 510320, China
Department of Molecular and Human Genetics, Baylor College of Medicine, Houston, TX 77030, USA

Li Ding, Xiao Wu, Lele Zhong, Pei Zhang, Yongzhong Lin and Ying Liu
Department of Neurology, the Second Hospital of Dalian Medical University, No. 467 Zhongshan Road, Shahekou District, Dalian City 116027, Liaoning Province, China

Zhongjun Chen
Neuro-Interventional Ward, Dalian Municipal Central Hospital of Dalian Medical University, Dalian City, China

Yan Sun
Anesthesiology Department, Jilin University, China
Japan Union Hospital, Changchun City, China

Haiping Bao
Department of Nerve Electrophysiology, the Second
Hospital of Dalian Medical University, Dalian City,
China

Jong Hyeon Ahn
Department of Neurology, Inha University Hospital,
Inha University College of Medicine, Incheon,
South Korea

Dae Joong Kim
Department of Anatomy, Inha University College
of Medicine, Incheon, South Korea

Jung-Joon Sung
Department of Neurology, Seoul National University
Hospital, Seoul, South Korea

Yoon-Ho Hong
Department of Neurology, Seoul National University
College of Medicine, Seoul National University
Seoul Metropolitan Government Boramae Medical
Center, Seoul, South Korea

Suk-Won Ahn
Department of Neurology, Chung-Ang University
Hospital, Chung-Ang University College of
Medicine, Seoul, South Korea

Jeong Jin Park
Department of Neurology, Konkuk University
Medical Center, Seoul, South Korea

Byung-Nam Yoon
Department of Neurology, Seoul Paik Hospital, Inje
University College of Medicine, Mareunnae-ro 9,
Jung-gu, Seoul 04551, Republic of Korea

Behrouz Rahmani
Section of Physiology, Department of Basic Sciences,
Faculty of Veterinary Medicine, University of
Tehran, Tehran, Iran
Neuroscience Research Center, Shahid Beheshti
University of Medical Sciences, Tehran, Iran

Abolhassan Ahmadiani and Sareh Asadi
Neuroscience Research Center, Shahid Beheshti
University of Medical Sciences, Tehran, Iran

Fatemeh Fekrmandi
Department of Radiation Oncology, University
Health Network, Princess Margaret Cancer Centre,
Toronto, Canada

Keivan Ahadi
Department of Orthopaedic Surgery, Milad
Hospital, Tehran, Iran

Tannaz Ahadi
Neuromusculoskeletal Research Centre, Department
of Physical Medicine and Rehabilitation, Iran
University of Medical Sciences, Tehran, Iran

Afagh Alavi
Genetics Research Center, University of Social
Welfare and Rehabilitation Sciences, Tehran, Iran

**Tatsuya Ueno, Rie Hagiwara, Tomoya Kon, Jin-
ichi Nunomura and Masahiko Tomiyama**
Department of Neurology, Aomori Prefectural
Central Hospital, 2-1-1 Higashi-Tsukurimichi,
Aomori 030-8551, Japan

Yukihiro Hasegawa
Department of Respiratory Medicine, Aomori
Prefectural Central Hospital, 2-1-1 Higashi-
Tsukurimichi, Aomori 030-8551, Japan

**Ozan E. Eren, Ruth Ruscheweyh, Florian Schöberl
and Andreas Straube**
Department of Neurology, University Hospital, LMU
Munich, Campus Großhadern, Marchioninistr. 15,
81377 Munich, Germany

Christoph Schankin
Department of Neurology, Inselspital, Bern
University Hospital, University of Bern, Bern,
Switzerland

**Kavin Vanikieti, Anuchit Poonyathalang and
Tanyatuth Padungkiatsagul**
Department of Ophthalmology, Faculty of Medicine
Ramathibodi Hospital, Mahidol University, 270
Rama VI Road, Bangkok 10400, Thailand

Panitha Jindahra
Department of Medicine, Faculty of Medicine
Ramathibodi Hospital, Mahidol University, 270
Rama VI Road, Bangkok 10400, Thailand

Piyaphon Cheecharoen and Patchalin Patputtipong
Department of Radiology, Faculty of Medicine
Ramathibodi Hospital, Mahidol University, 270
Rama VI Road, Bangkok 10400, Thailand

Gesa Meyer-Hamme, Thomas Friedemann and Sven Schroeder
HanseMerkur Center for Traditional Chinese Medicine at the University Medical Center Hamburg-Eppendorf, Martinistrasse 52, House O55, 20246 Hamburg, Germany

Henry Johannes Greten
Heidelberg School of Chinese Medicine, Karlsruher Str. 12, 69126 Heidelberg, Germany
Department of Neurophysiology, Instituto di Ciencias Biomedicas Abel Salazar, University of Porto, Rua de Jorge Viterbo Ferreira n. 228, 4050, –313 Porto, Portugal

Rosemarie Plaetke
Department of Medical Biometry and Epidemiology, University Medical Center Hamburg-Eppendorf, Martinistrasse 52, 20246 Hamburg, Germany

Christian Gerloff
Department of Neurology, University Medical Center Hamburg-Eppendorf, Martinistrasse 52, 20246 Hamburg, Germany

Pengfei Li
Department of Plastic and Aesthetic Center, The First Affiliated Hospital, College of Medicine, Zhejiang University, #79 Qingchun Road, Hangzhou, Zhejiang Province 310003, People's Republic of China

Danfeng Lou
Department of Infectious Diseases, Shulan(Hangzhou) Hospital, #848 Dongxin Road, Hangzhou, Zhejiang Province 310000, People's Republic of China

Hui Lu
Department of Hand Surgery, The First Affiliated Hospital, College of Medicine, Zhejiang University, #79 Qingchun Road, Hangzhou, Zhejiang Province 310003, People's Republic of China

Seok-Jin Choi
Department of Neurology, Inha University Hospital, Incheon, Republic of Korea

Boram Kim, Sung-Min Kim and Jung-Joon Sung
Department of Neurology, Seoul National University Hospital, 101, Daehak-Ro Jongno-Gu, Seoul 03080, Republic of Korea

Haeng-Jin Lee and Seong-Joon Kim
Department of Ophthalmology, Seoul National University Hospital, Seoul, Republic of Korea

Index

www.ingramcontent.com/pod-product-compliance
Lightning Source LLC
Chambersburg PA
CBHW082023190326
41458CB00010B/3255